Spinal Oncology

Editors

MARK H. BILSKY
ILYA LAUFER

NEUROSURGERY CLINICS OF NORTH AMERICA

www.neurosurgery.theclinics.com

Consulting Editors

RUSSELL R. LONSER
DANIEL K. RESNICK

April 2020 • Volume 31 • Number 2

ELSEVIER

1600 John F. Kennedy Boulevard • Suite 1800 • Philadelphia, Pennsylvania, 19103-2899

http://www.theclinics.com

NEUROSURGERY CLINICS OF NORTH AMERICA Volume 31, Number 2
April 2020 ISSN 1042-3680, ISBN-13: 978-0-323-73286-4

Editor: Katerina Heidhausen
Developmental Editor: Laura Fisher

Neurosurgery Clinics of North America (ISSN 1042-3680) is published quarterly by Elsevier Inc., 360 Park Avenue South, New York, NY 10010-1710. Months of issue are January, April, July, and October. Business and Editorial Offices: 1600 John F. Kennedy Blvd., Suite 1800, Philadelphia, PA 19103-2899. Customer Service Office: 11830 Westline Industrial Drive, St. Louis, MO 63146. Periodicals postage paid at New York, NY, and additional mailing offices. Subscription prices are $434.00 per year (US individuals), $785.00 per year (US institutions), $470.00 per year (Canadian individuals), $974.00 per year (Canadian institutions), $534.00 per year (international individuals), $974.00 per year (international institutions), $100.00 per year (US students), $255.00 per year (international students), and $100.00 per year (Canadian students). International air speed delivery is included in all *Clinics* subscription prices. All prices are subject to change without notice. **POSTMASTER:** Send address changes to *Neurosurgery Clinics of North America*, Elsevier Periodicals Customer Service, 11830 Westline Industrial Drive, St. Louis, MO 63146. **Customer Service: 1-800-654-2452 (US and Canada). From outside the US and Canada, call: 1-314-453-7041. Fax: 1-314-453-5170. E-mail: JournalsCustomerService-usa@elsevier.com (for print support) and journalsonline-support-usa@elsevier.com (for online support).**

Reprints. For copies of 100 or more, of articles in this publication, please contact the Commercial Reprints Department, Elsevier Inc., 360 Park Avenue South, New York, NY 10010-1710. Tel. 212-633-3874; Fax: 212-633-3820; E-mail: reprints@elsevier.com.

Neurosurgery Clinics of North America is covered in *MEDLINE/PubMed (Index Medicus), EMBASE/Excerpta Medica, and Current Contents/Clinical Medicine (CC/CM).*

Contributors

CONSULTING EDITORS

RUSSELL R. LONSER, MD
Professor and Chair, Department of Neurological Surgery, The Ohio State University Wexner Medical Center, Columbus, Ohio, USA

DANIEL K. RESNICK, MD, MS
Professor and Vice Chairman, Program Director, Department of Neurosurgery, University of Wisconsin-Madison School of Medicine and Public Health, Madison, Wisconsin, USA

EDITORS

MARK H. BILSKY, MD
William E. Snee Endowed Chair in Spine Oncology, Vice Chairman of Clinical Affairs, Neurosurgery, Memorial Sloan Kettering Cancer Center, Department of Neurological Surgery, Professor of Neurosurgery Weill Medical College of Cornell University, New York, New York, USA

ILYA LAUFER, MS, MD
Neurosurgeon and Director of the Minimally Invasive Spine Tumor Surgery Program, Department of Neurosurgery, Memorial Sloan Kettering Cancer Center, New York, New York, USA

AUTHORS

CHRISTOPHER P. AMES, MD
Professor of Clinical Neurological Surgery and Orthopaedic Surgery, Department of Neurological Surgery, University of California, San Francisco Medical Center, San Francisco, California, USA

ORI BARZILAI, MD
Department of Neurosurgery, Memorial Sloan Kettering Cancer Center, New York, New York, USA

MARK H. BILSKY, MD
William E. Snee Endowed Chair in Spine Oncology, Vice Chairman of Clinical Affairs, Neurosurgery, Memorial Sloan Kettering Cancer Center, Department of Neurological Surgery, Professor of Neurosurgery Weill Medical College of Cornell University, New York, New York, USA

MICHIEL E.R. BONGERS, MD
Research Fellow, Orthopaedic Oncology Service, Massachusetts General Hospital, Harvard Medical School, Boston, Massachusetts, USA

STEVEN D. CHANG, MD
Department of Neurosurgery, Stanford University, Stanford, California, USA

XUGUANG CHEN, MD
Department of Radiation Oncology, Johns Hopkins University, Baltimore, Maryland, USA

NICOLAS DEA, MD, MSc, FRCSC
Clinical Associate Professor of Neurosurgery, Division of Spine Surgery, Vancouver General Hospital and the University of British Columbia, Blusson Spinal Cord Center, Vancouver, British Columbia, Canada

THOMAS F. DeLANEY, MD
Andres Soriano Professor, Department of Radiation Oncology, Massachusetts General Hospital, Harvard Medical School, Boston, Massachusetts, USA

JEFF EHRESMAN, BS
Department of Neurosurgery, Johns Hopkins School of Medicine, Baltimore, Maryland, USA

PETER C. GERSZTEN, MD
Department of Neurosurgery, University of Pittsburgh Medical Center, Pittsburgh, Pennsylvania, USA

AMOL J. GHIA, MD
Department of Radiation Oncology, Associate Professor, Director of Spine Stereotactic Radiosurgery in the Central Nervous System, The University of Texas MD Anderson Cancer Center, Houston, Texas, USA

IBRAHIM HUSSAIN, MD
Department of Neurosurgery, Memorial Sloan Kettering Cancer Center, Department of Neurological Surgery, Weill Cornell Medical College, New York, New York, USA

WILLIAM C. JACKSON, MD
Department of Radiation Oncology, University of Michigan, Ann Arbor, Michigan, USA

DAVID J. KONIECZKOWSKI, MD, PhD
Chief Resident, Harvard Radiation Oncology Program, Massachusetts General Hospital, Boston, Massachusetts, USA

ILYA LAUFER, MS, MD
Neurosurgeon and Director of the Minimally Invasive Spine Tumor Surgery Program, Department of Neurosurgery, Memorial Sloan Kettering Cancer Center, New York, New York, USA

MICHAEL LIM, MD
Department of Neurosurgery, Johns Hopkins School of Medicine, Baltimore, Maryland, USA

DIMITRIOS MATHIOS, MD
Department of Neurosurgery, Johns Hopkins School of Medicine, Baltimore, Maryland, USA

ANTONIO MEOLA, MD, PhD
Department of Neurosurgery, Stanford University, Stanford, California, USA

FABIO Y. MORAES, MD
Department of Oncology, Division of Radiation Oncology, Queen's University, Kingston Health Sciences Centre, Kingston, Ontario, Canada

ZIEV B. MOSES, MD
Department of Neurosurgery, Rush University Medical Center, Chicago, Illinois, USA

NELSON MOSS, MD
Department of Neurosurgery, Memorial Sloan Kettering Cancer Center, New York, New York, USA

WILLIAM CHRISTOPHER NEWMAN, MD
Fellow in Neurosurgical Oncology, Department of Neurosurgery, Memorial Sloan Kettering Cancer Center, New York, New York, USA

JOHN E. O'TOOLE, MD, MS
Professor, Department of Neurosurgery, Co-Director, Coleman Foundation Comprehensive Spine Tumor Clinic, Rush University Medical Center, Chicago, Illinois, USA

MOHAMMAD ZEESHAN OZAIR, PhD, MD
Laboratory of Stem Cell Biology and Molecular Embryology, The Rockefeller University, New York, New York, USA

WHITNEY E. PARKER, MD, PhD
Department of Neurosurgery, Memorial Sloan Kettering Cancer Center, Department of Neurological Surgery, Weill Cornell Medical College, New York, New York, USA

ZACH PENNINGTON, BS
Department of Neurosurgery, Johns Hopkins School of Medicine, Baltimore, Maryland, USA

KRISTEN REDMOND, MD
Department of Radiation Oncology, Johns Hopkins University, Baltimore, Maryland, USA

ADAM M. ROBIN, MS, MD
Department of Neurosurgery, Henry Ford Hospital, Detroit, Michigan, USA

ROBERT ROTHROCK, MD
Department of Neurosurgery, Mount Sinai Hospital, New York, New York, USA

ADAM SCHMITT, MD
Department of Radiation Oncology, Memorial Sloan Kettering Cancer Center, New York, New York, USA

JOSEPH H. SCHWAB, MD, MS
Associate Professor in Orthopaedic Surgery, Orthopaedic Oncology Service, Massachusetts General Hospital, Harvard Medical School, Boston, Massachusetts, USA

DANIEL M. SCIUBBA, MD
Department of Neurosurgery, Johns Hopkins School of Medicine, Baltimore, Maryland, USA

PAVAN PINKESH SHAH, BS
Department of Neurosurgery, Johns Hopkins School of Medicine, Baltimore, Maryland, USA

SCOTT SOLTYS, MD
Department of Radiation Oncology, Stanford University, Stanford, California, USA

DANIEL E. SPRATT, MD
Department of Radiation Oncology, University of Michigan, Ann Arbor, Michigan, USA

NICHOLAS J. SZERLIP, MD
Department of Neurosurgery, University of Michigan, Ann Arbor, Michigan, USA

CLAUDIO E. TATSUI, MD
Department of Neurosurgery, Associate Professor, The University of Texas MD Anderson Cancer Center, Houston, Texas, USA

RAFAEL A. VEGA, MD, PhD
Division of Neurosurgery, Assistant Professor, Director of Neurosurgical Oncology, Beth Israel Deaconess Medical Center, Harvard Medical School, Boston, Massachusetts, USA

YOSHIYA (JOSH) YAMADA, MD, FRCPC
Attending Radiation Oncologist, Department of Radiation Oncology, Memorial Sloan Kettering Cancer Center, New York, New York, USA

MICHAEL YAN, MD
Department of Oncology, Division of Radiation Oncology, Queen's University, Kingston Health Sciences Centre, Kingston, Ontario, Canada

Contents

Preface **xi**

Mark H. Bilsky and Ilya Laufer

Neurologic, Oncologic, Mechanical, and Systemic and Other Decision Frameworks for Spinal Disease **151**

William Christopher Newman, Ilya Laufer, and Mark H. Bilsky

The incidence of metastatic spinal disease is increasing as systemic treatment options are improving and concurrently increasing the life expectancy of patients, and the interventions are becoming increasingly complex. Treatment decisions are also complicated by the increasing armamentarium of surgical treatment options. Decision-making frameworks such as NOMS (neurologic, oncologic, mechanical, and systemic) help guide practitioners in their decision making and provide a structure that would be readily adaptable to the evolving landscape of systemic, surgical, and radiation treatments. This article describes these decision-making frameworks, discusses their relative benefits and shortcomings, and details our approach to treating these complex patients.

Evolving Role of Stereotactic Body Radiation Therapy in the Management of Spine Metastases: Defining Dose and Dose Constraints **167**

Fabio Y. Moraes, Xuguang Chen, Michael Yan, Daniel E. Spratt, Kristen Redmond, William C. Jackson, and Yoshiya (Josh) Yamada

When treating solid tumor spine metastases, stereotactic high-dose-per-fraction radiation, given in a single fraction or in a hypofractionated approach, has proved to be a highly effective and safe therapeutic option for any tumor histology, in the setting of de novo therapy, as salvage treatment of local progression after previous radiation, and in the postoperative setting. There are variations in practice based on the clinical presentation, goals of therapy, as well as institutional preferences. As a biologically potent therapy, a thoughtful and careful attention to detail with patient selection, treatment planning, and delivery is crucial for treatment success.

Hybrid Therapy for Spinal Metastases **191**

Robert Rothrock, Zach Pennington, Jeff Ehresman, Mark H. Bilsky, Ori Barzilai, Nicholas J. Szerlip, and Daniel M. Sciubba

The combination of separation surgery and stereotactic body radiotherapy optimizes the treatment of metastatic spine tumors. The integration of SBRT into treatment paradigms produces superb local control rates and consequently has diminished the role of surgery from principle treatment to one of adjuvant therapy. Under this paradigm, hybrid therapy for the treatment of metastatic spine tumors employs separation surgery to decompress the spinal cord and stabilize the spine while creating a safe target for ablative SBRT. Hybrid therapy is well tolerated, allows an early return to systemic therapy, and provides durable, local tumor control compared with more aggressive traditional approaches.

NEUROSURGERY CLINICS OF NORTH AMERICA

FORTHCOMING ISSUES

July 2020
Epilepsy Surgery: The Network Approach
R. Mark Richardson and Vasileios Kokkinos, *Editors*

October 2020
Metastases to the Central Nervous System
Edjah K. Nduom and Jeff Olson, *Editors*

RECENT ISSUES

January 2020
New Technologies in Spine Surgery
Nathaniel P. Brooks and Michael Y. Wang, *Editors*

October 2019
Pituitary Adenomas
Manish K. Aghi and Lewis S. Blevins, *Editors*

SERIES OF RELATED INTEREST

Neurologic Clinics
http://www.neurologicclinics.com
Neuroimaging Clinics
http://www.neuroimaging.theclinics.com/

THE CLINICS ARE AVAILABLE ONLINE!
Access your subscription at:
www.theclinics.com

Preface

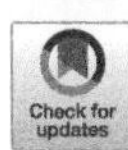

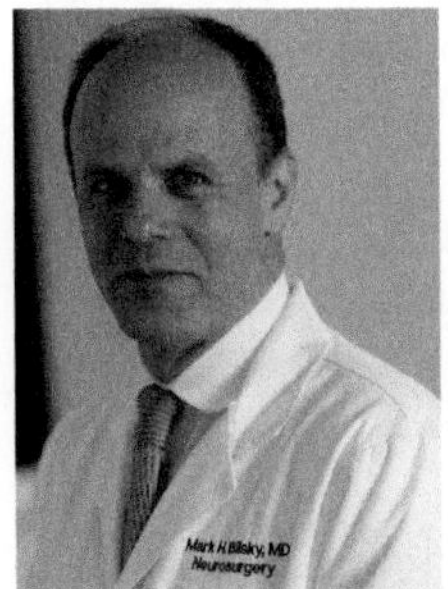

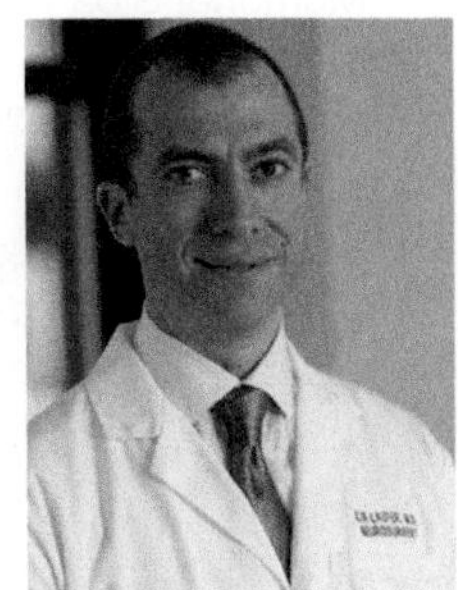

Mark H. Bilsky, MD   Ilya Laufer, MS, MD

Editors

This issue of *Neurosurgery Clinics of North America* explores major advances in surgery, radiation, and systemic therapy that have fundamentally changed outcomes for both malignant and benign spine tumors. The past decade has witnessed a transition from aggressive surgery to multidisciplinary integrated approaches that have significantly improved local tumor control and even survival for metastatic and primary malignant and benign metastatic tumors while substantially reducing morbidity. It is critically important for those treating spine tumors to recognize the major shifts in the approaches to all spine tumors.

Metastases represent the most common tumor pathologic condition that all spine surgeons see routinely in their practices. Multiple technologies have impacted outcomes, including most prominently, stereotactic body radiotherapy (SBRT), as well as minimally invasive spine techniques and targeted systemic therapies. Decision making for metastatic tumors has transitioned from simple decisions regarding the need for surgery or conventional external beam radiation therapy to complex decisions requiring the integration of multimodality therapy. In the articles on metastatic spine tumors, current decision frameworks and algorithms, such as NOMS, LMNOP, and MOSS, are presented to provide guidance for practitioners. The remaining articles discuss the specific treatment modalities that have impacted outcomes, including the rationale for SBRT used as definitive therapy or as a postoperative adjuvant therapy following separation surgery (also known as hybrid therapy) or spine laser interstitial thermotherapy.

As opposed to metastatic tumors, primary malignant bone tumors are exceedingly rare. A number of primary neoplasms occur in the spine, including giant cell tumors, aneurysmal bone cysts, and chondrosarcoma; however, for spine oncologists, chordoma has been a major focus in terms of treatment advances and research. This focus is justified because chordoma is unique to the neural axis, which can occur anywhere from the skull base to the sacrum. For the past 2 decades, chordoma treatment has largely been dominated by descriptions of surgical techniques (ie, en bloc resection). Although technically masterful, surgery alone has demonstrated relatively poor local control rates leading to a search for alternatives. This issue explores not only surgical techniques but also outcomes data regarding the integration of advanced radiation techniques (ie, proton beam, carbon ion, and SBRT) used as definitive, neoadjuvant, or postoperative adjuvant therapy. In addition, active investigations into the molecular drivers and the development of systemic therapy are presented.

Benign neurogenic spine tumors and meningioma are principally treated with open surgical resection, but reductions in morbidity and improved local control rates are being impacted by minimally invasive techniques, the integration of radiation therapy, and even systemic therapy, particularly for syndromic-associated tumors. All of these modalities are explored in separate articles, but perhaps the most impactful new strategies for treatment are the integration of the Da Vinci robot for resection of paraspinal schwannomas and biologics for tumors associated with Neurofibromatosis type 1 (NF-1) and NF-2.

Finally, technical advances in the resection of intramedullary tumors are reported, including d-wave motor monitoring and 5-aminolevulinic

Neurosurg Clin N Am 31 (2020) xi–xii
https://doi.org/10.1016/j.nec.2020.01.001
1042-3680/20/© 2020 Published by Elsevier Inc.

acid, to improve the tumor resection. Whereas these techniques have not fundamentally changed outcomes, they may help improve the safety and completeness of tumor resection.

Mark H. Bilsky, MD
Memorial Sloan Kettering Cancer Center
1275 York Avenue, c705
New York, NY 10065, USA

Ilya Laufer, MS, MD
Neuro Advanced Care Unit
Department of Neurosurgery
Memorial Sloan Kettering Cancer Center
1275 York Avenue, C707
New York, NY 10065, USA

E-mail addresses:
bilskym@mskcc.org (M.H. Bilsky)
lauferi@mskcc.org (I. Laufer)

Neurologic, Oncologic, Mechanical, and Systemic and Other Decision Frameworks for Spinal Disease

William Christopher Newman, MD, Ilya Laufer, MS, MD, Mark H. Bilsky, MD*

KEYWORDS

• NOMS • Metastatic epidural spinal cord compression • Stereotactic body radiotherapy • Stereotactic radiosurgery • LMNOP • Spinal Instability Neoplastic Score

KEY POINTS

- NOMS (neurologic, oncologic, mechanical, and systemic) is an assessment framework for incorporating a patient's systemic disease burden, neurologic status, spinal stability, and primary cancer diagnosis into a treatment decision.
- Clinicians can use the NOMS considerations to determine the optimal treatment integrating current evidence-based medicine, technological advances, and institutional preferences. The NOMS decision framework at any point in time can incorporate new systemic, radiation, and surgical treatment options as they become available without changing the 4 sentinel decision points.
- Rigid prognostic and treatment recommendation systems are limited in their long-term utility by their inability to account for the impact of novel treatments.

INTRODUCTION

In the United States, approximately 300,000 adults have bone metastases, and approximately 20% to 40% of those metastases involve the spine.[1–4] Similar to other osseous lesions, spine metastases often present with pain; however, for spine metastases, the presenting pain syndromes are dictated based on the location of the tumor within the spine. The most common presenting symptom is biological or tumor-related pain that is nocturnal or early morning pain that resolves as the patient ambulates; however, mechanical or axial load pain is also very common, resulting typically from vertebral body and facet fractures. Epidural tumor resulting in spinal cord compression can lead to radiculopathy, myelopathy, and ultimately paralysis.[4] The prevalence of metastatic spine disease has increased partly as an ascertainment issue with the widespread availability of advanced diagnostic imaging such as MRI and [18F]fluorodeoxyglucose PET. In addition, systemic therapies, including both biologics and checkpoint inhibitors, have led to improved survivals for virtually every tumor histology; however, these agents rarely affect bone disease, which inevitably leads to an increase in spine metastases as patients achieve better visceral-tumor control.

The treatment goals for patients with spine metastases are palliative and are focused on maintaining or restoring neurologic function, alleviating pain, achieving spinal stability, preserving quality of life, and preventing local recurrence. Historically, spinal metastases have been treated with invasive surgical procedures (ie, spondylectomy, corpectomy) with the goal of decompression of neural elements and gross total removal followed by palliative conventional external beam radiotherapy (EBRT). However, aggressive tumor

Memorial Sloan Kettering Cancer Center, 1275 York Avenue, c705, New York, NY 10021, USA
* Corresponding author.
E-mail address: bilskym@mskcc.org

Neurosurg Clin N Am 31 (2020) 151–166
https://doi.org/10.1016/j.nec.2019.11.005

excision places patients at risk of significant morbidity and, in the absence of effective adjuvant tumor-directed therapy, provides poor long-term local tumor control.[5–7] Although less morbid, management with conventional EBRT alone provides short-term pain control in patients with spinal metastases but does not provide durable local tumor control.[8,9]

It is from this need for durable local tumor control as well as less morbid surgical interventions that technological advances such as spine stereotactic body radiotherapy (SBRT) or stereotactic radiosurgery (SRS), as well as techniques for minimally invasive spinal decompression and stabilization, have arisen. These techniques have allowed the delivery of ablative doses of radiation to the tumor without causing significant toxicity to adjacent critical structures, such as the spinal cord, resulting in outstanding local tumor control.[10] The ability to obtain durable local tumor control with radiation therapy has allowed the goal of surgical intervention to shift from complete surgical resection to that of separation surgery, a term emphasizing the need for limited tumor resection in order to provide a small space between the tumor and the spinal cord so an ablative dose of stereotactic radiosurgery can be delivered to the entire tumor volume while respecting the constraints of spinal cord tolerance.

In the setting of increasingly effective systemic therapies whereby long-term survival is measured in years and not months, and an evolving armamentarium of surgery-based and radiation-based treatments, the fundamental question of how to select the appropriate treatment of this increasingly complex and diverse patient population is critical. To aid physicians in patient evaluation and treatment decisions, several patient description instruments, treatment algorithms, and decision frameworks have been developed. The scoring systems and algorithms range in the degree of complexity and prescriptiveness. Although there is a benefit to providing clear guidance about the treatment decisions, the rapid pace of medical advances threatens to render such algorithms obsolete within a few years of their creation. For example, the Tomita[11] and the revised Tokuhashi scores[12] incorporated the evidence available at the time of their creation to guide the selection of surgical techniques and define treatment goals, but they are unable to incorporate the modern treatment options, such as SBRT, or determine prognosis in the modern era of targeted therapies. To overcome the shortcomings of fixed algorithmic scoring systems, NOMS (neurologic, oncologic, mechanical, and systemic) was created as a dynamic decision framework that has gained wide acceptance in the assessment of patients with spinal metastatic tumors. The NOMS framework incorporates neurologic, oncologic, mechanical, and systemic assessments of the patients to determine the optimal treatment approach.[13] This framework is easily adapted to the surgical, radiation, and medical treatment options available in the individual medical centers and incorporates novel technologies as they become available. Since its design, there have been several new treatment algorithms that have been championed, all of which incorporate these 4 fundamental assessments and are predicated on the integration of SBRT.

This article describes the patient evaluation instruments germane to the neurologic, oncologic, mechanical, and systemic components of NOMS and the surgical and radiation oncology advances that have changed the management paradigms of patients with spinal metastatic disease. It also evaluates the benefits and shortcomings of existing treatment algorithms and the limitations inherent to prognostic scoring systems.

Neurologic, Oncologic, Mechanical, and Systemic

Neurologic assessment: clinical and radiographic

Clinical assessment The patient's neurologic status is an important component of the clinical assessment because this indicates the impact of the epidural spinal cord compression (ESCC). The patient's neurologic status can be broken down into motor and sensory components and is often assessed using either the Medical Research Council (MRC) scale for muscle strength or American Spinal Injury Association Impairment Scale (AIS). The MRC is a scale that grades muscle strength ranging from 0 to 5, with 0 being absent strength and 5 being full strength (**Table 1**). The AIS rates the degree of spinal cord injury from E to A, with American Spinal Injury Association (ASIA) E being neurologically normal and ASIA A being a complete spinal cord injury with no preservation of motor or sensory sacral segment function (**Table 2**).

Although the aforementioned scales are the most commonly used, patient clinical findings concerning for myelopathy are also important considerations. These findings include difficulty with fine motor hand coordination, bowel and bladder incontinence, or progressive gait impairment. In addition, findings of radiculopathy caused by nerve root compression are also considered in

Table 1
Medical Research Council scale for muscle strength

Score	Description
0	No muscle contraction
1	Flicker or trace muscle movement
2	Active movement with gravity eliminated
3	Active movement against gravity, but not against resistance of the examiner
4	Active movement against gravity and resistance, but not full strength
5	Full strength, normal power

the neurologic assessment. Ambulation represents a critical component of neurologic examination, and loss of ambulation from metastatic epidural spinal cord compression (MESCC) serves as an important determinant of the timing of surgery and predictor of postoperative neurologic outcome.

Table 2
American Spinal Injury Association scale grades

ASIA Grade	Description
A	Complete injury with no preservation of motor or sensory function in sacral segments
B	Incomplete injury with sensory but not motor function preserved below the neurologic level, including the sacral segments
C	Incomplete injury with preservation of motor function below the neurologic level and more than half of key muscle groups with less than grade 3 strength
D	Incomplete injury with preservation of motor function below the neurologic level and more than half of key muscle groups with greater than or equal to grade 3 strength
E	Normal sensory and motor functions

Radiographic assessment ESCC score, also known as the Bilsky score, uses MRI to define the degree of ESCC caused by extramedullary spine tumors. The Bilsky score is a 6-point scale ranging from 0 to 3, with scores of 0 to 1c constituting low-grade compression and scores of 2 and 3 constituting high-grade compression (**Fig. 1**).[14] The scoring system was developed to standardize reporting in the literature but also to critically examine SBRT outcomes based on a consistent assessment of spinal cord compression. Although neurologic status is an important part of the decision-making algorithm in planning treatments, most patients undergo spinal imaging before they develop neurologic deficits. Therefore, the Bilsky score provides the description of radiographic ESCC that covers the full range of symptomatic and asymptomatic tumors. The epidural tumor extension must be advanced before the patients develop neurologic deficits, and this usually only occurs in patients with ESCC3.

Oncologic assessment

Prediction of tumor response to systemic and radiation therapy guides the oncologic assessment. Traditionally, the oncologic assessment was largely guided by the primary tumor type. Tumors such as multiple myeloma, lymphoma, and small cell tumors generally rapidly respond to systemic and radiation therapy and rarely require surgical decompression. In contrast, solid tumors show a wide range of sensitivity and response to systemic and radiation therapy (**Table 3**).[15] Therefore, for solid tumor metastases, the need for surgical decompression is determined by the extent of spinal cord compression and symptoms. Hormone-responsive tumors such as breast and prostate cancer generally respond readily to conventional EBRT (cEBRT) and, in the absence of neurologic deficits and mechanical instability, can be treated with cEBRT. In contrast, other solid tumor metastases, particularly sarcomas, melanoma, renal cell, non–small cell lung, and colorectal carcinomas are radioresistant to cEBRT (see **Table 3**). SBRT overcomes radioresistance and provides durable tumor control. As better understanding is gained of the molecular basis of radiation response, the oncologic assessment requires consideration of the molecular profile of the tumor to help predict treatment response, in addition to the primary tumor histologic type.

Mechanical assessment

Spinal instability is a key indication for surgical intervention in metastatic spine disease. Patients with mechanically unstable fractures caused by tumors require stabilization, because radiotherapy

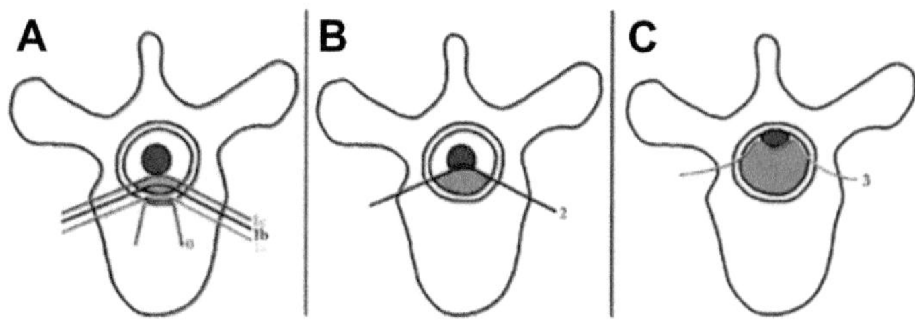

Fig. 1. ESCC scale. Grades 0 to 1c signify a range from bone only involvement at one end to deformation of the thecal sac without spinal cord compression. Grades 2 and 3 are considered high-grade spinal cord compression and can be differentiated based the presence of cerebrospinal fluid around the spinal cord on T2-weighted MRI. (*From* Bilsky MH, Laufer I, Fourney DR, et al. Reliability analysis of the epidural spinal cord compression scale. J Neurosurg Spine. 2010;13(3):324–8; with permission.)

and systemic therapy cannot restore mechanical stability. Observation of the patient's movement serves as the critical component of stability assessment. Patients experiencing severe pain elicited by position changes in the setting of a fracture generally require fracture stabilization and experience significant pain relief after surgery. The Spinal Instability Neoplastic Score (SINS) was developed to help gauge the degree of spinal instability and help clinicians determine the need for surgical referral and potential surgical intervention.[16] The SINS is based on 6 components: location (junctional, mobile spine, semirigid spine, or rigid spin segments), pain, type of osseous lesion (lytic, blastic, or mixed), radiographic spinal alignment (kyphosis, scoliosis, subluxation, and so forth), degree of vertebral body collapse, and involvement of the posterolateral elements (**Table 4**). These components are given weighted scores and the sum of these scores classifies a lesion as stable, unstable, or indeterminate, with unstable lesions needing instrumented fixation and the indeterminate lesions requiring surgical evaluation in order to determine the need for stabilization.

Table 3
Primary tumor relative radiosensitivity

Study	Lymphoma, Seminoma, Myeloma	Breast	Prostate	Sarcoma	Melanoma	Gastro intestinal	NSCLC	Renal
Gilbert et al,[38]	F	U	U	U	U	U	U	U
Maranzano et al,[9] 2005	F	F	F	U	U	U	U	U
Rades & Abrahm,[27] 2010	F	I	I	I	U	I	U	I
Rades & Abrahm,[27] 2010	F	F	F	U	U	U	U	U
Katagiri et al,[8] 1998	F	F	F	U	U	U	U	U
Maranzano et al,[9] 2005	F	F	F	U	U	U	U	U
Rades & Abrahm,[27] 2010	F	I	I	I	U	I	U	I

Abbreviations: F, favorable; I, intermediate; NSCLC, non–small cell lung cancer; U, unfavorable radiosensitivity.
From Gerszten PC, Mendel E, Yamada Y. Radiotherapy and radiosurgery for metastatic spine disease: what are the options, indications, and outcomes? Spine 2009;34(22 Suppl):S84; with permission.

Table 4
Spinal Instability Neoplastic Score component scoring

SINS Component	Description	Score
Location	Junctional (occiput–C2, C7–T2, T11–L1, L5–S1)	3
	Mobile spine (C3–C6, L2–L4)	2
	Semirigid (T3–T10)	1
	Rigid (S2–S5)	0
Pain	Yes	3
	Occasional pain but not mechanical	1
	Pain-free lesion	0
Bone lesion	Lytic	2
	Mixed (lytic/blastic)	1
	Blastic	0
Radiographic spinal alignment	Subluxation/translation present	4
	De novo deformity (kyphosis/scoliosis)	2
	Normal alignment	0
Vertebral body collapse	>50% collapse	3
	<50% collapse	2
	No collapse with >50% body involved	1
	None of the above	0
Posterolateral involvement of spinal elements	Bilateral	3
	Unilateral	1
	None of the above	0
Total	Stable	0–6
	Indeterminate	7–12
	Unstable	13–18

Systemic assessment

Functional status Treatment of metastatic disease is delivered with the intent to provide durable palliation. In this setting, understanding the long-term benefits of any intervention are especially important because the cost of time-consuming or highly invasive procedures with long recovery times must be weighed against the patient's life expectancy and ability to recover meaningfully within that time. For example, a patient with a high degree of frailty or disability may not live long enough to benefit from an aggressive surgical intervention or might be at very high risk of perioperative complications.

The 2 mainstays of measuring a patient's overall functional status are the Karnofsky Performance Status (KPS) and the Eastern Cooperative Oncology Group (ECOG) scale.[17,18] The KPS is scored from 0 to 100, with a score of 0 representing a dead patient, 40 representing severe disability requiring special care and assistance, 70 representing the lower limit for complete self-care, and 100 being a completely asymptomatic patient (**Table 5**). The ECOG scale ranges from 0 to 5, with 0 representing being fully active and with no signs of disease-associated restriction, 2 representing being ambulatory and capable of self-care without the ability to perform work activities, and 4 representing complete disability. Similar to KPS, a maximum score of 5 on the ECOG signifies death.

In patients with poor performance status (ie, KPS $\leq$ 40), treatments such as spine SBRT are less likely to provide clinically significant benefits compared with less complex, less costly, and less time-intensive interventions such as EBRT.[19] Moreover, in patients with poor performance status, consideration should be given to the discussion of goals of care as opposed to continued aggressive management. Of note, KPS greater than or equal to 70 is often used as an entry criterion into many clinical trials and other large studies.

Survival prognosis Over time, there have been many tools used for prognostic stratification of patients with metastatic spine disease, but the most common include the Tomita score[11] and the revised Tokuhashi.[20] The Tomita score is a retrospective preoperative assessment based on 6 factors analyzed in 67 patients with spinal metastases. Patients were given a summative score ranging from 2 to 10 based on the grade of the malignancy (ie, rate of growth), presence of visceral metastases, and extent of bone metastases. This score then dictated the treatment

Table 5
Karnofsky performance scale index

Karnofsky Score	Description
100	Normal; no complaints and no evidence of disease
90	Minor symptoms; able to carry on normal activities of life
80	Normal activity with effort; more than minimal symptoms of disease
70	Able to provide self-care; unable to perform normal activities or active work
60	Requires occasional assistance but able to care for most personal needs
50	Requires significant assistance and frequent medical care
40	Disabled and requiring specialized care
30	Severely disabled and requiring hospitalization or active supportive treatment
20	Extremely sick and requiring hospitalization with active supportive treatment
10	Moribund
0	Dead

strategy that was chosen, with scores of 2 to 3 being recommended a wide or marginal excision for long-term local control, scores of 4 to 5 being recommended marginal or intralesional excision, scores of 6 to 7 justifying palliative surgery, and 8 to 10 indicating nonoperative supportive care.[11]

The Tokuhashi score takes into account the general condition of the patient, the number of extraspinal bone metastases, the number of spine metastases, the presence of metastases to the major internal organs, the presence of a neurologic deficit, and the primary cancer diagnosis.[12] The 2017 revision to the Tokuhashi score takes into account all of the same factors as the 2005 revision but updates the 1-year survival prognosis based on the primary tumor diagnosis.[20] This update allows for a reflection of current systemic treatment effectiveness and its impact on life expectancy. The authors of the 2017 revision found a statistically significant improvement in predictive accuracy with this update.

A modern iteration of survival prediction instruments was developed and validated by the Skeletal Oncology Research Group (SORG).[21] The SORG nomogram accurately predicts the 3-month and 12-month survivals and has been externally validated. Machine learning modeling provided a further refinement of the SORG survival prediction instrument, adding several laboratory values to the assessment.

Although survival prediction provides important information to the surgeon and the patient, its utility in clinical decisions requires further elucidation. Clearly, extensive surgery should be avoided in patients with limited survival, whereas the goals of therapy for patients with long expected survival must incorporate durable local tumor control. Although many of the systems share common prognostic components, such as the functional status, the extent of metastatic tumor dissemination, and tumor type, they all require constant updating as the systemic therapy evolves and patient survival improves with it. This issue is best exemplified by the Tokuhashi scoring system's need for a 2005 and then a 2017 update with statistically significant increases in accuracy between each. These static tools only capture the potential interventions of a given time point, and, as treatment strategies become less morbid and more effective, the ability of sicker patients to tolerate these procedures increases. This increased tolerability is something that can only be reflected in these prognostic scoring systems through frequent updating, a characteristic that often renders these models obsolete after their publication.

The components of NOMS continue to represent the 4 key considerations required for the evaluation of patients with metastatic tumors. Although the assessment instruments evolved over time and will continue to change, the 4 components have withstood the test of time. Since the inception of NOMS, the treatment options have also greatly evolved. The dynamic nature of this framework allows NOMS to incorporate the technological and medical advances into the treatment recommendations and to remain current as the assessment instruments and treatment options change. The evolution of radiotherapy and surgical technique represent the key technological advances that have transformed the treatment recommendations.

Technological Advances

Radiotherapy evolution

Conventionally fractionated EBRT has been used to treat spinal metastases for decades. As previously mentioned, tumors showed a wide range of responses to cEBRT. The difference among tumors of different histology has been extensively studied, with tumors labeled on the spectrum from exquisitely radiosensitive to highly radioresistant. Renal cell carcinoma (RCC) represents one of the prototypical radioresistant metastases in the spine, known to quickly recur after cEBRT. The resistance of RCC tumors to cEBRT led surgeons to undertake gross total tumor excision in order to achieve local control, counting on surgery when radiotherapy was ineffective. However, such RCC excisions, often undertaken in the en bloc fashion, were associated with very extensive surgery, prolonged recovery, and the potential for severe complications.

The development of SBRT has allowed the delivery of high dose per fraction radiation to spine tumors at tumoricidal doses while minimizing toxicity to adjacent structures. Data support the concept that high dose per fraction tumor radiation (ie, >10 Gy per fraction) is tumoricidal through both double-stranded DNA damage as well as vascular injury mechanisms.[22] In SBRT, patients receive high-dose single or hypofractionated, highly conformal radiation at tumor-ablative doses.[23] This approach is compared with conventional EBRT, in which significantly lower radiation doses per fraction are delivered over 10 to 20 treatments.

There are several important benefits that SBRT provides. First, in patients who have tumors with low-grade epidural extension (ie, ESCC 0–1c), definitive treatment can be provided with SBRT alone with durable symptomatic responses and high rates of local control. SBRT provides this local control irrespective of the primary tumor histology and volume. Four-year local control rates of 98% were reported after high-dose single-fraction SBRT in a large case series that included numerous tumors that would have been resistant to cEBRT, including RCC.[24] Several series specifically examined SBRT outcomes in patients with RCC, confirming excellent local control. In this way, SBRT has helped eliminate the need for more invasive surgical techniques such as en bloc spondylectomies for solitary metastases. Note that this durable response is independent of tumor histology.[24–26] Second, SBRT allows the patient to spend less time being treated (typically 1-3 fractions) compared with conventional EBRT, in which the patients return for treatment over the course of weeks. Third, SBRT delivers high doses of radiation while sparing adjacent healthy tissues, such as the spinal cord, nerve roots, or the esophagus. Fourth, SBRT can be used as salvage treatment in patients who have failed prior conventional EBRT. In general, nearly all patients with spinal metastases undergo radiotherapy at some point during their treatment unless their performance status is too poor, they have a highly chemosensitive malignancy (ie, hematologic malignancy), or their life expectancy is too short.[27]

Surgery evolution

Although patients with low-grade ESCC can undergo SBRT as the definitive treatment of their spinal metastasis, patients with high-grade ESCC require surgical decompression before SBRT. However, even among patients who require surgery, SBRT has altered the treatment strategy. Because SBRT provides safe and durable local control, the goal of surgery shifted from gross total excision to spinal cord decompression only. Complete tumor excision usually requires a vertebrectomy and vertebral body reconstruction, followed by postoperative radiotherapy. In contrast, tumor excision for the spinal cord decompression can be limited to the removal of the epidural tumor alone, while preserving the vertebral body and shortening the operative time and decreasing morbidity. Thus, the purpose of surgery shifted to the creation of safe conditions for SBRT rather than an attempt at surgical cures. This combination of separation surgery with SBRT provides safe and durable local control among patients with high-grade ESCC.

Improvements in spinal instrumentation and the development of minimally invasive surgical (MIS) techniques have also greatly changed surgical indications and outcomes. Before popularization of instrumented spinal stabilization, patients with MESCC underwent laminectomy without stabilization. Such surgery frequently failed to provide satisfactory functional outcomes, with cEBRT alone providing comparable functional results. However, improved understanding of spinal instability and stabilization techniques allowed surgeons to safely stabilize the spinal column, showing superiority of surgery compared with cEBRT for patients with symptomatic MESCC.

Further improvements in spinal technology allow surgeons to perform instrumented stabilization and decompression using MIS techniques. MIS techniques are muscle sparing and do not require significant subperiosteal dissections and displacement or destruction of muscle tissue. Instead, techniques such as percutaneous instrumentation, miniopen approaches for decompression, and tumor removal through tubular or expandable retractors minimize muscle disruption, use smaller incisions, are less morbid, and often enable patients to receive radiation sooner after surgery with fewer wound complications and better quality-of-life outcomes.[28–32] Even less invasive approaches using laser interstitial thermal ablation of tumors are being used increasingly.[33,34] The lower systemic stress of MIS broadened the patient population considered for stabilization by decreasing surgical morbidity and expediting recovery. As the surgical armamentarium expands and procedural morbidity decreases, the decision framework for which procedures to offer to which patients must adapt to this changing landscape.

TREATMENT ALGORITHMS AND MANAGEMENT FRAMEWORKS

Neurologic, Oncologic, Mechanical, and Systemic

The NOMS framework incorporates 4 fundamental patient factors (neurologic, oncologic, mechanical instability, and systemic disease) into patient decision making with the goal of determining the appropriateness of radiation, surgery, systemic therapy, or a combination thereof.[13] In brief, the neurologic consideration is an assessment of the degree of ESCC and resultant myelopathy or radiculopathy. The oncologic consideration refers to the expected tumoral response to available treatments, such as EBRT, SBRT, or systemic treatment options. Mechanical instability considers the extent to which spinal metastases have compromised the integrity of the spine and predisposed it to pathologic movements. The fourth factor considers the extent of systemic disease as well as the overall health of the patient in order to determine whether the patient can tolerate the proposed treatment. In total, these factors create a comprehensive overview of the patient that frames treatment decision making in the context of the patient's overall well-being and disease status.

Although the NOMS framework may seem to be a very general framework, this is at the core of its strength. By remaining general and not attaching itself to any 1 treatment modality or scoring system, the NOMS framework allows itself to remain up to date with advances in oncology. Whether it is the advent of biologics and checkpoint inhibitors in systemic treatments or the decreased morbidity of MIS techniques and cement augmentation allowing shorter posterior fixation constructs and quicker recoveries in patients previously thought too systemically ill to undergo surgery, the NOMS framework is capable of incorporating these advances into its decision-making algorithm. Similarly, when new grading systems such as SINS, which better defined and made more consistent the classification of spinal instability, are developed, they can be seamlessly integrated into the decision framework. Or, as the role of radiation therapy alone in the management of higher-grade ESCC becomes better studied, NOMS can incorporate this into its decision-making paradigm. Most importantly, if these classification schemas become obsolete and are replaced by more accurate tools, NOMS seamlessly is able to shed itself of the old algorithm and dynamically adapt without changing its core components. Although this is a strength of NOMS decision framework compared with a static algorithm, frequent updates to decision making require focused attention by surgeons and radiation oncologists.

Location of Disease, Mechanical Instability, Neurology, Oncology, Patient Fitness, Prognosis, Response to Prior Therapy

The LMNOP (location of disease, mechanical instability, neurology, oncology, patient fitness, prognosis, response to prior therapy) framework was devised as a modification of the NOMS framework that more explicitly incorporated the extent of spinal disease (ie, number and location of levels involved), the use of the SINS grading system, and response to prior systemic therapy in what the investigators described as a "principle-based approach."[35] In the original article, the investigators detailed the range of options available for treatment of lesions at levels ranging from the occiput to the sacrum, but did not provide prescriptive information regarding how to choose 1 of the available treatment options (ie, anterior, posterior, lateral, or a combination). Their description of the mechanical instability component is based on SINS.

The components of neurology and oncology are largely the same in LMNOP as they are in NOMS, focusing on the patient's neurologic status or signs of myelopathy and the degree of radiosensitivity, respectively. The final aspect of the framework, the patient characteristics, is a more explicit explanation of the systemic component of NOMS. Patient fitness, prognosis, prior responses to therapy, and even patient wishes all combine to create the image as to what types of interventions the patient physiologically can tolerate as well as what interventions are consistent with their goals of care. As described earlier in relation to NOMS, this last component is often assessed in conjunction with the patient's oncologist.

Medical/Mental, Oncological, Stenosis, Stability

The MOSS (medical/mental, oncological, stenosis, stability) framework originated from Marco and colleagues[36] in a 2018 article that attributed the need for a new algorithm to the shortcomings of the NOMS framework. In particular, they describe NOMS as a static framework that aggressively advocates surgical intervention and relies too heavily on SINS grading without being prescriptive enough with respect to which surgical avenue to pursue. The most important contribution of MOSS reflecting the powerful philosophy advocated by Rex Marco is that systemic disease and patient preference are the most critical components of metastatic assessment in directing treatment. In MOSS, the medical/mental component is similar to the systemic component of NOMS with the patient's physiologic reserve, performance status (quantified using ECOG or KPS), and personal wishes being factored into the ultimate decision making. The oncologic component focuses on tumor histology (specifically radiosensitivity) as well as staging and prognosis. Similar to NOMS, tumor histology is used to determine the effectiveness of radiation therapy and whether or not surgical adjuncts are needed. Patient prognosis regarding life expectancy and disease burden is used similarly to the systemic aspect of NOMS, but with the key difference that the investigators advocate the use of the revised prognostic scoring system of Tokuhashi and colleagues[12] for estimating patient prognosis when input from oncologists is unavailable.

The stenosis component focuses on the ambulatory and neurologic status of the patient and then factors in the degree of ESCC to determine the need for surgical decompression versus radiosurgical treatment. Lastly, the stability component is guided by a different definition of stability without integrating the SINS score. The MOSS framework defines physiologic instability as a spine that, when physiologically loaded, cannot maintain its normal configuration and manifests pain syndromes or neurologic symptoms.[37] No other explicit defining criteria are offered. In patients who are unstable with a life expectancy of greater than 3 months and tumors recalcitrant to available adjuvant therapies, the authors advocate consideration of surgical stabilization.

Comparison of Treatment Frameworks

The modern treatment frameworks (ie NOMS, LMPNOP, and MOSS) that incorporate SBRT are very similar in terms of treatment recommendations. NOMS was first reported in 2004 and, although the 4 sentinel decision points remain the same, the decisions have changed with the incorporation of new techniques and evidence-based medicine. The LMNOP framework uses the same criteria as NOMS but explicitly includes references to SINS grading and makes more explicit the systemic disease component of NOMS through its patient fitness, prognosis, and prior therapy component. In all, by adding the additional components, LMNOP makes more explicit the fundamental principles of NOMS but does not add to or redefine the assessment framework that was previously proposed. Each paradigm is flexible enough to allow for the inclusion of new grading systems as well as the incorporation of novel treatment options that may make systemic therapies or radiation treatments more effective or render surgical interventions less morbid.

According to its investigators, MOSS was developed to overcome the deficiencies of NOMS but closer examination reveals some misinterpretation of the NOMS concepts. The MOSS investigators interpret that the mechanical evaluation in NOMS is firmly rooted in SINS. Although SINS indeed serves as a useful instrument in stability evaluation, the mechanical component may be assessed in various ways. NOMS was developed and published a decade before SINS and can incorporate other methods of stability assessment. Fundamentally, the definition of stability provided in MOSS is very similar to the definition of neoplastic spinal instability provided that lies at the foundation of SINS. In addition, MOSS investigators view surgery as a highly morbid intervention. This perception is rapidly changing with increasing MIS options. Overall, MOSS uses the same general principles as NOMS but places a lesser emphasis on the potential benefits of surgical interventions and describes it as an intervention for when no other options are available. In many ways, MOSS has not left room in its decision-making tree for novel percutaneous or cement augmented techniques that minimize morbidity, improve quality of life, and enable patients to get postoperative radiation treatments quickly.[32] In addition, the rational integration of effective radiotherapy serves as one of the foundations of NOMS treatment recommendations, in agreement with the idea that alternative treatments should be considered before the recommendation of surgery.

NOMS remains the most dynamic assessment framework. The additional discrete assessments proposed by other systems are already incorporated into the 4 NOMS components. Furthermore, it is important to distinguish the assessment framework from the treatment recommendations. The critical assessments of the neurologic function, tumor type, mechanical stability, overall functional status, and expected survival have passed the test of time, as shown by their numerous permutations in all of the evaluation systems mentioned earlier. The treatment recommendations based on these 4 assessments change as medicine evolves. Furthermore, the treatments must be tailored to the individual treatment situation based on the locally available technology and physician and patient preference. Rigid treatment recommendation systems fail to accommodate such treatment evolution and availability. The 4 parameters of NOMS are easily recalled, consider the overall condition of the patient, and allow for the seamless integration of treatment advances into the decision-making process. For this reason, in our clinical practice, the authors continue to use the NOMS framework for treatment decision making.

CASE EXAMPLES

Case 1

A 51-year-old woman with history of metastatic colorectal cancer presented with progressive lower back pain exacerbated by changing position from sitting to standing. On neurologic examination, she was full strength with no sensory deficits and normal deep tendon reflexes. MRI of her lumbar spine showed an L3 compression fracture and an L5 burst fracture with extension into the right-sided posterior elements as well as destructive lytic changes, without epidural tumor extension (**Fig. 2**A, B).

Neurologic, oncologic, mechanical, and systemic assessment

Neurologic: patient was neurologically intact with ESCC grade 0.

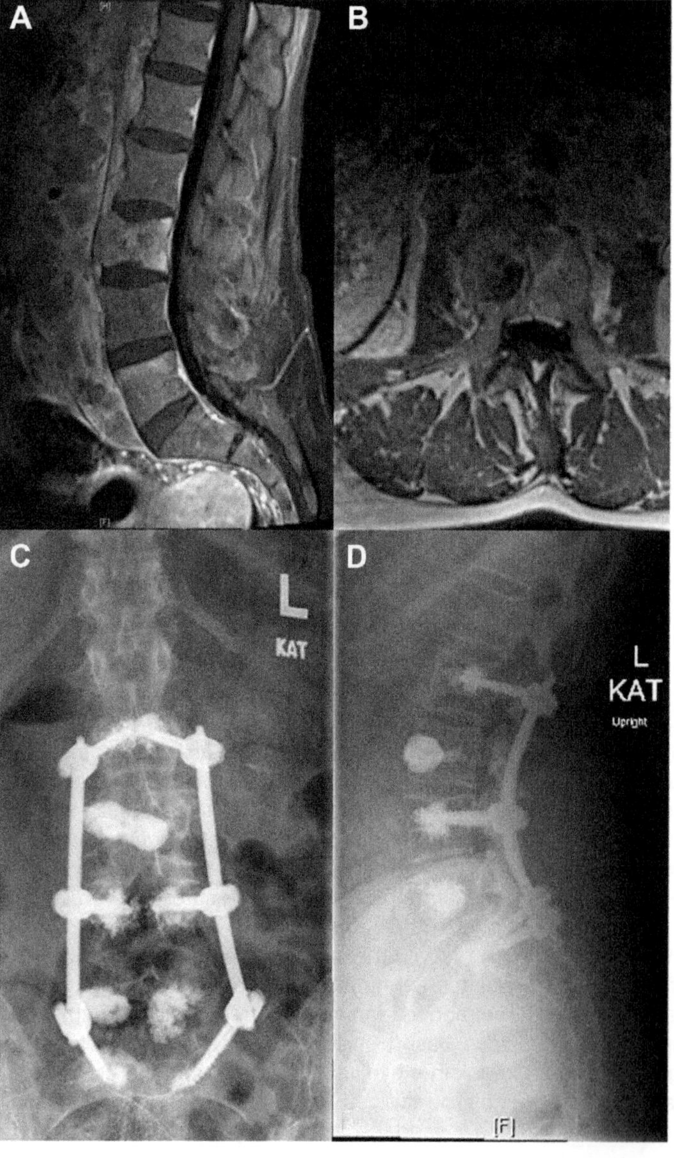

Fig. 2. T1 postcontrast sagittal (*A*) and axial (*B*) MRI showing fractures of the L3 and L5 vertebral bodies without extension of disease into the spinal canal. Postoperative anteroposterior (AP) (*C*) and lateral (*D*) radiographs show the L2-S1 construct with cement augmentation and kyphoplasties at the L3 and L5 levels.

Oncologic: colon cancer is a radioresistant cancer.

Mechanical: the patient had evidence of mechanical instability manifested by worsening pain with changes in position. Her SINS was 9.

Systemic: the patient's systemic disease was well controlled and she had no other significant medical comorbidities.

The patient has mechanical instability and radioresistant tumor without spinal cord compression. Therefore, the patient requires stabilization and does not require decompression. The radioresistant tumor should be treated with SBRT to achieve durable local control. The patient underwent percutaneous L2-S1 percutaneous instrumented stabilization. Screw cement augmentation was performed at the L2, L4, and S1 screws and vertebral body augmentation using balloon-assisted kyphoplasty technique at L3 and L5 (**Fig. 2**C, D). Stabilization was recommended based on the pain pattern consistent with mechanical instability, supported by the SINS score. In the absence of spinal cord compression and mechanical radiculopathy, there was no need for decompression of the neural elements. Because of the radioresistant nature of colon cancer, SBRT was the preferred adjuvant therapy. In addition, her systemic assessment revealed limited cancer dissemination and few medical comorbidities, suggesting reasonable expected survival and low risk of perioperative complication. She then received 24 Gy in a single fraction to the L3 and L5 levels within 1 month of her surgery.

Case 2

A 55-year-old woman with history of metastatic non–small cell lung adenocarcinoma (T1A, N0, M0) presented to clinic with an incidentally found T8 vertebral body metastasis (**Fig. 3**A,B). She had pain that increased in severity in the middle of the night and morning but was not exacerbated by movement or changing positions. On clinical examination, she was neurologically intact with normal deep tendon reflexes. She was not on any systemic treatment at the time of spinal metastasis diagnosis.

Neurologic, oncologic, mechanical, and systemic assessment

Neurologic: patient was neurologically intact with no invasion of tumor into the canal (ESCC grade 1b).

Oncologic: EGFR-mutant cell lung adenocarcinoma is a radioresistant cancer.

Mechanical: the patient had no subjective complaints of mechanical instability and only complains of biological pain. Her SINS score was 4.

Systemic: the patient's systemic disease was limited, she had newly diagnosed metastatic cancer with good expected response to targeted therapy, limited systemic dissemination, and she had no other significant medical comorbidities.

Based on the NOMS assessment, the authors recommended this patient for palliative radiotherapy treatment. In the absence of mechanical instability or spinal cord compression, the patient did not require surgery. She did require radiotherapy in order to achieve local tumor control. Her tumor was radioresistant to cEBRT, therefore SBRT was recommended. She is systemically well controlled and in good health, so continuing with treatment was reasonable. She received 27 Gy over 3 fractions of image-guided intensity modulated radiation therapy (**Fig. 3**C) with subsequent improvement in her biological pain. At 4-year follow-up, she had no recurrence of her disease.

Case 3

A 50-year-old man with a history of BRAF mutant thyroid cancer and metastases to his chest wall and spine presented to the emergency department with 1 week of progressive mechanical back pain and intermittent, position-dependent bilateral lower extremity paresthesias. Neurologically, the patient was grossly intact with 1+ patellar and biceps reflexes and normal gait. MRI showed a T4 metastasis with ESCC grade 3 circumferential spinal cord compression (**Fig. 4**A, B).

Neurologic, oncologic, mechanical, and systemic assessment

Neurologic: the patient had neurologic deficits caused by spinal cord compression manifested as intermittent position-dependent paresthesias. Based on imaging, he had grade 3 ESCC at the T4 level (see **Fig. 4**A, B).

Oncologic: thyroid cancer is not radiosensitive.

Mechanical: the patient had subjective complaints of mechanical instability. His SINS score was 10 (1 point for location, 3 points for pain, 2 points for being a lytic lesion, 0 points for normal alignment, 1 point for <50% vertebral body collapse, and 3 points for bilateral posterolateral element involvement).

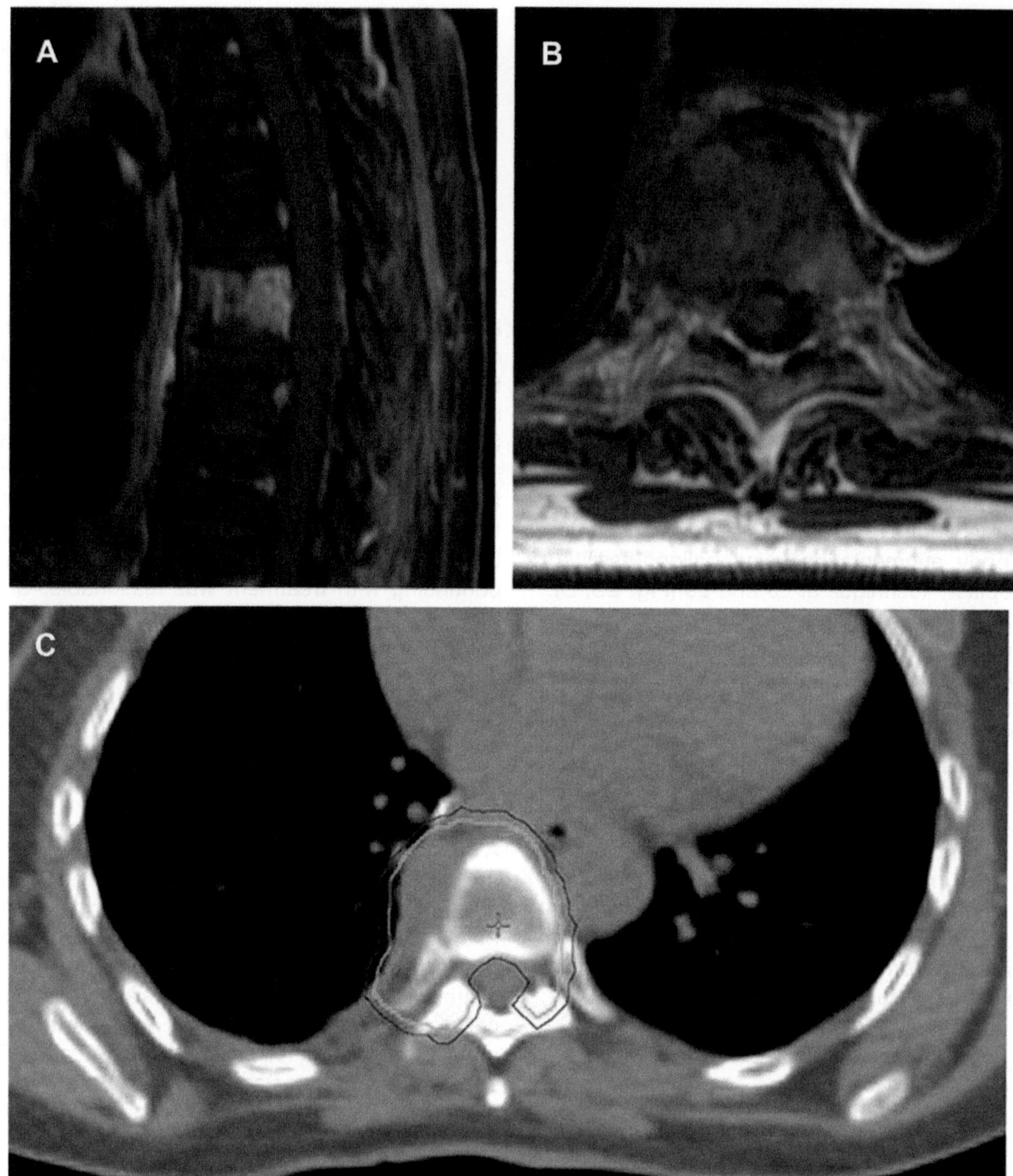

Fig. 3. T1 postcontrast MRI sagittal image (*A*) showing T8 vertebral body involvement with corresponding post-contrast axial image (*B*) through T8 showing left-sided pedicle involvement with no extension into the epidural space. (*C*) Radiation dose planning showing the contouring of the vertebral body and adjacent posterior elements as well as the adjacent lung mass.

Systemic: the patient's systemic disease was well controlled and he was not on systemic therapy.

Based on the NOMS assessment, the authors recommended the patient for a preoperative embolization followed by open surgical stabilization with cement augmentation and spinal cord decompression. Based on the patient's neurologic symptoms and focal area of high-grade cord compression, laminectomies were performed from T3 to T5 as part of separation surgery. Instrumented fixation was performed from T2 to T7 with cement augmentation (**Fig. 4**C, D). Postoperatively, the patient underwent SBRT for treatment of the affected levels.

Case 4

The patient is a 61-year-old woman with metastatic RCC admitted to the hospital with movement-exacerbated neck pain and found to have a C4

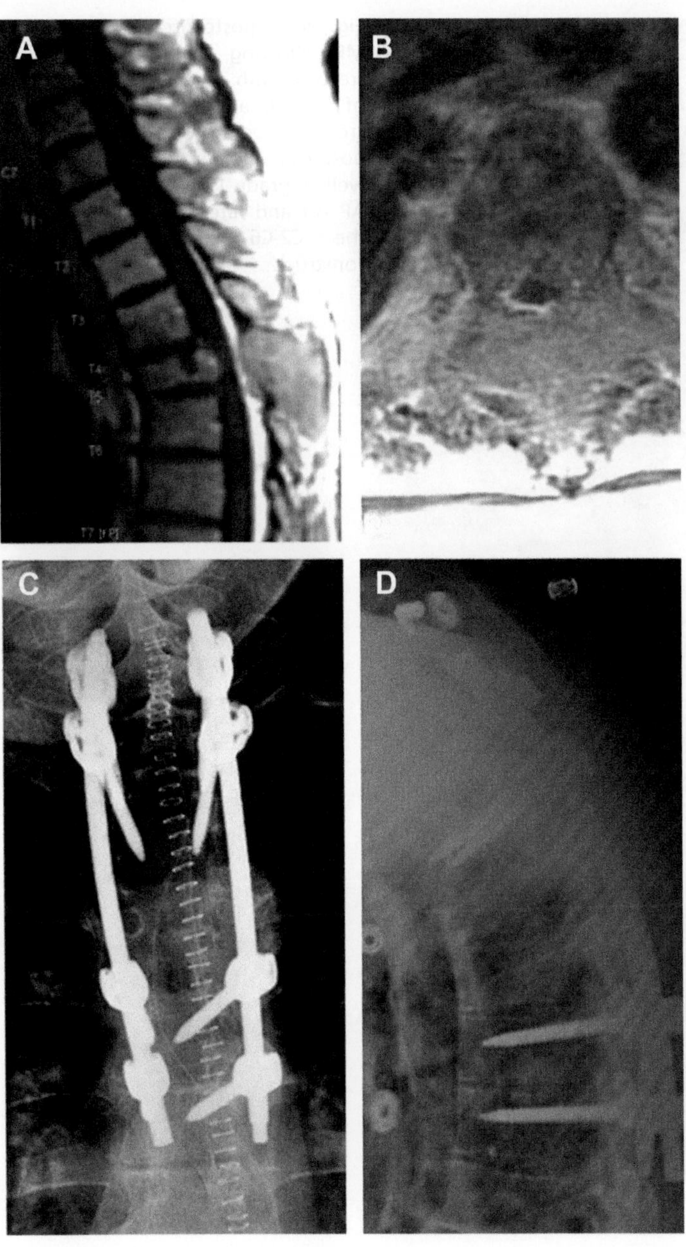

Fig. 4. T1-postcontrast sagittal (*A*) MRI showing T4 pathologic fracture with tumor involvement of the posterior elements as well as an axial image (*B*) showing circumferential ESCC. AP (*C*) and lateral (*D*) postoperative images showing the T2-T7 posterior segmental fixation construct with cement augmentation.

metastasis with a burst fracture and extension into the posterior elements (**Fig. 5**A, B). On examination, she is neurologically intact with normal deep tendon reflexes and normal gait. She has neck pain with active cervical range of motion. MRI showed the aforementioned burst fracture with greater than 50% loss of vertebral height and grade 1C ESCC.

Neurologic, oncologic, mechanical, and systemic assessment

Neurologic: the patient had no neurologic deficits. Based on imaging, she had grade 1C ESCC C4 (see **Fig. 5**B).

Oncologic: RCC is not radiosensitive and is highly vascular.

Mechanical: the patient had subjective complaints of mechanical instability. Her SINS score was 11 (2 points for location, 3 points for pain, 2 points for being a lytic lesion, 0 points for normal alignment, 2 points for >50% vertebral body collapse, and 2 points for unilateral posterolateral element involvement).

Systemic: the patient's systemic disease was well controlled and she was not on systemic therapy.

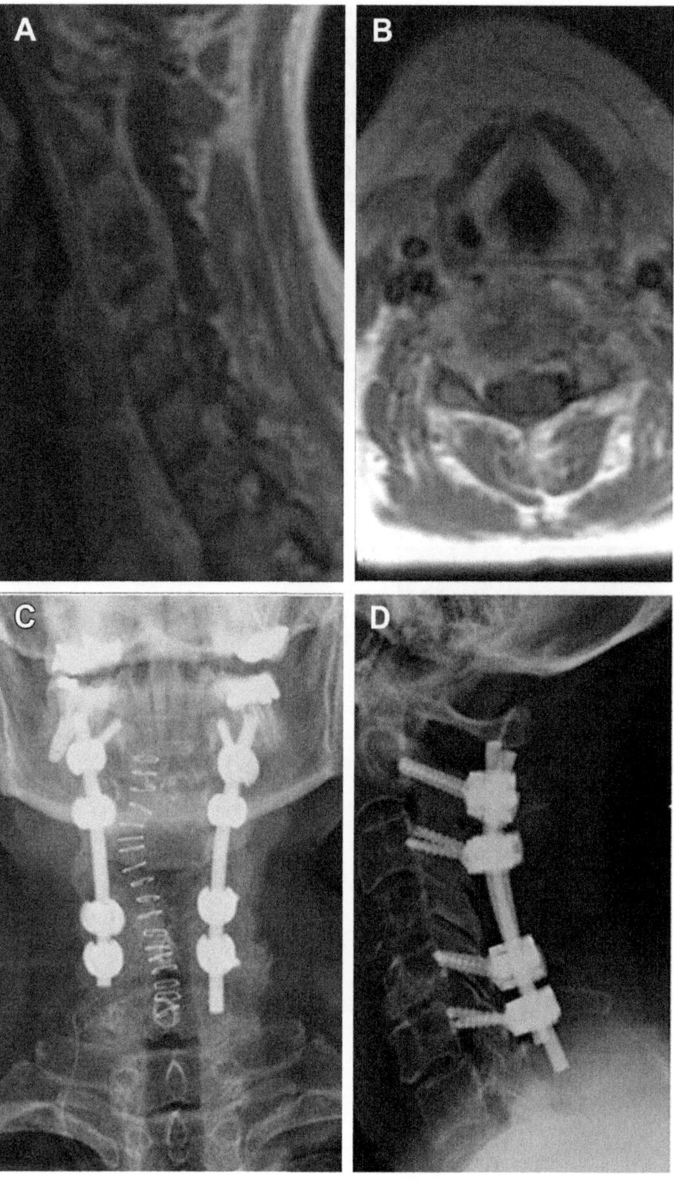

Fig. 5. T1-postcontrast sagittal (*A*) MRI showing C4 pathologic burst fracture with greater than 50% loss of height, and corresponding axial cross section (*B*) showing unilateral posterior element involvement as well as grade 1C ESCC. Postoperative AP (*C*) and lateral (*D*) images show the C2-C6 posterior segmental construct.

Based on the NOMS assessment, the authors recommended the patient for preoperative embolization followed by open surgical decompression and stabilization. Decompression was performed from C3 to C5 in order to increase separation between the spinal cord and the radiation target and minimize spinal cord radiation dose. Posterior instrumented fixation was performed from C2 to C6 (**Fig. 5**C, D). Postoperatively, she received hypofractionated SBRT with 27 Gy delivered over 3 fractions. At her 4-year follow-up, she had had no recurrence of disease at this site.

DISCLOSURE

Dr I. Laufer is consultant for Depuy/Synthes, Globus, and Spine Wave. Dr M.H. Bilsky is consultant for Varian, Royalties Depuy/Synthes, and Globus. Dr W.C. Newman has nothing to disclose.

REFERENCES

1. Hernandez RK, Adhia A, Wade SW, et al. Prevalence of bone metastases and bone-targeting agent use among solid tumor patients in the United States. Clin Epidemiol 2015;7:335–45.

2. North RB, LaRocca VR, Schwartz J, et al. Surgical management of spinal metastases: analysis of prognostic factors during a 10-year experience. J Neurosurg Spine 2005;2(5):564–73.
3. Sinson GP, Zager EL. Metastases and spinal cord compression. N Engl J Med 1992;327(27):1953–4 [author reply: 1954–5].
4. Wong DA, Fornasier VL, MacNab I. Spinal metastases: the obvious, the occult, and the impostors. Spine 1990;15(1):1–4.
5. Boriani S, Gasbarrini A, Bandiera S, et al. En bloc resections in the spine: the experience of 220 patients during 25 years. World Neurosurg 2017;98:217–29.
6. Sakaura H, Hosono N, Mukai Y, et al. Outcome of total en bloc spondylectomy for solitary metastasis of the thoracolumbar spine. J Spinal Disord Tech 2004; 17(4):297–300.
7. Tomita K, Kawahara N, Baba H, et al. Total en bloc spondylectomy for solitary spinal metastases. Int Orthop 1994;18(5):291–8.
8. Katagiri H, Takahashi M, Inagaki J, et al. Clinical results of nonsurgical treatment for spinal metastases. Int J Radiat Oncol Biol Phys 1998;42(5):1127–32.
9. Maranzano E, Bellavita R, Rossi R, et al. Short-course versus split-course radiotherapy in metastatic spinal cord compression: results of a phase III, randomized, multicenter trial. J Clin Oncol 2005; 23(15):3358–65.
10. Greco C, Pares O, Pimentel N, et al. Spinal metastases: from conventional fractionated radiotherapy to single-dose SBRT. Rep Pract Oncol Radiother 2015;20(6):454–63.
11. Tomita K, Kawahara N, Kobayashi T, et al. Surgical strategy for spinal metastases. Spine 2001;26(3): 298–306.
12. Tokuhashi Y, Matsuzaki H, Oda H, et al. A revised scoring system for preoperative evaluation of metastatic spine tumor prognosis. Spine 2005;30(19): 2186–91.
13. Laufer I, Rubin DG, Lis E, et al. The NOMS framework: approach to the treatment of spinal metastatic tumors. Oncologist 2013;18(6):744–51.
14. Bilsky MH, Laufer I, Fourney DR, et al. Reliability analysis of the epidural spinal cord compression scale. J Neurosurg Spine 2010;13(3):324–8.
15. Gerszten PC, Mendel E, Yamada Y. Radiotherapy and radiosurgery for metastatic spine disease: what are the options, indications, and outcomes? Spine 2009;34(22 Suppl):S78–92.
16. Fisher CG, DiPaola CP, Ryken TC, et al. A novel classification system for spinal instability in neoplastic disease: an evidence-based approach and expert consensus from the Spine Oncology Study Group. Spine 2010;35(22):E1221–9.
17. Bollen L, van der Linden YM, Pondaag W, et al. Prognostic factors associated with survival in patients with symptomatic spinal bone metastases: a retrospective cohort study of 1,043 patients. Neuro Oncol 2014;16(7):991–8.
18. Switlyk MD, Kongsgaard U, Skjeldal S, et al. Prognostic factors in patients with symptomatic spinal metastases and normal neurological function. Clin Oncol (R Coll Radiol) 2015;27(4):213–21.
19. Spratt DE, Beeler WH, de Moraes FY, et al. An integrated multidisciplinary algorithm for the management of spinal metastases: an International Spine Oncology Consortium report. Lancet Oncol 2017; 18(12):e720–30.
20. Morgen SS, Fruergaard S, Gehrchen M, et al. A revision of the Tokuhashi revised score improves the prognostic ability in patients with metastatic spinal cord compression. J Cancer Res Clin Oncol 2018;144(1):33–8.
21. Paulino Pereira NR, Mclaughlin L, Janssen SJ, et al. The SORG nomogram accurately predicts 3- and 12-months survival for operable spine metastatic disease: external validation. J Surg Oncol 2017; 115(8):1019–27.
22. Song CW, Kim M-S, Cho LC, et al. Radiobiological basis of SBRT and SRS. Int J Clin Oncol 2014; 19(4):570–8.
23. Chan NK, Abdullah KG, Lubelski D, et al. Stereotactic radiosurgery for metastatic spine tumors. J Neurosurg Sci 2014;58(1):37–44.
24. Yamada Y, Katsoulakis E, Laufer I, et al. The impact of histology and delivered dose on local control of spinal metastases treated with stereotactic radiosurgery. Neurosurg Focus 2017;42(1):E6.
25. Gerszten PC, Burton SA, Ozhasoglu C, et al. Radiosurgery for spinal metastases: clinical experience in 500 cases from a single institution. Spine 2007; 32(2):193–9.
26. Yamada Y, Lovelock DM, Yenice KM, et al. Multifractionated image-guided and stereotactic intensity-modulated radiotherapy of paraspinal tumors: a preliminary report. Int J Radiat Oncol Biol Phys 2005; 62(1):53–61.
27. Rades D, Abrahm JL. The role of radiotherapy for metastatic epidural spinal cord compression. Nat Rev Clin Oncol 2010;7(10):590–8.
28. Disa JJ, Smith AW, Bilsky MH. Management of radiated reoperative wounds of the cervicothoracic spine: the role of the trapezius turnover flap. Ann Plast Surg 2001;47(4):394–7.
29. Yang Z, Yang Y, Zhang Y, et al. Minimal access versus open spinal surgery in treating painful spine metastasis: a systematic review. World J Surg Oncol 2015;13:68.
30. Donnelly DJ, Abd-El-Barr MM, Lu Y. Minimally invasive muscle sparing posterior-only approach for lumbar circumferential decompression and stabilization to treat spine metastasis–technical report. World Neurosurg 2015;84(5):1484–90.
31. Kumar N, Malhotra R, Maharajan K, et al. Metastatic spine tumor surgery: a comparative study of

minimally invasive approach using percutaneous pedicle screws fixation versus open approach. Clin Spine Surg 2017;30(8):E1015–21.

32. Barzilai O, Amato M-K, McLaughlin L, et al. Hybrid surgery-radiosurgery therapy for metastatic epidural spinal cord compression: a prospective evaluation using patient-reported outcomes. Neurooncol Pract 2018;5(2):104–13.
33. Tatsui CE, Stafford RJ, Li J, et al. Utilization of laser interstitial thermotherapy guided by real-time thermal MRI as an alternative to separation surgery in the management of spinal metastasis. J Neurosurg Spine 2015;23(4):400–11.
34. Tatsui CE, Lee S-H, Amini B, et al. Spinal laser interstitial thermal therapy: a novel alternative to surgery for metastatic epidural spinal cord compression. Neurosurgery 2016;79(Suppl 1):S73–82.
35. Ivanishvili Z, Fourney DR. Incorporating the spine instability neoplastic score into a treatment strategy for spinal metastasis: LMNOP. Global Spine J 2014; 4(2):129–36.
36. Marco Rex AW, Brindise J, Dong D. MOSS: A patient-centered approach. In: Metastatic Spine Disease: A guide to diagnosis and Management. Ed. Springer: Rex W Marco; 2018.
37. Panjabi MM. Clinical spinal instability and low back pain. J Electromyogr Kinesiol 2003;13(4):371–9.
38. Gilbert RW, Kim JH, Posner JB. Epidural spinal cord compression from metastatic tumor: Diagnosis and treatment. Ann Neurol 1978;3(1): 40–51.

Evolving Role of Stereotactic Body Radiation Therapy in the Management of Spine Metastases

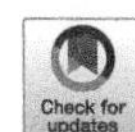

Defining Dose and Dose Constraints

Fabio Y. Moraes, MD[a,1], Xuguang Chen, MD[b,2], Michael Yan, MD[a,1], Daniel E. Spratt, MD[c,3], Kristen Redmond, MD[b,2], William C. Jackson, MD[c,3], Yoshiya (Josh) Yamada, MD, FRCPC[d,*]

KEYWORDS

- Stereotactic spine radiosurgery • Hypofractionated stereotactic body radiation therapy
- Treatment planning • Reirradiation of spine metastases • Spine radiosurgery dose constraints
- Spine SBRT

KEY POINTS

- High-dose spine stereotactic radiosurgery provides durable tumor control.
- Hypofractionated stereotactic body radiation therapy (SBRT) is an effective treatment strategy for spine metastases.
- Reirradiation with spine SBRT is well tolerated and provides meaningful local control.
- Postoperative SBRT is both safe and effective.
- Despite variations in institutional practice, outcomes for spine SBRT are excellent.

INTRODUCTION

Stereotactic body radiation therapy (SBRT) of the spine is an effective oncologic tool for treating vertebral column solid tumor bone metastases, and excellent outcomes have been described for its use as definitive or adjuvant therapy, as primary or salvage treatment, and both in terms of local tumor control as well as toxicity. Spine radiosurgery has now been incorporated for several years into the National Comprehensive Cancer Network (NCCN) guidelines version 3.2019[1] for managing spine metastases.

Since it was first described by Hamilton and colleagues[2] in 1995, spine SBRT has evolved into a unique discipline that has been facilitated by technologic innovations such as on-board imaging with cone beam computed tomography (CBCT) and highly conformal radiation treatment plans using intensity modulated techniques (intensity-modulated radiation therapy) that provide high-

[a] Department of Oncology, Division of Radiation Oncology, Queen's University, Kingston Health Sciences Centre, Kingston, Ontario, Canada; [b] Department of Radiation Oncology, Johns Hopkins University, Baltimore, MD, USA; [c] Department of Radiation Oncology, University of Michigan, Ann Arbor, MI, USA; [d] Department of Radiation Oncology, Memorial Sloan Kettering Cancer Center, New York, NY, USA

[1] Present address: 25 King St W, Kingston, ON K7L 5P9, Canada

[2] Present address: 401 N Broadway Ste 1440, Baltimore, MD 21287, United States

[3] Present address: 1500 E Medical Center Dr, Ann Arbor, MI 48109

* Corresponding author. 1275 York Avenue, New York, New York 10065, USA

E-mail address: yamadaj@mskcc.org

Neurosurg Clin N Am 31 (2020) 167–189

https://doi.org/10.1016/j.nec.2019.12.001

1042-3680/20/

precision treatment that delivers very-high-dose-per-fraction radiation within tumors but limits the dose of radiation to nearby normal tissue structures such as the spinal cord or esophagus to safe limits. However, the practice of spine SBRT continues to evolve and there is no consensus on radiation dose to normal tissues as well as tumor, and a range of doses are used by experienced spine SBRT centers across the country.

First, a discussion of the literature relevant to spine SBRT in terms of tumor control and symptom response, as well as toxicity and normal tissue dose constraints is provided. Then 3 clinical scenarios that were submitted to 4 experts in spine SBRT are discussed in a tumor board format, and their approach for treatment is detailed to show the variation in practice that currently exists.

TUMOR CONTROL/SYMPTOM RESPONSE

Single-Fraction Stereotactic Body Radiation Therapy

Single-fraction (SF) SBRT is often referred to as spine radiosurgery, originally drawing from the extensive experience of cranial radiosurgery for brain metastases. It is a similar paradigm to cranial radiosurgery, in which space-occupying lesions are embedded into critical normal tissue, but, by delivering a very high dose in an SF, results in treated tumor control of 80% to 90% but using high-precision treatment techniques to limit the dose given to the surrounding brain to very safe levels.[3]

There seems to be a dose-response relationship in terms of local control of spine metastases, even in the setting of radiosurgery. Folkert and colleagues,[4] in the largest reported experience for sarcoma metastases, showed a clear dose-response relationship for local control of this radioresistant group of tumors, with high-dose SF SBRT providing the highest degree of long-term tumor control. An analysis of patterns of failure of 66 sarcoma metastases of the spine treated with radiosurgery also noted improved local control with dose escalation.[5] Similar findings have been reported for renal cell carcinomas.[6] Spine radiosurgery given in the very highest doses is likely an ablative therapy, resulting in a high likelihood of very durable tumor control. In a large single-institution retrospective study of more than 800 treated lesions, the cumulative incidence of local failure in patients given 2400 cGy in an SF was 2.1% at 4 years, whereas lower doses in an SF resulted in a significantly higher probability of local failure of 20% ($P<.001$).[7] Neither tumor size nor histology were significant predictors of local failure. The only significant factor associated with local failure was the delivered dose of radiation.

Although single-arm prospective and retrospective series suggest that outcomes following SF SBFT may be superior to conventional external-beam radiation therapy (cEBRT), the first randomized controlled trial, Radiation Therapy Oncology Group (RTOG) 0631, was recently conducted to compare SF SBRT 16 to 18 Gy with cEBRT 8 Gy in 1 fraction for patients with 1 to 3 sites of spinal metastasis.[8] The preliminary results of this phase III trial, reported only in abstract form at the American Society for Radiation Oncology (ASTRO) 2019 annual meeting, showed no significant difference in the proportion of patients with pain response (40% vs 58%) or change in pain score (−3.00 vs −3.83) at 3 months following treatment between the SF SBRT and cEBRT groups.[8] Further follow-up may be required to discern a clinically significant difference between the 2 treatment arms, because a 3-month end point is likely insufficient to show a tangible difference between the 2 groups. The ongoing Canadian SC-24 trial, which randomizes patients to cEBRT of 20 Gy in 5 fractions versus SBRT of 24 Gy in 2 fractions, will be important in better understanding the efficacy of these 2 treatment modalities.[9] A German randomized phase 2 trial of 30 Gy in 10 fractions versus 24 Gy in an SF has also reported preliminary results, finding superior palliative response in patients receiving 24 Gy in an SF.[10] More mature results from this trial are also eagerly awaited.

There Are Mechanisms of Response Unique to Very-High-Dose-per-Fraction Radiation Therapy

SF SBRT may potentially enhance cell killing by engaging antitumor immunity.[11] Ablative doses of 15 to 25 Gy cause a significant increase in CD8+ T-cell priming in the draining lymph node tissue.[12] The in vivo effect of SF 18-Gy SBRT in spinal metastasis was recently shown by the report of Steverink and colleagues,[13] which showed significantly increased necrosis and apoptosis in tumor cells and reduction in CD31+ vessel count after SBRT. In addition, high-dose radiation greater than 15 Gy may activate alternative tumoricidal pathways and lead to ablation of tumor vasculature, resulting in early apoptosis of tumor cells.[14]

Hypofractionated Stereotactic Body Radiation Therapy

Hypofractionated (HF) SBRT exploits normal cell repair between fractions to reduce the risk of injury to adjacent critical organs such as the spinal cord, esophagus, and uninvolved bone. For this reason, hypofractionation is favored by some clinicians, because of the belief that toxicity is reduced with this strategies. For example, hypofractionation in the case of salvage radiation of previously irradiated tissues or large treatment volumes may help mitigate the risk of significant toxicity. HF SBRT may also be associated with lower rates of vertebral compression fractures, because dose per fraction has been consistently shown to correlate with post-SBRT fracture risk.[15] In terms of tumor control, reoxygenation and redistribution of cell cycle between fractions may enhance tumor killing by subsequent fractions.[16] Although the optimal dose fractionation schedule for enhancing checkpoint blockade is unknown, there is also emerging preclinical evidence suggesting that fractionated SBRT is better at stimulating a systemic immune response against untreated tumors.[17] Therefore, HF SBRT may have a better therapeutic ratio with improved normal tissue protection and tumor killing.

The doses and fractionation schedules used for HF SBRT are highly variable and no prospective studies to date have compared outcomes between them. The most common regimens used include 24 to 27 Gy in 2 to 3 fractions and 30 to 35 Gy in 5 fractions. Pain relief from these regimens is comparable with SF SBRT (77%–87%), as shown in **Table 1**.[18,19] Short-term and intermediate-term local control also ranges between 84% and 94% (see **Table 1**), similar to lower-dose SF treatments.[18,20] It is more difficult to ascertain whether there is a correlation between local control and prescription dose in the HF setting given the vastly different treatment regimens and overall similar control rate.

Current Evidence of Direct Comparison Between Single-Fraction and Hypofractionated Stereotactic Body Radiation Therapy

Based on the studies summarized in **Table 1**, SF and HF SBRT provide excellent pain relief and tumor control. In practice, the choice between SF and HF SBRT is often institution dependent and may be determined by several clinical factors. One such factor is the presence of epidural disease and spinal cord compression, which may limit tumor coverage with SF SBRT given the need to minimize spinal cord dose.[16] In these situations, separation surgery has been advocated as a neoadjuvant maneuver to provide enough distance from the spinal cord to the gross tumor in order to deliver an effective dose of radiation while maintaining the spinal cord dose at safe levels.[21] Nevertheless, SF SBRT has been used in small series for the treatment of metastatic epidural spinal cord compression with low complication rates.[22,23] The size of the target lesion is also of concern, with bigger lesions favoring HF regimens because of the amount of normal tissue within the radiation field. There is some suggestion that bigger lesions may be associated with poorer local control, although this was not the case in the largest reported series.[4,24]

Direct comparisons between SF and HF SBRT have yielded conflicting data. Heron and colleagues[25] compared HF (9–35 Gy in 3–5 fractions) with SF regimens (6–20 Gy) and concluded that HF regimens yielded superior local control (96% vs 70% at 2 years), with the caveat that SF doses in the study were low (mean, 16.3 Gy). A retrospective review of 332 spinal metastases treated with SF (18–24 Gy) versus HF (27 Gy in 3 fractions) SBRT found no association between fractionation scheme and local control.[24] A multi-institutional randomized controlled trial is directly comparing SF 24 Gy versus HF SBRT 27 Gy in 3 fractions in oligometastatic patients, with locoregional control as the primary end point.[26] This trial has been reported in abstract form, showing a significant benefit for both local control and freedom from new distant metastases (DMs) in favor of 24-Gy SF SBRT versus HF SBRT 9 Gy in 3 fractions. The 3-year incidence of local recurrence was 6.1% of the lesions compared with 23% for the high-dose SF SBRT and HF regimens, respectively ($P<.0005$), and the 3-year incidence of DM progression was 4.1% compared with 17.5% for the SF SBRT and HF SBRT regimens, respectively ($P<.02$).[27]

Clinically, SF SBRT yielded excellent pain relief in up to 75% to 85% of patients in large reported series (see **Table 1**). There may be a dose response between local control and prescription dose, because several series using 18 Gy or less report tumor control of 85% to 88%,[28–30] whereas series with a prescription dose of 24 Gy often report a control rate of 92% to 98%.[7,31]

In contrast, radioresistant tumors may benefit most from SF SBRT. **Table 2** summarizes studies that reported outcomes of radioresistant histologies.[4,7,24,31–38] SF SBRT had crude local control rates of 52% to 97%, with a weighted average of 87% over 859 lesions, whereas control rates from HF SBRT range from 57% to 90%, with a slightly lower weighted average of 80% over 319 lesions. Two single-institution studies comparing SF (mostly 24 Gy) and HF (mostly 27–30 Gy in 3 fractions) SBRT yielded superior 1-year local control for SF SBRT in both renal cell carcinoma (95% vs 71%) and sarcoma (91% vs 84%).[4,6] Note that low-dose SF SBRT at 16 to 18 Gy yielded local control of only 52% to 75% in radioresistant histologies (see **Table 2**), suggesting that dose escalation may be needed for these tumors.

Table 1
Select studies of single-fraction and hypofractionated stereotactic body radiation therapy for de novo spine metastasis

Author, Year	Study Design	Patients/ Lesions (N)	Histology	Prior RT (%)	Total Dose	Fractions (N)	Pain Relief (%)	Local Control (%)	Follow-up (mo)
Ryu et al,[28] 2004	Retrospective	49/61	Mixed	0	NA (12–16)	1	85	95	9 (6–24)
Gerszten et al,[32] 2007	Prospective	NA/156	Mixed	0	20 (12.5–25)	1	86 (in entire 500-lesion cohort)	90	21 (3–53)
Chang et al,[40] 2012	Retrospective	NA/131	Mixed	0	27 (mean SF equivalent 19.9 Gy)	3	83	85	22 (NA)
Garg et al,[31] 2012	Prospective	61/63	Mixed	0	24 (16–24)	1	NA	92	20 (1–52)
Guckenberger et al,[18] 2014	Retrospective	30one-third87	Mixed	0	24 (8–60)	3 (1–20)	77	84	12 (0–105)
Pichon[20]	Prospective	30/49	Mixed	0	27	3	NA (39 complete response)	94	19 (4–38)
Yamada et al,[7] 2017	Retrospective	657/811	Mixed	0	24 (18–26)	1	NA	96	27 (2–141)
Sprave et al,[10] 2018	Prospective	27/30	Mixed	0	24	1	74	NA	8 (NA)
Ghia et al,[29] 2018	Prospective	28/28	Radioresistant	0	18 (18–24)	1	NA	86	17 (3–54)
Guckenberger et al,[19] 2018	Prospective	54/60	Mixed	0	35 or 48.5	5 or 10	87 (30 complete response)	87	12 (1–47)
Tseng et al,[81] 2018	Retrospective	145/279	Mixed	0	24	2	NA	86	15 (1–72)
Ozdemir et al,[30] 2019	Retrospective	78/125	Mixed	0	18 (16–18)	1	NA	88	13 (NA)
Ryu[88]	Prospective	NA	Mixed	0	NA (16–18)	1	40	NA	NA

Total dose, number of fractions, and follow-up are presented in median (range) unless specified.
Abbreviations: NA, not available; RT, radiotherapy.

Table 2
Select studies on spine stereotactic body radiation therapy in radioresistant histologies with sample size greater than 20

Author, Year	Study Design	Histology/ Number of Lesions	Prior RT (%)	Total Dose	Fractions (N)	Local Control (%)	Follow-up (mo)
Gerszten et al,[32] 2007	Prospective	RCC/93 Melanoma/38	NA (69 overall)	20 (12.5–25)	1	RCC 87 Melanoma 75	21 (3–53)
Staehler et al,[33] 2011	Prospective	RCC/105	NA	20 (19–20)	1	90	15 (1–42)
Garg et al,[31] 2012	Prospective	RCC/33	0	24 (16–24)	1	91	20 (1–52)
Miller et al,[34] 2016	Retrospective	RCC/151	24	16 (10–18)	1	75	12 (1–83)
Miller et al,[35] 2017	Retrospective	Sarcoma/40	40	16	1	52	15 (2–95)
Yamada et al,[7] 2017	Retrospective	RCC/170 Sarcoma/113 Melanoma/48	0	24 (18–26)	1	RCC 97 Sarcoma 97 Melanoma 94	27 (2–141)
Folkert et al,[4] 2014	Retrospective	Sarcoma/120	10	24 (24–36)	1 (1–6)	82	12 (1–81)
Sellin et al,[36] 2015	Retrospective	RCC/40	0	24 (24–30)	1 (1–5)	57	49 (38–76)
Bishop et al,[24] 2015	Retrospective	RCC/125 Sarcoma/27	NA	24 (18–27)	1 (1–3)	RCC 90 Sarcoma 78	19 (0–111)
Meyer et al,[37] 2018	Retrospective	RCC/75	NA	Mean BED3 63.3	NA	80	13 (0–59)
McGee et al,[38] 2019	Prospective	Mixed radioresistant/ 41	NA	18 (14–18)	1	78	9 (NA)

Abbreviation: RCC, renal cell carcinoma.

Dosimetric Parameters to Improve Local Control

Adequate dose coverage of the tumor instead of prescription dose may be essential in maintaining high rates of tumor control, especially in spine SBRT, in which the part of the tumor closest to the spinal cord is routinely underdosed. One study found that a minimum dose (D_{min}) to the gross tumor volume (GTV) greater than 15 Gy in 1 fraction was associated with superior local control.[39] Another study found that the biologically effective dose (BED) at α/β of 10 (BED10) of the GTV D_{min} greater than 33.4 Gy (1-fraction equivalent 14 Gy) was associated with 1-year local control of 94% versus 80% for D_{min} BED10 less than 33.4 Gy.[24] Yamada and colleagues[7] reviewed 811 spinal lesions, of which 82% had radioresistant histologies, treated with SF SBRT and found that GTV D_{95} (D_{min} to 95% volume) greater than 18.3 Gy was associated with 2% local failure, compared with 14% with GTV D_{95} less than 18.3 Gy. Therefore, it seems GTV coverage is crucial in successful SBRT, and the D_{min} coverage may be D_{min} of 15 Gy and D_{95} of 18.3 Gy in 1 fraction.

Special Consideration: Reirradiation

Because of the rapid dose decrease, spine SBRT may be most advantageous in the setting of reirradiation where the spinal cord has received a substantial dose previously. **Table 3** summarizes evidence supporting the use of SBRT in treating spinal metastases that have progressed after prior radiation.[32,40–48] The overall pain control rate was 65% to 86%, and crude local control rate was

Table 3
Select studies of spine stereotactic body radiation therapy in reirradiation

Author, Year	Study Design	Patients/ Lesions (N)	Histology	Prior RT (%)	Total Dose	Fractions (N)	Pain Relief (%)	Local Control (%)	Follow-up (mo)
Gerszten et al,[32] 2007	Retrospective	NA/344	Mixed	100%	20 (12.5–25)	1	86 (in entire 500-lesion cohort)	88	21 (3–53)
Sahgal et al,[41] 2009	Retrospective	39/60	Mixed	62%	24	3	NA	87	8 (1–48)
Choi et al,[42] 2010	Retrospective	42/51	Mixed	100%	20 (10–30)	2 (1–5)	65	74	7 (2–47)
Mahadevan et al,[43] 2011	Retrospective	60/81	Mixed	100%	24 (24–35)	3 (3–5)	65	93	12 (4–36)
Garg et al,[44] 2011	Prospective	59/63	Mixed	100%	NA (27–30)	NA (3–5)	NA	76	18 (NA)
Nikolajek et al,[45] 2011	Retrospective	54/70	Mixed	100%	18 (10–28)	1	86	87	14 (3–48)
Chang et al,[40] 2012	Retrospective	NA/54	Mixed	100%	27 (mean SF equivalent 20.6)	3 (NA)	78	81	22 (NA)
Thibault et al,[46] 2015	Retrospective	40/56	Mixed	100%	30 (20–35)	NA (2–5)	NA	78	7 (1–39)
Hashmi et a,[47] 2016	Retrospective	215/247	Mixed	100%	18 (16–24)	1 (1–3)	74	87	8
Boyce-Fappiano et al,[48] 2017	Retrospective	162/237	Mixed	100%	16 (16–35)	1 (1–5)	81	71	10

71% to 93%. The weighted local control rate of the 1263 retreated lesions was 83%. The study by Choi and colleagues[42] suggests that SF-equivalent dose of 15 Gy or greater is associated with improved local control. Therefore, similar dosimetric parameters for D_{min} and D_{95} may be applicable in the reirradiation setting to ensure adequate tumor coverage and improve local control.

Special Consideration: Postoperative Stereotactic Body Radiation Therapy

Surgical stabilization and tumor resection are often indicated in patients with spinal metastases causing mechanical instability, spinal cord compression, or rapidly progressive neurologic deficits. SBRT may be able to overcome the hypoxic environment of the postoperative bed, thereby improving local control. Furthermore, separation surgery may allow dose escalation to the gross tumor by removing the epidural portion of the tumor and creating space between the target and the spinal cord, the major dose-limiting organ.[49] In addition, pre-SBRT cement augmentation may be indicated in the case of symptomatic vertebral compression fracture, and its use has been tested in the prophylactic setting as well, showing pain relief in 95% of patients and local control of 90%.[50] **Table 4** summarizes outcomes of the largest studies of postoperative SBRT to date.[50–59] The weighted local control rate of the total 720 lesions treated was 81%.

There are data suggesting that higher dose per fraction may offer superior local control in the postoperative setting. Moulding and colleagues[51] reported 21 patients treated with decompression surgery followed by SF SBRT, and observed superior 1-year tumor control with 24 Gy compared with 18 to 23 Gy (94% vs 81%). A large retrospective study of both SF and HF SBRT showed better 1-year local control with SF (24 Gy) and high-dose HF (24–30 Gy in 3 fractions) regimens compared with low-dose HF, 91% and 96% versus 77%, respectively.[52] This finding is consistent with a recent prospective study showing 91% local control with high-dose HF SBRT (30 Gy in 5 fractions), compared with only 77% with low-dose SF SBRT (16 Gy).[55,59] Nevertheless, the optimal dosing of postoperative SBRT has yet to be established, and high-dose SF and HF regimens both offer excellent local control.

TOXICITIES OF SPINAL STEREOTACTIC BODY RADIATION THERAPY

Normal tissue dose constraints as defined by Emami and colleagues[60] and subsequently the quantitative analyses of normal tissue effects in the clinic (QUANTEC) collaboration were not developed to predict toxicity risks in the setting of ablative radiotherapy.[60–62] In addition, ablative doses may result in novel toxicities, such as vertebral compression fractures (VCFs), not previously observed with conventional schedules. Analysis of modern spinal SBRT cohort studies helps provide a better estimate of normal tissue tolerances with this emerging technique. The key evidence regarding major spinal SBRT toxicities and dose constraint recommendations in the de novo setting are discussed here.

RADIATION MYELOPATHY

Radiation myelopathy (RM) is defined as the presentation of neurologic symptoms localized to the region of irradiated cord or cauda equina in the absence of tumor progression. It is one of the most dreaded complications of spinal SBRT, with the potential for significant morbidity, such as paraplegia or quadriplegia or loss of autonomic processes, depending on injury location.[63] RM has been shown to manifest between 6 and 24 months after conventional radiotherapy, with a median latent time of 18 months.[64,65] In ablative cohorts, the median latency was only 12 months. A previous comprehensive review of 1388 spinal SBRT patients reported a 0.4% incidence of RM at a mean follow-up of 15 months.[66] Traditionally viewed as a serial organ at risk (OAR), the maximum point dose (D_{max}) is often used to define radiotherapy tolerance in these organs. However, there is evolving evidence of volumetric considerations, although these are not yet clearly defined.[63,67]

Spinal Cord

Several detailed dosimetric analyses have been conducted to better delineate the ablative dose tolerance of the spinal cord. Sahgal and colleagues[68] reported a multi-institutional dosimetric comparison of 9 patients who experienced RM matched with 66 control patients. The median equivalent dose in 2 Gy fractions (EQD2) doses to the cord were 74 Gy and 36 Gy respectively in the RM and control cohorts. A systematic review corroborated these doses, with median EQD2 of 74 Gy and 38 Gy in RM and non-RM cohorts respectively in the summarized analysis of the 7 included series.[69] From Sahgal and colleagues'[68] study, a logistic regression model was generated that estimated the probability of RM as a function of D_{max}.

Similarly, Katsoulakis and colleagues[70] observed 2 cases of RM in a cohort of 228 patients treated with SF spinal SBRT. However, dosimetric analyses determined that the cord doses were

Table 4
Select studies of postoperative spine stereotactic body radiation therapy with sample size greater than 20

Author, Year	Study Design	Patients/ Lesions (N)	Histology	Prior RT (%)	Total Dose Median (Range)	Median No of Fractions (Range)	Pain Relief (%)	Local Control (%)	Median Follow-up, Range (mo)
Moulding et al,[51] 2010	Retrospective	21/21	Mixed	0	24 (18–24)	1	NA	81	10 (1–55)
Laufer et al,[52] 2013	Retrospective	186/186	Mixed	49	NA (18–36)	1–6	NA	82	8 (1–66)
Tao et al,[53] 2016	Prospective	66/69	Mixed	48	27 (16–30)	3 (1–5)	NA	67	30 (1–145)
Chan et al,[54] 2016	Retrospective	70/75	Mixed	35	NA (18–40)	3 (1–5)	NA	65	11 (1–49)
Miller et al,[55] 2017	Retrospective	83/83	Mixed	41	16 (12–16)	1	NA	77	9 (1–87)
Barzilai et al,[56] 2018	Retrospective	111/111	Mixed	NA	27 (24–27)	3 (1–5)	NA	94	7 (4–12)
Ito et al,[57] 2018	Retrospective	28/28	Mixed	100	24	2	NA	75	13 (4–38)
Wardak et al,[50] 2019	Prospective	29/29	Mixed	NA	20	1	95	96	10 (0–63)
Alghamdi et al,[58] 2019	Retrospective	47/83	Mixed	53	24 (24–30)	2 (1–4)	NA	82	12 (1–54)
Redmond et al,[59] 2019	Prospective	33/35	Mixed	0	30	5	67	91	10 (1–47)

lower in these patients than the median D_{max} of 13.85 Gy. Through dose volume atlas of myelopathy incidence modeling, it was determined that a D_{max} of 14 Gy was an acceptable constraint. A third model generated by Grimm and colleagues[71] used data from the early Stanford experience for both de novo and reirradiated patients.[72] A probit model was generated and compared with literature values to put forth both low-risk (1%) and high-risk (3%) estimates of the spinal cord constraint.

Elements of each model were combined in the Hypofractionated Treatment Effects in Clinic (HyTEC) report in the construction of their constraint guidelines, which are shown in **Table 5**.[63]

Table 5
Organ at risk dose constraints

Toxicity End Point	Evidence (Year)	OAR Dose[a]	Toxicity Incidence (%)	Constraint Recommendations[a]
Neurologic Injury				
Spinal cord myelopathy	HyTEC Report[63] Sahgal et al,[68] 2013 Katsoulakis et al,[70] 2017	As per HyTEC report regression model	<5	1 fx, 12.4–14 Gy 2 fx, 17 Gy 3 fx, 20.3 Gy 4 fx, 23 Gy 5 fx, 25.3 Gy
Cauda equina[b]	RTOG 0653[73]	16 Gy/1 fx	0	1 fx, 16 Gy
Plexopathy				
Brachial	Forquer et al,[76] 2009 Chang et al,[75] 2014	30–70 Gy/3–4 fx 35 Gy/4 fx	<19 <30	1 fx, 15 Gy 2 fx, 20 Gy 3 fx, 23 Gy 4 fx, 27–35 Gy[c] 5 fx, 33 Gy
Lumbrosacral[d]	Stubblefield et al,[78] 2017 Zeng et al,[77] 2019	18–26 Gy/1 fx 16.5 Gy/2 fx	<6 <4.5	1 fx, 18–26 Gy 2 fx, <16.5 Gy
VCF	Sahgal et al,[15] 2013 Thibault et al,[80] 2017 Faruqi et al,[82] 2018	8–35 Gy/1–5 fx	14	Keep <20 Gy/fx Consider more conservative constraints for high-risk lesions[e]
Esophageal toxicity	Sharma et al,[74] 2017 Cox et al,[83] 2012 Harder et al,[85] 2017 Wu et al,[86] 2014	14 Gy/1 fx ($D_{2.5cc}$) As per Harder et al[85] model ($D_{1.5cc}$) As per Wu et al[86] regression model (D_{5cc} or D_{max})	<5 <10.6 <20	1 fx, $D_{2.5cc}$ <14 Gy 3 fx, $D_{1.5cc}$ <14.3 Gy or D_{5cc} <16.8 Gy or D_{max} <27.6 Gy 4 fx, D_{5cc} <18.1 Gy or D_{max} <30.2 Gy 5 fx, $D_{1.5cc}$ <16 Gy or D_{5cc} <19 Gy or D_{max} <32.2 Gy Caution when concurrent chemotherapy is given

SBRT dose constraints are derived and integrated from best available dosimetric evidence sources.
Abbreviation: fx, fraction.
[a] All listed doses are D_{max} unless noted otherwise.
[b] Likely similar to spinal cord constraint; there is a general lack of dosimetric literature evidence. Note that RTOG 0653 constraints were met in 74% of cases.
[c] Upper limit derived from Chang and colleagues[75] with higher plexopathy threshold (30% vs 19%).
[d] Likely similar to brachial plexus constraint; there is a general lack of dosimetric literature evidence.
[e] Risk factors: greater than 50% vertebral body involvement, lytic appearance, lumbar/sacral involvement, baseline VCF, and spinal malalignment.

Cauda Equina

Anatomically, the cauda equina (CE) begins around L1/L2 as the spinal cord ends. Although a central nervous structure, it cannot be assumed to have the same SBRT tolerance as the spinal cord.[63] The literature is sparse in defining CE tolerance. In the RTOG 0631 phase 2 trial of 16 Gy in an SF spinal SBRT, with a CE constraint of 16 Gy, there was no observed RM.[73]

PLEXOPATHY

Like the spinal cord, damage to the nerve bundles of the brachial and sacral plexuses can result in neurologic symptoms termed brachial plexopathy (BP) and lumbrosacral plexopathy (LSP) respectively. The brachial plexus originates from C5 to T1 nerve roots, whereas the lumbrosacral plexus originates from L4 to S4.

Brachial Plexopathy

A dosimetric analysis of 56 (60 segments) spine SBRT patients receiving SF treatment revealed no events of BP with a mean D_{max} of 17 Gy.[74]

However, much of the literature for plexus tolerances originates from apical lung studies. Chang and colleagues[75] discovered a 30% (3 out of 10) incidence rate of BP in patients with apical tumors treated with 50 Gy in 4 fractions, with the affected patients having plexus D_{max} greater than 35 Gy. A series from Indiana University of 37 patients with apical non–small cell lung cancer (NSCLC) revealed a 19% BP rate (7 of 37 patients) with 3 to 4 fractions of SBRT. The median plexus D_{max} was 25 Gy in those without BP, and 30 Gy in those who experienced it. Using 2-year Kaplan-Meier estimates of BP risk, the investigators derived BP constraints for isoeffect dose levels.[76]

Lumbrosacral Plexopathy

The evidence surrounding the ablative tolerance of the sacral plexus tolerance are lacking. Zeng and colleagues[77] retrospectively reviewed a series of 22 patients receiving sacral SBRT with 24 Gy in 2 fractions. The median D_{max} was 16.5 Gy. One patient experienced sacral plexopathy at 8 months, with a sacral plexus D_{max} of 30 Gy. A retrospective series of 47 sacral SBRT patients receiving SF treatment from 18 to 26 Gy reported the incidence of nerve injury by spinal level. Overall, 6 injuries occurred out of 98 spinal segments treated (6%) from L4 to sacrum.[78]

VERTEBRAL COMPRESSION FRACTURE

VCF is one of the more common toxicities following spinal SBRT. It was first described by Rose and colleagues[79] in a cohort of 62 patients receiving SF SBRT 18 to 24 Gy. They observed a significant VCF incidence of 39%, with lesion location (between T10 and sacrum), lytic appearance, and percentage body involvement being independent predictors of the end point. A large multi-institutional study of 252 patients and 410 spinal segments reported an overall 14% VCF incidence with a median latency of 2.5 months. Dose per fraction (>20 Gy), baseline compression fracture greater than 50% of height, lytic tumor, and spinal malalignment were all found to be significantly associated with VCF risk.[15] A computed tomography (CT)–based segmental analysis of 100 spine SBRT lesions confirmed that lytic appearance and dose per fraction were independent predictors of VCF risk, with a threshold of greater than 11.6% vertebral body involvement and greater than 20 Gy per fraction respectively.[80]

Given the rates of VCF with SF regimens, fractionated schedules gained interest. Tseng and colleagues[81] reported the outcomes of a prospective study of 145 patients and 279 de novo spinal metastases treated with 24 Gy in 2 fractions. They reported a VCF incidence of 13%, with a total of 39.4% of these patients requiring salvage intervention (4.7% of all patients). A recent systematic review of 11 studies totaling 2911 spine segments treated reported a similar VCF incidence of 14%, with a median latency of 2.6 months. Again, lytic disease, higher dose per fraction, spinal deformity, baseline VCF, and greater than 40% to 50% vertebral body involvement were predictive of VCF. The overall salvage rate was 37%.[82]

ESOPHAGEAL TOXICITY

The esophagus lies anterior to the thoracic vertebral bodies and is at risk of receiving high doses in spinal SBRT. Both acute and late toxicities have been observed in the literature. A Cleveland Clinic series of 56 patients (60 segments) receiving SF cervical/thoracic spine SBRT resulted in a 13% esophageal toxicity rate. The esophageal mean D_{max} was 14 Gy.[74] The largest dedicated series focusing on esophageal toxicity reported the outcomes of 182 patients (204 segments) receiving a median dose of 24 Gy/1 fraction. The crude incidence of esophageal toxicity was 7% (n = 14). Through logistic regression modeling, it was determined that $D_{2.5cc}$ less than 14 Gy resulted in less than 5% risk of grade 3 esophageal toxicity.[83]

Several dosimetric models have been constructed to determine esophageal ablative dose constraints. Nuyttens and colleagues[84] determined that, for 5-fraction SBRT, a D_{1cc} of 32.9 Gy and a D_{max} of 43.4 Gy were associated with a 50% risk of grade 2 esophageal toxicity. A series of 150 patients (190 segments) determined that $D_{1.5cc}$ was the strongest predictor of grade 2+ toxicity, putting forth dose constraint recommendations for 3-fraction and 5-fraction SBRT.[85] In addition, Wu and colleagues[86] assessed 125 SBRT patients and derived logistic regression models for D_{5cc} and D_{max} that determined dose constraints for 3, 4, and 5 fractions in which the risk of grade 2+ toxicity was limited to less than 20%.

SUMMARY

Spine SBRT is an indispensable treatment modality for spinal metastases offering excellent durable local control, especially in the settings of radioresistant tumor, reirradiation, and postoperative ablation. With the exception of 1 phase III trial that has been reported in abstract form only, reporting a benefit of 24 Gy in 1 fraction compared with 9 Gy in 3 fractions, no single regimen has been shown in a randomized fashion to be superior. Both SF and HF regimens are safe (robust OAR constraints are available) and well supported by evidence, and minimum dosimetric parameters required for improved local control include GTV D_{min} greater than 15 Gy and D_{95} greater than 18.3 Gy. Ongoing prospective, randomized studies will shed more light on the role of SBRT in the management of spinal metastasis and the optimal prescription dose for spine SBRT.

CLINICAL CASE DISCUSSIONS

The following case discussions are presented from 4 different institutions with significant spine SBRT experience. A clinical summary with relevant diagnostic imaging is provided, followed by a short description and commentary of key relevant points and recommendations for management from each institution.

CASE 1. DE NOVO SPINE METASTASIS

Clinical summary:

- A 62-year-old man with newly diagnosed renal cell carcinoma
- Mild back pain, not mechanical
- No prior cancer history, no prior radiotherapy
- Vertebral body and early epidural disease only lytic lesion at T12 (see next image)
- Spinal Instability Neoplastic Score (SINS) 6
- Several small lung nodules
- Planned for nivolumab and ipilimumab systemic therapy
- No comorbidities
- Karnofsky Performance Score (KPS) 90

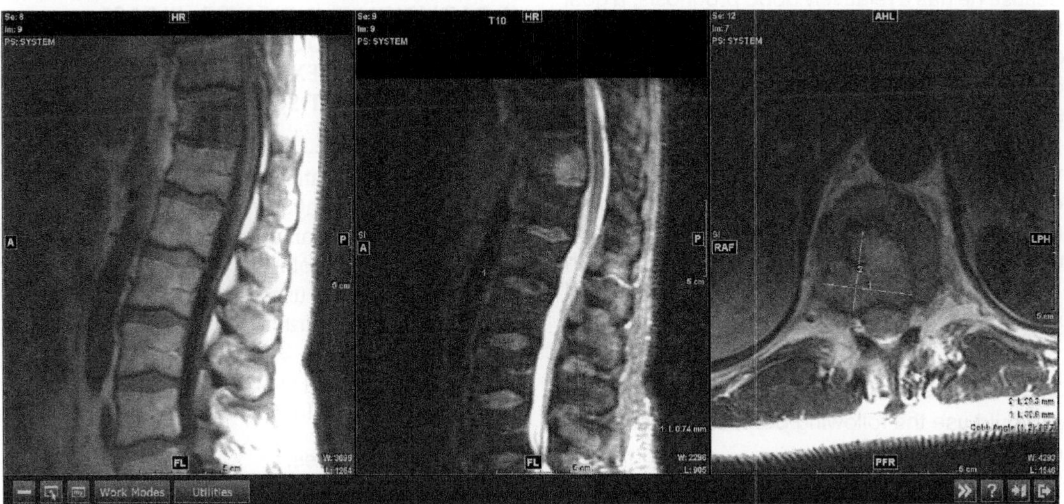

IS SURGERY INDICATED?

Institution A

Surgery is generally indicated in patients with high-grade spinal cord compression and neurologic deficits or with mechanical instability that is not amenable to cement augmentation. Given the low-grade epidural disease (Bilsky 1a) and stable SINS (6), surgery is not indicated in this patient.

Institution B

Given his mechanical stability and low-grade epidural involvement without spinal cord compression, surgery is not indicated.

Institution C

Given the case presented has low-grade epidural disease (Bilsky 1a) and stable SINS (6), we would not offer any invasive procedure that includes surgery.

Institution D

This patient has no indications for surgery. The patient is mechanically stable, has only early epidural disease, and there no need for further tumor tissue.

IS RADIATION TREATMENT INDICATED?

Institution A

This patient has limited spine disease, pain, and epidural extension, so I would recommend radiotherapy. In addition, SBRT might potentiate the effect of immunotherapy.

Institution B

Because he has a relatively good prognosis, a goal of treatment should be durable local control to prevent future metastatic epidural spinal cord compression. With a radioresistant histology such as renal cell carcinoma, we would recommend SBRT or stereotactic radiosurgery (SRS) rather than conventionally fractionated radiation therapy, because the latter has a low probability of providing durable local control. In cases with epidural involvement such as this, we favor treatment with 3 fractions (SBRT). For cases without epidural extension, we favor treatment with an SF (SRS).

Institution C

We would use the following process for treatment decision:

Step 1: complete clinical history and a good physical examination; patient has good performance status (PS) and a nonmechanical pain.

Step 2: review the systemic burden of disease (CT chest, abdomen, and pelvis): assuming the patient is oligometastatic helps our decision. We would also acquire full spine MRI.

Step 3: review whether any effective systemic treatments are available: ipilimumab and nivolumab.

Step 4: NOMS (neurologic, oncologic, mechanical, and systemic)

N: T12 lesion; Bilsky grade 1a or 1b epidural disease without spinal cord compression.

O: Renal cell carcinoma; unfavorable histology.

M: T12 lesion and the pain is not mechanical. SINS is 6: characterize mechanical stability.

S: As previously discussed, surgery is not indicated.

Summary: patient is presenting with limited spine disease (T12), nonmechanical pain, and low-grade epidural extension, and has potential survival of 6 months or more, so I would recommend stereotactic ablative body radiotherapy.

Institution D

This patient can be evaluated according to the NOMS framework. Neurologically/oncologically the patient is neurologically intact with limited epidural radioresistant disease and no prior radiation therapy to the site of interest. Mechanically the spine is stable, not requiring stabilization, and systemically the patient still has a favorable expectation of a good prognosis. Therefore, radiosurgery alone would be the recommended therapy in order to provide durable and effective tumor control and palliation that will have the least negative impact on quality of life.

IF RADIATION IS INDICATED, PLEASE RECOMMEND A DOSE FRACTIONATION SCHEDULE, AND EXPLAIN WHY YOU CHOSE THAT TREATMENT SCHEDULE

Institution A

I would treat this patient with 24 Gy in 2 fractions. My default fractionation is 2 fractions given data suggesting comparable rates of local control as SF regimens, but a potentially lower risk of vertebral body fracture. If I am unable to meet my constraints outlined here in 2 fractions, I would fractionate further into 27 Gy in 3 fractions. However, given the limited disease, I suspect that I would be able to meet constraints for a 2-fraction paradigm.

Planning objectives:

- Cord plus 2 mm: maximum point dose less than 17 Gy
- Esophagus: less than 20 Gy
- Greater than 95% coverage of GTV
- Greater than 85% coverage of planning target volume (PTV)
- Typical prescription isodose line 55% to 65%

Institution B

For treatment planning, in cases with any degree of epidural involvement, if feasible, we perform a myelogram immediately before CT-based simulation (myelogram for spinal cord delineation), because we have previously shown that this approach more accurately delineates the spinal cord compared with registering T2-weighted MRI, thereby improving PTV coverage and reducing spinal cord dose.[87]

We use the Elekta BodyFIX immobilization system when treating spine lesions at T5 and down.

After myelogram simulation, we register T1-weighted postcontrast MRI and T2-weighted MRI to aid in delineation of tumor extent/involvement.

We follow the International Spine Radiosurgery Consortium consensus guidelines for target volume delineation.[88] In this case, the tumor involves most of the vertebral body and is slightly lateralized to the right, and we would therefore cover the entire vertebral body and right-sided (ipsilateral) pedicle and transverse process in our clinical target volume (CTV).

We add a 2-mm symmetric expansion to the CTV for creation of a PTV and use a 1 mm planning organ at risk volume (PRV) on the spinal cord when the spinal cord has been defined on a myelosim.

Our preferred 3-fraction spine SBRT regimen is 9 Gy in 3 fractions to 27 Gy,[89] delivered every other day.

Our planning objectives and normal tissue constraints are as follows:

Structure	Parameter	Constraint
PTV	$D_{95\%}$ (%)	$\geq$100%
PTV	$D_{1\%}$ (%)	$\leq$130%
Spinal cord	$D_{0.1cc}$ (Gy)	$\leq$22 Gy
Spinal cord 1-mm PRV	$D_{0.1cc}$ (Gy)	$\leq$24 Gy
Liver	D_{700cc} (Gy)	$\leq$15 Gy
Great vessels (thoracic aorta)	$D_{01.cc}$ (Gy)	$\leq$30 Gy

Institution C

Our group default would be to treat this patient with 24 Gy in 2 fractions: good local control and lower risk of toxicity. I would offer 24 Gy in an SF because of the data showing higher rates of local control despite the potentially higher risk of vertebral compression fracture.

At our center, to be eligible for an SF, patients need to fit all the following criteria.

Criteria for SF spine SBRT:

- Only 1 vertebral level involved
- Performance status 0 to 2
- No rapid neurologic decline
- Involved vertebral level is below T4
- No prior radiotherapy to vertebral level involved
- Patient is ambulatory
- Greater than or equal to 3-mm gap between the spinal cord and edge of epidural/spinal lesion
- No spinal instability caused by compression fracture
- Less than 50% loss of vertebral body height
- No bony retropulsion causing neurologic abnormality
- Paraspinal/spinal mass less than 5 cm in greatest dimension

The presented case fits the criteria.

OVERALL STEREOTACTIC ABLATIVE BODY RADIOTHERAPY GUIDANCE

- Reinforce thermoplastic mask for lesion at T4 and higher
- Elekta BodyFIX immobilization system when treating spine lesions at T5 and down
- GTV: MRI-guided GTV
- CTV: following the international guidelines
- PTV: 2-mm to 3-mm uniform expansion around CTV
- Organs at risk
- Spinal cord PRV (2.0-mm uniform margin around spinal cord), thecal sac, relevant OARs (eg, esophagus, kidneys, lungs)
- Dose prescribed to PTV mean dose
- Treatment isocentre: near center of PTV in superior-inferior (SI) and anterior-posterior (AP) and laterally; consider CBCT clearance
- Inverse planning objectives set for dose sculptors such as rings around target (to reduce dose around target) and thecal sac (and/or spinal cord PRV)
- Planning aim: maximize PTV V100% without violating thecal sac/spinal cord PRV limit

DOSE: 24 GY IN 2 FRACTIONS

Structure	Parameter	Constraint
PTV	$D_{95\%}$ (%)	$\geq$100%
PTV	$D_{1\%}$ (%)	$\leq$130%
Spinal cord 2-mm PRV	$D_{0.35cc}$ (Gy)	$\leq$17 Gy
Liver	Mean	$\leq$8 Gy
Esophagus	$D_{0.35cc}$ (Gy)	$\leq$20 Gy

Institution D

This case is appropriate for radiosurgery. Twenty-four gray in an SF is able to provide durable long-term local control superior to any hypofractionation schedule reported in the literature. Although there is a higher likelihood of vertebral body fracture with 24 Gy in 1 fraction (8% requiring an intervention because of fracture), the cumulative incidence of local failure was 2.3% at 4 years at our institution, including radioresistant disease such as renal cell carcinoma. The very high local control benefit may offset the risk of fracture in the long term, because even hypofractionation does not eliminate the risk of postradiation vertebral body fracture. Giving the same dose in 2 fractions seems to result in a higher cumulative rate of local failure. Overall, 17% showed local failure at 2 years but approximately 30% risk of local relapse in the case of mild epidural disease. This finding suggests that 24 Gy for 1 fraction is a more ablative treatment of solid tumor spinal metastases than hypofractionated treatment schedules.

Twenty-four gray for 1 fraction planning objectives

PTV Coverage	Ideal: V100%>90% and V95%>95% Acceptable: V100%>80% and V95%>90%
PTV inhomogeneity	Maximum point dose: 110%–130% Global D_{max} must be within PTV
High dose 2 spillage	Hotspots >115% should be within PTV, hotspots >105% outside of PTV should be limited to 5 cc

Percent of the target volume receiving 100% of the prescribed dose.

NORMAL TISSUE CONSTRAINTS

Structure	Parameter	Dose
Spinal cord (myelogram defined)	D_{max}	14 Gy
	$D_{0.35cc}$	10 Gy
	Dose transecting cord	10 Gy
Cauda (myelogram defined)	D_{max}	18 Gy
	$D_{0.35cc}$	14 Gy
Bowel/stomach	D_{max}	15 Gy (stomach) 16 Gy (bowel)
	D_{5cc}	12 Gy

CASE 2. REIRRADIATION

Clinical summary:

- A 68-year-old man with stage IV prostate cancer, limited metastatic disease, diagnosed 6 years ago, developed spinal metastases 2 years ago and was treated with 3000 cGy/ 10 fractions T1 to T7 at that time, and is currently on hormonal therapy.
- Three-month history of progressive nonmechanical midback pain, worse at night, graded 7 out of 10. MRI shows progressive T4, T5, T6 disease. Disease involves vertebral body and spinous process at T4, circumferential disease at T5 with epidural and extraosseus paraspinal disease, and vertebral body–only disease at T6.
- Has several other osseous metastases but is otherwise stable and not symptomatic; prostate-specific antigen level has increased from 8.0 to 12.0 ng/mL.
- Still working full time as a nuclear physicist.

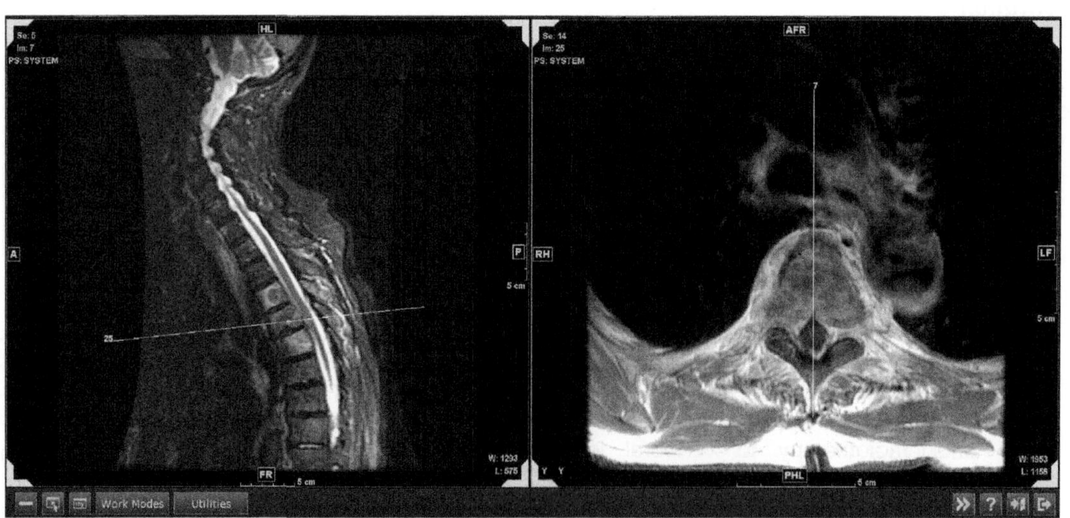

IS SURGERY INDICATED?

Institution A

Given that the patient does not have evidence of mechanical instability and has low-grade epidural disease (Bilsky 1b), we would recommend reirradiation with SBRT rather than surgical intervention.

Institution B

No. Surgery is not indicated but should be discussed: low-grade epidural disease (Bilsky 1b), no mechanical instability, SINS 7 (neurosurgery should be consulted), and nonmechanical pain.

Institution C

Although a SINS is not provided, based on the clinical scenario and provided imaging, we estimate that his SINS is 7, driven by his nonmechanical pain, less than 50% vertebral body collapse at T5, and involvement of bilateral posterolateral spinal elements. Because a score of 7 denotes indeterminate stability, we would recommend neurosurgical consultation for further assessment of stability; however, based on the information provided, we do not anticipate that surgical stabilization would be recommended in this case.

Institution D

This patient has multilevel sclerotic bone disease with early epidural disease without symptoms associated with mechanical instability. The midthoracic spine, buttressed by multiple levels of ribs, is a less common site of instability. The probability of need for mechanical stabilization is low in this case.

IS RADIATION TREATMENT INDICATED?

Institution A

Yes. This patient has both 7 out of 10 pain and Bilsky grade 2 disease and, as such, I would recommend reirradiation using SBRT.

Institution B

Based on NOMS criteria:

N: low-grade epidural disease (Bilsky 1b).
O: prostate cancer (favorable to intermediate histology).
M: SINS is 7 (indeterminate stability: neurosurgery should be consulted but we do not anticipate stabilization will be needed).
S: good performance status and prognosis; potential survival greater than 6 months.
SBRT would provide symptom relief and durable local control.

Institution C

N: the patient has grade 1a or 1b epidural disease based on the available imaging.
O: the patient has prostate cancer, which is considered a favorable intermediate histology.
M: although a SINS is not provided, based on the clinical scenario and provided imaging, we estimate that his SINS is 7, driven by his nonmechanical pain, less than 50% vertebral body collapse at T5, and involvement of bilateral posterolateral spinal elements. Because a score of 7 denotes indeterminate stability, we would recommend neurosurgical consultation for further assessment of stability; however, based on the information provided, we do not anticipate that surgical stabilization would be recommended in this case.
S: the patient has a good performance status and may still live several years with metastatic prostate cancer, and, as such, one goal of treatment in addition to symptom relief should be durable local control to prevent future metastatic epidural spinal cord compression given the current presence of epidural disease. Because he is likely mechanical stable and has minimal epidural involvement, we would not favor surgical treatment in his case. Our recommendation therefore would be for reirradiation to T4 through T6. We would recommend treatment with spine SBRT to allow maximum dose to the tumor while sparing the spinal cord given the prior conventionally fractionated radiation therapy. We do not favor SF SRS in the setting of reirradiation or in cases with epidural extension.

Institution D

Following the NOMS framework:

N: neurologically intact with early epidural disease.
O: although prostate cancer is generally considered radiosensitive, it has recurred after a prior course of radiation and hence can be considered resistant to radiation.
M: mechanically intact.
S: overall good prognosis and will benefit from treatment that provides dural tumor control.

IF RADIATION IS INDICATED, PLEASE RECOMMEND A DOSE FRACTIONATION SCHEDULE, AND EXPLAIN WHY YOU CHOSE THAT TREATMENT SCHEDULE

Institution A

This patient has been previously treated with radiation therapy and the target volume would include

3 vertebral levels. Therefore, I would prescribe 27 Gy in 3 fractions using SBRT.

Institution B

SBRT 27 Gy in 3 fractions (delivered every other day); previously treated with radiation therapy (2 years ago).

Institution C

Our preferred retreatment regimen for reirradiation is 3 fractions of spine SBRT, 9 Gy in 3 fractions to 27 Gy, delivered every other day.

Institution D

Unless on a protocol for SF radiosurgery, this patient would be recommended to undergo salvage SBRT with 9 Gy given in 3 fractions on 3 consecutive days.

PLEASE INCLUDE YOUR TREATMENT PLANNING OBJECTIVES FOR EACH SITUATION, WITH NORMAL TISSUE CONSTRAINTS

Institution A

For the spinal cord constraint in the reirradiation setting, I usually allow a cumulative BED3 of 75 Gy accounting for 25% repair if there has been greater than 6 months between courses and 50% repair if there has been greater than 1 year between courses. This patient received 30 Gy in 10 fractions, which was completed 2 years prior. This treatment was a BED3 of 60 Gy, $0.5 \times 60 = 30$ Gy effective BED3 from the prior course. I would allow $75 - 40 = 35$ Gy BED3 in the current plan, which would equate to a spinal cord constraint to the cord plus 2 mm of approximately 16.2 Gy in 3 fractions. In the reirradiation setting, I would aim for greater than 90% coverage of the GTV and 85% coverage of the PTV. I typically prescribe to the 55% to 65% isodose line.

Institution B

For the spinal cord constraint PRV 2 mm in the reirradiation setting:

We allow 14.5 Gy in 3 fractions if no epidural component or 17.4 Gy in 3 fractions if epidural component is present.
In the reirradiation setting, we allow underdosing the CTV/tumor near the spinal cord.
We aim for greater than 90% coverage of the GTV and 85% coverage of the PTV.

Institution C

OAR Name	α/β (Gy)	Dose Limit Maximum to 0.1 cc (EQD2) (Gy)	Previous Dose Discount (%) (0% Means no Discount) For >3 y, 50% Discount Suggested			
			< 3 mo	3–6 mo	6 mo – 1 y	1–3 y
Esophagus	2.5	70	0	10	25	50
Great vessels	2.5	100	0	10	25	50
Heart	2.5	70	0	10	25	50
Spinal cord	2.5	50	0	10	25	50
Trachea/ bronchus	2.5	70	0	10	25	50

Because it has been 2 years since his prior irradiation, we would forgive 50% of the previous dose for the OARs listed earlier. We would use equivalent dose in 2-Gy fraction limits to the spinal cord, limiting the dose to less than 50 Gy. This approach will result in underdosing of the tumor near the spinal cord, which is acceptable in this setting.

Institution D

The following dose criteria are used for 3-fraction hypofractionated reirradiation:

Structure	Dose Constraint	Dose (Gy)	Comment
Spinal cord (myelogram defined)	D_{max}	14.5	D_{max} limit dose. The guideline dose is 13.9 Gy
	$D_{0.35cc}$	10	—
Esophagus	D_{max}	20.4	—
Trachea	Prescription	—	No hot spots

CASE 3. POSTOPERATIVE CASE

Clinical summary:

- A 60-year-old man with stage IV renal cell carcinoma
- New-onset back pain, worse with movement, 8 out of 10 severity for 1 week
- MRI shows high-grade cord compression at T6
- Tumor involves the vertebral body, and left pedicle and lamina
- Working full time, KPS 80
- No contraindications to surgery
- No prior radiotherapy to this area

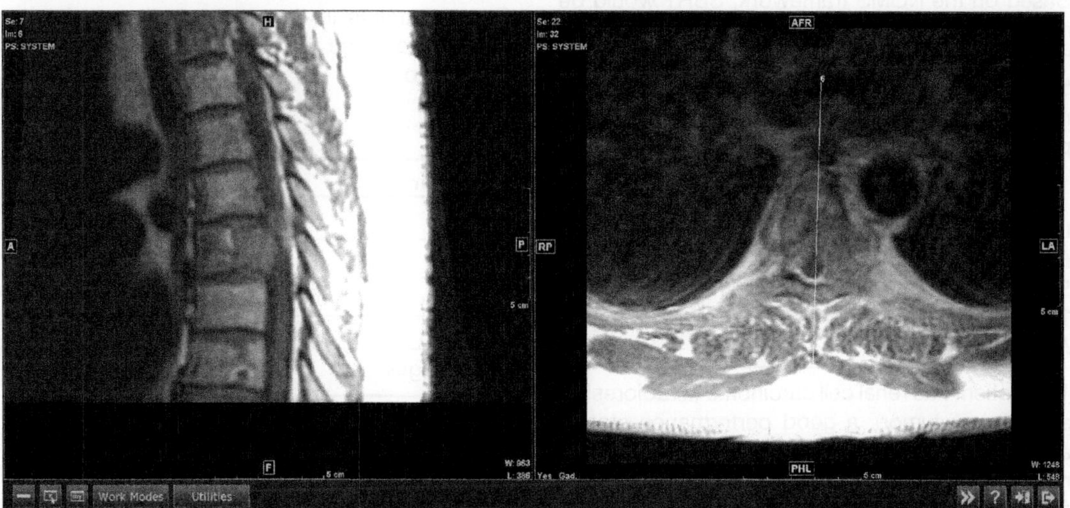

IS SURGERY INDICATED?

Institution A

Given the Bilsky grade 2 high-grade epidural disease as well as mechanical back pain, I would recommend separation surgery and decompression of the spinal cord.

Institution B

Patient presenting with mechanical pain and a high-grade epidural disease (Bilsky grade 2). Thus, we would assess for separation surgery and decompression of the spinal cord.

Institution C

Given his reasonable performance status, estimated life expectancy greater than 6 months, and high-grade metastatic epidural spinal cord compression from a radioresistant histology, we would recommend treatment with a separation surgery and stabilization followed by postoperative spine SBRT in attempt to achieve durable local control. Separation surgery is indicated to create at least a 2-mm separation between the thecal sac and spinal cord to allow for safe postoperative spine SBRT.

Institution D

Using the NOMS framework, this patient has radioresistant Bilsky grade 2 epidural disease (neurologic/oncologic). The patient also has severe mechanical back pain (mechanical). Because the patient is medical fit for surgery (systemic), separation surgery is indicated to decompress the epidural space and provide mechanical stabilization.

IS RADIATION TREATMENT INDICATED?

Institution A

Yes, I would recommend postoperative radiation therapy in order to decrease the rate of local recurrence following surgery.

Institution B

This is a 60-year-old man with metastatic renal cell carcinoma. He has a good performance status (KPS 80) and is still working full time. No history of no prior radiation therapy to this area. Potential survival greater than 6 months.

N: Bilsky grade 2 epidural disease at T6.
O: renal cell carcinoma (unfavorable histology).
M: mechanical pain but we cannot define stability (SIN cannot be determined).
S: recommend treatment with a separation surgery and stabilization followed by postoperative spine SBRT. Treatment is designed to achieved durable local control.

Institution C

Although we are not given the extent of the patient's systemic burden and his remaining systemic treatment options, we assume based on his good overall performance status that the patient has an expected survival of greater than 6 months, if not years. Thus, given his symptomatic metastatic epidural spinal cord compression, we would recommend treatment at T6.

Institution D

Based on the NOMS framework, SBRT would be recommended because renal cell carcinoma is a histology relatively resistant to conventional radiation therapy and will benefit with more durable tumor control with a high-dose-per-fraction paradigm.

IF RADIATION IS INDICATED, PLEASE RECOMMEND A DOSE FRACTIONATION SCHEDULE, AND EXPLAIN WHY YOU CHOSE THAT TREATMENT SCHEDULE

Institution A

This patient has renal cell carcinoma (a radioresistant primary tumor), a good performance status, and limited spine involvement. Therefore, I would recommend SBRT. I would prescribe 24 Gy in 2 fractions.

Institution B

Our group default would be to treat this patient with 24 Gy in 2 fractions: good local control, convenience, and lower risk of toxicity.

Institution C

Our preferred 3-fraction postoperative spine SBRT regimen is 9 Gy in 3 fractions to 27 Gy, delivered every other day.

Institution D

Because this patient has not had radiation to this area, and the prognosis is still favorable, we would recommend 24 Gy in an SF provided sufficient separation (approximately 2 mm) between the epidural tumor edge and spinal cord was achieved with separation surgery. If sufficient separation was not achievable, then we would consider a hypofractionated regimen such as 10 Gy in 3 fractions.

PLEASE INCLUDE YOUR TREATMENT PLANNING OBJECTIVES FOR EACH SITUATION, WITH NORMAL TISSUE CONSTRAINTS

Institution A

Cord plus 2 mm: maximum point dose less than 17 Gy
Esophagus: less than 20 Gy
Greater than 95% coverage of GTV
Greater than 85% coverage of PTV
Typical prescription isodose line 55% to 65%

Institution B

Our constraints in the postoperative setting are identical to those for intact vertebrae and would be as follows:

Structure	Parameter	Constraint
PTV	$D_{95\%}$ (%)	≥100%
PTV	$D_{1\%}$ (%)	≤130%
Spinal cord 2-mm PRV	$D_{0.35cc}$ (Gy)	≤17 Gy
Liver	Mean	≤8 Gy
Esophagus	$D_{0.35cc}$ (Gy)	≤20 Gy

Institution C

Our planning objectives and normal tissue constraints are outlined in the following table in the midthorax/upper thorax:

Structure	Parameter	Constraint
PTV	$D_{95\%}$ (%)	≥100%
PTV	$D_{1\%}$ (%)	≤130%
Spinal cord	$D_{0.1cc}$ (Gy)	≤22 Gy
Spinal cord PRV	$D_{0.1cc}$ (Gy)	≤24 Gy
Liver	D_{700cc} (Gy)	≤15 Gy
Great vessels	$D_{01.cc}$ (Gy)	≤30 Gy
Heart	$D_{01.cc}$ (Gy)	≤30 Gy
Esophagus	$D_{01.cc}$ (Gy)	≤27 Gy
Esophagus	$D_{5.0cc}$ (Gy)	≤16.5 Gy
Trachea	$D_{0,1cc}$ (Gy)	≤30 Gy

Institution D

24 Gy in 1 fraction planning objectives

PTV Coverage	Ideal: V100>90% and V95>95% Acceptable: V100>80% and V95>90%
PTV inhomogeneity	Maximum point dose: 110%–130% Global D_{max} must be within PTV
High dose spillage	Hotspots >115% should be within PTV, hotspots >105% outside of PTV should be limited to 5 cc

Normal tissue constraints

Structure	Parameter	Dose (Gy)
Spinal cord (myelogram defined)	D_{max}	14
	$D_{0.35cc}$	10
	Dose transecting cord	10
Cauda (myelogram defined)	D_{max}	18
	$D_{0.35cc}$	14
Bowel/stomach	D_{max}	15 (stomach) 16 (bowel)
	D_{5cc}	12

Three-fraction dose constraints

Structure	Dose Constraint	Dose (Gy)	Comment
Spinal cord (myelogram defined)	D_{max}	14.5	D_{max} limit dose. The guideline dose is 13.9 Gy
	$D_{0.35cc}$	10	—
Esophagus	D_{max}	20.4	—
Trachea	Prescription	—	No hot spots

CASE DISCUSSION SUMMARY

It is clear that there are similarities and variations in practice. There was 100% agreement with regard to when surgical intervention and/or radiation was recommended. Careful attention to target volumes and dose constraints of normal tissues is always crucial to successful treatment.

However, practices vary with regard to the dose and fractionation schedule recommended by each institution for any given scenario. Clinicians must weigh the potential risks and benefits of different fractionation schedules when recommending treatment options. For example, treatment schedules with higher doses per fraction likely provide a higher rate of durable local control but may also carry a higher risk of toxicity. The treatment should be matched to the goals of care. If durable tumor control is the primary goal of therapy, such as in the case of oligometastatic breast cancer with an excellent long-term prognosis, then a high-dose radiosurgical approach may be most appropriate, even if there is a risk of vertebral body fracture. If palliation of pain for a recurrent metastasis is the primary objective, then high-dose radiosurgery may not be required. The therapeutic ratio should be maximized according to the therapeutic objective of treatment. Thus, variation between and within practices is appropriate, provided treatment is matched to the patient's needs and circumstances.

DISCLOSURE

No disclosures (F.Y. Morales, X. Chen, M. Yan, W.C. Jackson). Blue Earth Advisory Board, Janssen Advisory Board, AstraZeneca Advisory Board (D.E. Spratt). Accuray, research support, honorarium for educational session, travel, and lodging; BrainLAB, travel and lodging; Elekta, research support, travel, and lodging; Biomimetix, Data and Safety Monitoring Board (K. Redmond). BrainLAB, consultant; Vision RT, consultant; University of Wollongong, consulting professor; Chordoma Foundation, Medical Advisory Board (Y. Yamada).

REFERENCES

1. Available at: https://www.nccn.org/professionals/physician_gls/pdf/cns.pdf. Accessed September 30, 2019.
2. Hamilton AJ, Lulu BA, Fosmire H, et al. Preliminary clinical experience with linear accelerator-based spinal stereotactic radiosurgery. Neurosurgery 1995;36(2):311–9.
3. Moraes FY, Winter J, Atenafu EG, et al. Outcomes following stereotactic radiosurgery for small to medium-sized brain metastases are exceptionally dependent upon tumor size and prescribed dose. Neuro Oncol 2019;21(2):242–51.
4. Folkert MR, Bilsky MH, Tom AK, et al. Outcomes and toxicity for hypofractionated and single-fraction image-guided stereotactic radiosurgery for sarcomas

metastasizing to the spine. Int J Radiat Oncol Biol Phys 2014;88(5):1085–91.

5. Bishop AJ, Tao R, Guadagnolo BA, et al. Spine stereotactic radiosurgery for metastatic sarcoma: patterns of failure and radiation treatment volume considerations. J Neurosurg Spine 2017;27(3):303–11.
6. Ghia AJ, Chang EL, Bishop AJ, et al. Single-fraction versus multifraction spinal stereotactic radiosurgery for spinal metastases from renal cell carcinoma: secondary analysis of Phase I/II trials. J Neurosurg Spine 2016;24(5):829–36.
7. Yamada Y, Katsoulakis E, Laufer I, et al. The impact of histology and delivered dose on local control of spinal metastases treated with stereotactic radiosurgery. Neurosurg Focus 2017;42(1):E6.
8. Image-guided radiosurgery or stereotactic body radiation therapy in treating patients with localized spine metastasis. Available at: https://ClinicalTrials.gov/show/NCT00922974. Accessed September 30, 2019.
9. Study comparing stereotactic body radiotherapy vs conventional palliative radiotherapy (CRT) for spinal metastases. Available at: https://ClinicalTrials.gov/show/NCT02512965. Accessed September 30, 2019.
10. Sprave T, Verma V, Förster R, et al. Randomized phase II trial evaluating pain response in patients with spinal metastases following stereotactic body radiotherapy versus three-dimensional conformal radiotherapy. Radiother Oncol 2018;128(2):274–82.
11. Finkelstein SE, Timmerman R, McBride WH, et al. The confluence of stereotactic ablative radiotherapy and tumor immunology. Clin Dev Immunol 2011;2011:439752.
12. Lee Y, Auh SL, Wang Y, et al. Therapeutic effects of ablative radiation on local tumor require CD8+ T cells: changing strategies for cancer treatment. Blood 2009;114(3):589–95.
13. Steverink JG, Willems SM, Philippens MEP, et al. Early tissue effects of stereotactic body radiation therapy for spinal metastases. Int J Radiat Oncol Biol Phys 2018;100(5):1254–8.
14. Song CW, Kim MS, Cho LC, et al. Radiobiological basis of SBRT and SRS. Int J Clin Oncol 2014;19(4):570–8.
15. Sahgal A, Atenafu EG, Chao S, et al. Vertebral compression fracture after spine stereotactic body radiotherapy: a multi-institutional analysis with a focus on radiation dose and the spinal instability neoplastic score. J Clin Oncol 2013;31(27):3426–31.
16. Redmond KJ, Sahgal A, Foote M, et al. Single versus multiple session stereotactic body radiotherapy for spinal metastasis: the risk-benefit ratio. Future Oncol 2015;11(17):2405–15.
17. Dewan MZ, Galloway AE, Kawashima N, et al. Fractionated but not single-dose radiotherapy induces an immune-mediated abscopal effect when combined with anti-CTLA-4 antibody. Clin Cancer Res 2009;15(17):5379–88.
18. Guckenberger M, Mantel F, Gerszten PC, et al. Safety and efficacy of stereotactic body radiotherapy as primary treatment for vertebral metastases: a multi-institutional analysis. Radiat Oncol 2014;9:226.
19. Guckenberger M, Sweeney RA, Hawkins M, et al. Dose-intensified hypofractionated stereotactic body radiation therapy for painful spinal metastases: Results of a phase 2 study. Cancer 2018;124(9):2001–9.
20. Pichon B, Campion L, Delpon G, et al. High-dose hypofractionated radiation therapy for noncompressive vertebral metastases in combination with zoledronate: a phase 1 study. Int J Radiat Oncol Biol Phys 2016;96(4):840–7.
21. Moussazadeh N, Laufer I, Yamada Y, et al. Separation surgery for spinal metastases: effect of spinal radiosurgery on surgical treatment goals. Cancer Control 2014;21(2):168–74.
22. Ryu S, Rock J, Jain R, et al. Radiosurgical decompression of metastatic epidural compression. Cancer 2010;116(9):2250–7.
23. Lee I, Omodon M, Rock J, et al. Stereotactic radiosurgery for high-grade metastatic epidural cord compression. J Radiosurg SBRT 2014;3(1):51–8.
24. Bishop AJ, Tao R, Rebueno NC, et al. Outcomes for spine stereotactic body radiation therapy and an analysis of predictors of local recurrence. Int J Radiat Oncol Biol Phys 2015;92(5):1016–26.
25. Heron DE, Rajagopalan MS, Stone B, et al. Single-session and multisession CyberKnife radiosurgery for spine metastases-University of Pittsburgh and Georgetown University experience. J Neurosurg Spine 2012;17(1):11–8.
26. Randomized study comparing two dosing schedules for hypofractionated image-guided radiation therapy. Available at: https://ClinicalTrials.gov/show/NCT01223248. Accessed September 30, 2019.
27. Zelefsky MJ, Yamada Y, Lis E, et al. Phase III multicenter, prospective randomized trial comparing high dose single fraction radiation therapy to a 3-fraction sbrt regimen in the treatment of oligometastatic human cancer. Int J Radiat Oncol Biol Phys 2018;102(3, Supplement):S37–8.
28. Ryu S, Rock J, Rosenblum M, et al. Patterns of failure after single-dose radiosurgery for spinal metastasis. J Neurosurg 2004;101(Suppl 3):402–5.
29. Ghia AJ, Guha-Thakurta N, Hess K, et al. Phase 1 study of spinal cord constraint relaxation with single session spine stereotactic radiosurgery in the primary management of patients with inoperable, previously unirradiated metastatic epidural spinal cord

compression. Int J Radiat Oncol Biol Phys 2018; 102(5):1481–8.
30. Ozdemir Y, Torun N, Guler OC, et al. Local control and vertebral compression fractures following stereotactic body radiotherapy for spine metastases. J Bone Oncol 2019;15:100218.
31. Garg AK, Shiu AS, Yang J, et al. Phase 1/2 trial of single-session stereotactic body radiotherapy for previously unirradiated spinal metastases. Cancer 2012;118(20):5069–77.
32. Gerszten PC, Burton SA, Ozhasoglu C, et al. Radiosurgery for spinal metastases: clinical experience in 500 cases from a single institution. Spine (Phila Pa 1976) 2007;32(2):193–9.
33. Staehler M, Haseke N, Nuhn P, et al. Simultaneous anti-angiogenic therapy and single-fraction radiosurgery in clinically relevant metastases from renal cell carcinoma. BJU Int 2011;108(5):673–8.
34. Miller JA, Balagamwala EH, Angelov L, et al. Spine stereotactic radiosurgery with concurrent tyrosine kinase inhibitors for metastatic renal cell carcinoma. J Neurosurg Spine 2016;25(6):766–74.
35. Miller JA, Balagamwala EH, Angelov L, et al. Stereotactic radiosurgery for the treatment of primary and metastatic spinal sarcomas. Technol Cancer Res Treat 2017;16(3):276–84.
36. Sellin JN, Reichardt W, Bishop AJ, et al. Factors affecting survival in 37 consecutive patients undergoing de novo stereotactic radiosurgery for contiguous sites of vertebral body metastasis from renal cell carcinoma. J Neurosurg Spine 2015;22(1):52–9.
37. Meyer E, Pasquier D, Bernadou G, et al. Stereotactic radiation therapy in the strategy of treatment of metastatic renal cell carcinoma: a study of the Getug group. Eur J Cancer 2018;98:38–47.
38. McGee HM, Carpenter TJ, Ozbek U, et al. Analysis of local control and pain control after spine stereotactic radiosurgery reveals inferior outcomes for hepatocellular carcinoma compared with other radioresistant histologies. Pract Radiat Oncol 2019; 9(2):89–97.
39. Lovelock DM, Zhang Z, Jackson A, et al. Correlation of local failure with measures of dose insufficiency in the high-dose single-fraction treatment of bony metastases. Int J Radiat Oncol Biol Phys 2010;77(4): 1282–7.
40. Chang UK, Cho WI, Kim MS, et al. Local tumor control after retreatment of spinal metastasis using stereotactic body radiotherapy; comparison with initial treatment group. Acta Oncol 2012;51(5):589–95.
41. Sahgal A, Ames C, Chou D, et al. Stereotactic body radiotherapy is effective salvage therapy for patients with prior radiation of spinal metastases. Int J Radiat Oncol Biol Phys 2009;74(3):723–31.
42. Choi CY, Adler JR, Gibbs IC, et al. Stereotactic radiosurgery for treatment of spinal metastases recurring in close proximity to previously irradiated spinal cord. Int J Radiat Oncol Biol Phys 2010;78(2): 499–506.
43. Mahadevan A, Floyd S, Wong E, et al. Stereotactic body radiotherapy reirradiation for recurrent epidural spinal metastases. Int J Radiat Oncol Biol Phys 2011;81(5):1500–5.
44. Garg AK, Wang XS, Shiu AS, et al. Prospective evaluation of spinal reirradiation by using stereotactic body radiation therapy: The University of Texas MD Anderson Cancer Center experience. Cancer 2011;117(15):3509–16.
45. Nikolajek K, Kufeld M, Muacevic A, et al. Spinal radiosurgery–efficacy and safety after prior conventional radiotherapy. Radiat Oncol 2011;6:173.
46. Thibault I, Campbell M, Tseng CL, et al. Salvage Stereotactic Body Radiotherapy (SBRT) following in-field failure of initial SBRT for spinal metastases. Int J Radiat Oncol Biol Phys 2015;93(2):353–60.
47. Hashmi A, Guckenberger M, Kersh R, et al. Re-irradiation stereotactic body radiotherapy for spinal metastases: a multi-institutional outcome analysis. J Neurosurg Spine 2016;25(5):646–53.
48. Boyce-Fappiano D, Elibe E, Schultz L, et al. Analysis of the factors contributing to vertebral compression fractures after spine stereotactic radiosurgery. Int J Radiat Oncol Biol Phys 2017;97(2):236–45.
49. Redmond KJ, Lo SS, Fisher C, et al. Postoperative Stereotactic Body Radiation Therapy (SBRT) for spine metastases: a critical review to guide practice. Int J Radiat Oncol Biol Phys 2016;95(5): 1414–28.
50. Wardak Z, Bland R, Ahn C, et al. A phase 2 clinical trial of sabr followed by immediate vertebroplasty for spine metastases. Int J Radiat Oncol Biol Phys 2019; 104(1):83–9.
51. Moulding HD, Elder JB, Lis E, et al. Local disease control after decompressive surgery and adjuvant high-dose single-fraction radiosurgery for spine metastases. J Neurosurg Spine 2010;13(1):87–93.
52. Laufer I, Iorgulescu JB, Chapman T, et al. Local disease control for spinal metastases following "separation surgery" and adjuvant hypofractionated or high-dose single-fraction stereotactic radiosurgery: outcome analysis in 186 patients. J Neurosurg Spine 2013;18(3):207–14.
53. Tao R, Bishop AJ, Brownlee Z, et al. Stereotactic body radiation therapy for spinal metastases in the postoperative setting: a secondary analysis of mature phase 1-2 trials. Int J Radiat Oncol Biol Phys 2016;95(5):1405–13.
54. Chan MW, Thibault I, Atenafu EG, et al. Patterns of epidural progression following postoperative spine stereotactic body radiotherapy: implications for clinical target volume delineation. J Neurosurg Spine 2016;24(4):652–9.
55. Miller JA, Balagamwala EH, Berriochoa CA, et al. The impact of decompression with instrumentation

on local failure following spine stereotactic radiosurgery. J Neurosurg Spine 2017;27(4):436–43.
56. Barzilai O, Amato MK, McLaughlin L, et al. Hybrid surgery-radiosurgery therapy for metastatic epidural spinal cord compression: a prospective evaluation using patient-reported outcomes. Neurooncol Pract 2018;5(2):104–13.
57. Ito K, Nihei K, Shimizuguchi T, et al. Postoperative re-irradiation using stereotactic body radiotherapy for metastatic epidural spinal cord compression. J Neurosurg Spine 2018;29(3):332–8.
58. Alghamdi M, Sahgal A, Soliman H, et al. Postoperative stereotactic body radiotherapy for spinal metastases and the impact of epidural disease grade. Neurosurgery 2019;85(6):E1111–8.
59. Redmond KJ, Sciubba D, Khan M, et al. A Phase II study of post-operative Stereotactic Body Radiation Therapy (SBRT) for solid tumor spine metastases. Int J Radiat Oncol Biol Phys 2020;106(2):261–8.
60. Emami B, Lyman J, Brown A, et al. Tolerance of normal tissue to therapeutic irradiation. Int J Radiat Oncol Biol Phys 1991;21(1):109–22.
61. Marks LB, Yorke ED, Jackson A, et al. Use of normal tissue complication probability models in the clinic. Int J Radiat Oncol Biol Phys 2010;76(3 Suppl): S10–9.
62. Kirkpatrick JP, Meyer JJ, Marks LB. The linear-quadratic model is inappropriate to model high dose per fraction effects in radiosurgery. Semin Radiat Oncol 2008;18(4):240–3.
63. Sahgal A, Chang JH, Ma L, et al. Spinal cord dose tolerance to stereotactic body radiation therapy. Int J Radiat Oncol Biol Phys 2019. https://doi.org/10.1016/j.ijrobp.2019.09.038. [Epub ahead of print].
64. Habrand JL, Drouet F. Normal tissue tolerance to external beam radiation therapy: spinal cord. Cancer Radiother 2010;14(4–5):269–76 [in French].
65. Wong CS, Fehlings MG, Sahgal A. Pathobiology of radiation myelopathy and strategies to mitigate injury. Spinal Cord 2015;53(8):574–80.
66. Hall WA, Stapleford LJ, Hadjipanayis CG, et al. Stereotactic body radiosurgery for spinal metastatic disease: an evidence-based review. Int J Surg Oncol 2011;2011:979214.
67. Ryu S, Jin JY, Jin R, et al. Partial volume tolerance of the spinal cord and complications of single-dose radiosurgery. Cancer 2007;109(3):628–36.
68. Sahgal A, Weinberg V, Ma L, et al. Probabilities of radiation myelopathy specific to stereotactic body radiation therapy to guide safe practice. Int J Radiat Oncol Biol Phys 2013;85(2):341–7.
69. Chang JH, Shin JH, Yamada YJ, et al. Stereotactic body radiotherapy for spinal metastases: what are the risks and how do we minimize them? Spine (Phila Pa 1976) 2016;41(Suppl 20):S238–45.
70. Katsoulakis E, Jackson A, Cox B, et al. A detailed dosimetric analysis of spinal cord tolerance in high-dose spine radiosurgery. Int J Radiat Oncol Biol Phys 2017;99(3):598–607.
71. Grimm J, Sahgal A, Soltys SG, et al. Estimated risk level of unified stereotactic body radiation therapy dose tolerance limits for spinal cord. Semin Radiat Oncol 2016;26(2):165–71.
72. Gibbs IC, Kamnerdsupaphon P, Ryu MR, et al. Image-guided robotic radiosurgery for spinal metastases. Radiother Oncol 2007;82(2):185–90.
73. Ryu S, Pugh SL, Gerszten PC, et al. RTOG 0631 phase 2/3 study of image guided stereotactic radiosurgery for localized (1-3) spine metastases: phase 2 results. Pract Radiat Oncol 2014;4(2):76–81.
74. Sharma M, Bennett EE, Rahmathulla G, et al. Impact of cervicothoracic region stereotactic spine radiosurgery on adjacent organs at risk. Neurosurg Focus 2017;42(1):E14.
75. Chang JY, Li QQ, Xu QY, et al. Stereotactic ablative radiation therapy for centrally located early stage or isolated parenchymal recurrences of non-small cell lung cancer: how to fly in a "no fly zone. Int J Radiat Oncol Biol Phys 2014;88(5):1120–8.
76. Forquer JA, Fakiris AJ, Timmerman RD, et al. Brachial plexopathy from stereotactic body radiotherapy in early-stage NSCLC: dose-limiting toxicity in apical tumor sites. Radiother Oncol 2009;93(3):408–13.
77. Zeng KL, Myrehaug S, Soliman H, et al. Stereotactic body radiotherapy for spinal metastases at the extreme ends of the spine: imaging-based outcomes for cervical and sacral metastases. Neurosurgery 2019;85(5):605–12.
78. Stubblefield MD, Ibanez K, Riedel ER, et al. Peripheral nervous system injury after high-dose single-fraction image-guided stereotactic radiosurgery for spine tumors. Neurosurg Focus 2017;42(3):E12.
79. Rose PS, Laufer I, Boland PJ, et al. Risk of fracture after single fraction image-guided intensity-modulated radiation therapy to spinal metastases. J Clin Oncol 2009;27(30):5075–9.
80. Thibault I, Whyne CM, Zhou S, et al. Volume of lytic vertebral body metastatic disease quantified using computed tomography-based image segmentation predicts fracture risk after spine stereotactic body radiation therapy. Int J Radiat Oncol Biol Phys 2017;97(1):75–81.
81. Tseng CL, Soliman H, Myrehaug S, et al. Imaging-based outcomes for 24 Gy in 2 daily fractions for patients with de novo spinal metastases treated with spine Stereotactic Body Radiation Therapy (SBRT). Int J Radiat Oncol Biol Phys 2018;102(3): 499–507.
82. Faruqi S, Tseng CL, Whyne C, et al. Vertebral compression fracture after spine stereotactic body radiation therapy: a review of the pathophysiology and risk factors. Neurosurgery 2018;83(3):314–22.
83. Cox BW, Jackson A, Hunt M, et al. Esophageal toxicity from high-dose, single-fraction paraspinal

stereotactic radiosurgery. Int J Radiat Oncol Biol Phys 2012;83(5):e661–7.
84. Nuyttens JJ, Moiseenko V, McLaughlin M, et al. Esophageal dose tolerance in patients treated with stereotactic body radiation therapy. Semin Radiat Oncol 2016;26(2):120–8.
85. Harder EM, Chen ZJ, Park HS, et al. Dose-volume predictors of esophagitis after thoracic stereotactic body radiation therapy. Am J Clin Oncol 2017; 40(5):477–82.
86. Wu AJ, Williams E, Modh A, et al. Dosimetric predictors of esophageal toxicity after stereotactic body radiotherapy for central lung tumors. Radiother Oncol 2014;112(2):267–71.
87. Beeler WH, Paradis KC, Gemmete JJ, et al. Computed tomography myelosimulation versus magnetic resonance imaging registration to delineate the spinal cord during spine stereotactic radiosurgery. World Neurosurg 2019;122:e655–66.
88. Cox BW, Spratt DE, Lovelock M, et al. International Spine Radiosurgery Consortium consensus guidelines for target volume definition in spinal stereotactic radiosurgery. Int J Radiat Oncol Biol Phys 2012; 83(5):e597–605.
89. Husain ZA, Sahgal A, De Salles A, et al. Stereotactic body radiotherapy for de novo spinal metastases: systematic review. J Neurosurg Spine 2017;27(3): 295–302.

Hybrid Therapy for Spinal Metastases

Robert Rothrock, MD[a,1], Zach Pennington, BS[b,1], Jeff Ehresman, BS[b], Mark H. Bilsky, MD[c], Ori Barzilai, MD[c], Nicholas J. Szerlip, MD[d], Daniel M. Sciubba, MD[b,*]

KEYWORDS

• Spine • Metastases • Tumor • Radiosurgery • Separation surgery • Hybrid therapy • Radiation • Spinal cord

KEY POINTS

- Hybrid therapy describes separation surgery in tandem with early stereotactic radiation therapy (usually within 2 weeks) to provide durable local tumor control for spinal metastatic disease.
- The NOMS framework consists of 4 considerations (Neurologic, Oncologic, Mechanical, and Systemic) and facilitates treatment decision making in patients with metastatic spine tumors.
- Patients with symptomatic high-grade spinal cord compression from radioresistant tumors require surgical decompression before stereotactic body radiosurgery (SBRT).
- SBRT provides durable local control regardless of primary tumor histology or volume.
- There is level III evidence for improved local control and patient reported health-related quality of life outcomes with Hybrid therapy.

INTRODUCTION

Hybrid therapy is the combination of separation surgery followed by stereotactic body radiotherapy (SBRT). It represents a further step in the evolution of treatment for metastatic spine disease. The greatest advance in the treatment of metastatic spine tumors has been the development and integration of SBRT often delivered as a 24-Gy single fraction or 27 Gy in 3 fractions. SBRT can deliver an ablative dose of radiation to tumors traditionally considered resistant to conventional external beam radiation (cEBRT). Unfortunately, because of radiation constraints, "radioresistant" tumors causing high-grade epidural spinal cord compression (ESCC) cannot undergo definitive SBRT without first undergoing surgical decompression to provide a safer margin for radiation therapy.[1]

Overall, the goals of hybrid therapy for metastatic disease are 4-fold: (1) decompress the spinal cord to improve or maintain neurologic function, (2) provide mechanical stability, (3) achieve durable local tumor control, and (4) minimize treatment-related morbidity. Spinal cord decompression and stabilization are solely dependent on surgery, but local tumor control is completely predicated on the radiation response. Before the integration of SBRT into treatment paradigms, surgeons often used very aggressive surgical approaches to achieve en bloc or gross total resection of tumor because there was no expectation that cEBRT would provide durable tumor control when used as a postoperative adjuvant. These procedures often involved highly morbid anterior transcavitary or retroperitoneal approaches, multilevel vertebrectomies, extensive chest wall

[a] Department of Neurosurgery, Mount Sinai Hospital, New York, NY, USA; [b] Department of Neurosurgery, Johns Hopkins University School of Medicine, Baltimore, MD, USA; [c] Department of Neurosurgery, Memorial Sloan Kettering Cancer Center, New York, NY, USA; [d] Department of Neurosurgery, University of Michigan, Ann Arbor, MI, USA
[1] Co-first Authors: Robert Rothrock and Zach Pennington.
* Corresponding author. 600 North Wolfe Street, Meyer 5-185A, Baltimore, MD 21287.
E-mail address: dsciubb1@jhmi.edu

Neurosurg Clin N Am 31 (2020) 191–200
https://doi.org/10.1016/j.nec.2019.11.001

resections, prolonged surgical duration, and long recovery times for patients with multiple medical and oncologic comorbidities. The integration of SBRT as a postoperative adjuvant led to the development of separation surgery in which tumor resection is focused on decompressing the spinal cord to reconstitute the thecal sac providing a safe target for radiation without attempting a cytoreductive resection. Residual large paraspinal and vertebral body tumors do not need to be resected as they can be treated effectively with SBRT. Separation surgery is less morbid than traditional surgical approaches used for metastatic disease and potentially allows for an earlier return to systemic therapy.

DECISION MAKING

The NOMS framework was designed to facilitate decision making for patients with metastatic spine disease.[2] NOMS consists of 4 main elements; Neurologic, Oncologic, Mechanical, and Systemic. The Neurologic assessment considers myelopathy and functional radiculopathy as well as the radiographic degree of ESCC. The Oncologic assessment considers the modalities that affect local tumor control. Oncologic therapy includes chemotherapy, biologics and checkpoint inhibitors; however, with few exceptions, systemic therapies have not proven effective in treating osseous or epidural disease, so the oncologic assessment is predicated on radiosensitivity to cEBRT or SBRT. Mechanical stability is a separate assessment as radiation cannot stabilize an unstable spine, so patients are candidates a stabilizing intervention. Finally, the Systemic assessment evaluates the patient's systemic disease status and medical comorbidities to determine whether this patient is a candidate for the proposed treatment. The principle indications for surgery in the NOMS framework are high-grade ESCC (Neurologic) resulting from radioresistant tumor (Oncologic) and mechanical instability (Mechanical). Mechanical instability can often be treated with percutaneous cement augmentation or percutaneous pedicle screws. The focus of hybrid therapy (ie, the combination of separation surgery and SBRT) is the treatment of high-grade ESCC from radioresistant tumors.

SURGICAL INDICATIONS IN METASTATIC SPINE TUMORS

The rationale for hybrid therapy is based on numerous studies demonstrating both a benefit to surgical decompression of high-grade ESCC for radioresistant tumors as well as the ability to achieve durable local tumor control with SBRT. Several studies have demonstrated the benefits of surgery compared with cEBRT alone in the treatment of metastatic spine tumors.[3,4] The study by Patchell and colleagues[5] was fundamentally important in providing class 1 evidence establishing the benefits of surgery for high-grade ESCC from radioresistant tumors. This study was a prospective randomized trial comparing patients receiving conventionally cEBRT alone versus surgical decompression followed by cEBRT in solid tumors. Radiosensitive tumors, such as lymphoma and multiple myeloma were excluded. The prescribed dose of radiation was standardized in the trial to 30 Gy in 10 fractions in each arm. In every outcome variable, surgery improved outcomes, and, in fact, the study was terminated at the halfway point. The most important endpoint was ambulation, which was maintained or improved significantly in the surgical arm versus the radiation arm, 84% versus 57% (odds ratio 6.2 [95% CI, 2.0–19.8] $P = .001$), respectively.[5] Although it was not the primary outcome, an overall survival advantage was observed in the surgical arm of the study.

A major limitation of the Patchell study is the lack of longitudinal follow-up regarding local control (LC). Surgery is clearly superb at providing neurologic salvage and mechanical stability, but the question remains whether cEBRT can provide durable palliation. At the time this study was published, LC was not a priority as median survivals were often less than a year, and, for the predominant tumors in this study, non-small cell lung and colon carcinoma, was 4 months. However, newer systemic agents, that is, biologics and checkpoint inhibitors, have dramatically improved survival for virtually every tumor histology mandating more durable LC for spine tumors. This in part led to a transition from cEBRT to SBRT as a postoperative adjuvant.

In addition to providing durable tumor control, the second benefit of integrating SBRT as a postoperative adjuvant is the ability to limit the tumor resection to the epidural space, resulting in a transition from aggressive gross total or en bloc resections to separation surgery. The spinal cord is the most critical organ at risk (OAR), which limits high-dose SBRT to the dural margin without risking iatrogenic spinal cord injury. When the tumor is separated from the spinal cord by 2 to 3 mm, the entire tumor volume can be treated with an effective SBRT dose without exceeding the accepted spinal cord constraints. Currently, the minimum dose thought to provide tumor control is 15 Gy and the maximum dose to a single voxel on the spinal cord (cord Dmax) is 14 Gy[6]; thus, delivering a tumoricidal dose to the dural margin would result in undertreatment at the dural margin risking progressive spinal cord compression or overdosing the spinal cord resulting in radiation-induced myelitis. Ongoing trials are exploring higher-dose constraints for the spinal cord, that is cord Dmax 16 Gy, but this is unlikely to improve the ability to definitively treat high-grade ESCC as the reduction in epidural tumor regression often takes months for radioresistant histologies.[7] The oncologic goal of separation surgery is circumferential excision of epidural tumor to reconstitute the thecal sac and provide a 2-mm margin for the safe delivery of an ablative radiation dose. In the clinical setting, SBRT has been has been attempted in the treatment of high-grade ESCC but resulted in an unacceptable 20% risk of neurologic decompensation for radioresistant tumors.[8]

SEPARATION SURGERY

Preoperative Considerations

The preoperative workup and surgical considerations are critical to good outcomes from separation surgery. Many patients who have indications for hybrid therapy are excluded based on the extent of systemic disease, significant medical comorbidities, or the expectation of limited survival. By definition, most patients with cancer have an American Society of Anesthesiologists score of IV or greater, placing them at higher perioperative risk for mortality as validated by numerous clinical studies.[9–11] Patients with poor pulmonary function and significant liver tumor burden generally represent the highest-risk patient populations. Many algorithms have been developed to predict perioperative mortality and survival. Currently, the best algorithm may be the Skeletal Oncology Research Group (SORG) nomogram, which has been validated in the era of extended survivals provided by improved systemic biologic and checkpoint inhibitors.[12] Finally, screening high-risk patients for deep venous thrombosis (DVT) may help prevent pulmonary embolism. In a study by Zacharia and colleagues,[13] lower extremity screening Dopplers demonstrated that 24% of nonambulatory patient harbored a DVT versus 6% of ambulatory patients. High-risk patients are routinely screened with Dopplers in the perioperative period and inferior vena cava (IVC) filters are placed to prevent pulmonary embolism due to a need to withhold full dose anticoagulation for 2 to 3 weeks postoperatively.

Identification of hypervascular tumors is important for consideration of appropriate candidates for preoperative embolization. Standard MRI criteria indicating hypervascularity are intratumoral bleed, diffuse contrast enhancement, and large flow voids; however, these findings are unreliable. Recently, dynamic contrast-enhanced MRI has demonstrated high sensitivity and specificity for hypervascularity but is difficult to obtain on an urgent basis.[14] From a practical standpoint, tumor histology is the best predictor of tumor hypervascularity. The most common hypervascular tumors are renal cell carcinoma, papillary and follicular thyroid carcinoma, and leiomyosarcoma; however, the laundry list is long. Predictors of hypervascularity based on tumor histology include prefixes, such as "angio" or "hemangio" or the vascularity of the organ of tumor origin (eg, kidney). The most hypervascular tumor in a series reported by Nair and colleagues[15] was solitary fibrous tumor, which seems to follow none of the rules except for the revelation that it was formerly called "hemangiopericytoma." In newly diagnosed tumors without a known histology, clues to hypervascularity can often be garnered from the systemic workup, such as a large kidney mass. Complete embolization of the blood supply can be achieved in over 85% of thoracic and lumbar tumors, but less than 40% of cervical tumors.[16] The most common limitation to total embolization is the presence of a radiculomedullary or brainstem feeder.

Technical Considerations

Our technique for separation surgery has been described previously, step-by-step, elsewhere.[17] Although surgeons may have different preferences, the general surgical approach for separation surgery is usually similar.

Setup: following induction of general anesthesia, including venodyne boots, A-line and Foley catheter insertion, patients are placed prone with pressure points padded. Intraoperative neurophysiological monitoring is routinely used, including electromyography, somatosensory-evoked potentials (SSEPs), and motor-evoked potentials (MEPs), and electrodes are inserted before positioning. Preflip baseline signals are only obtained when there is concern for the possibility of neurologic insult from patient positioning secondary to gross instability. The incision site is prepped and draped in standard fashion. Fluoroscopy is used to localize the incision and the posterior bony elements are exposed in standard fashion. Notably, Cobb periosteal elevators are avoided to minimize the risk of downward pressure to the unstable and compressed spinal cord.

Posterior Instrumentation

Our practice is to place instrumentation before decompression and resection of the epidural tumor due to the risk of working over an open spinal canal, with the exception of patients with acute neurologic decompensation who may benefit from immediate decompression. Pedicle or lateral mass screws can be placed via anatomic freehand technique or by the use of various navigational guidance systems.[18] Rods are contoured to approximate the anatomic kyphosis or lordosis depending on the spinal segment and are placed and secured before decompression without limiting the necessary surgical exposure. Traditionally, pedicle or lateral mass screws are placed a minimum of 2 levels superior and inferior to the index tumor level. Long segmental fixation provides support for extensive posterior element osteotomies. In addition, long constructs are used to distribute the load in omnipresent osteoporotic bone and to obviate the consequences of adjacent segment bone progression (**Fig. 1**). However, both problems can be overcome with the use of cement-augmented screws. Cement augmentation is currently being explored to reduce the levels of fixation to a single level adjacent to the index level. Cement augmentation of the screws or the anterior column can aid in bony purchase and decrease the risk of hardware failure.[19] Cement injection via vertebroplasty or fenestrated screws provides a reliable way to cement-augment the osseous-screw purchase in patients with cancer (**Fig. 2**).[20]

Anterior Reconstruction

If greater than 50% of the vertebral body is resected during tumor resection, anterior column support is achieved by inserting polymethylmethacrylate (PMMA) into the anterior vertebral body defect.[21] The PMMA is injected into the defect and compressed against the endplates with a Penfield 3. If the cortical bone at the index level has been destroyed, Steinman pins are driven into the adjacent endplates and used as a rebar to prevent rotation of the cement. PMMA is ideally suited for tumor reconstruction as it can be placed in the middle of a vertebral body without the need to engage an intact endplate. Importantly, as it does not affect SBRT dosimetry[22] cages can be used, but they typically require a larger approach corridor than PMMA and require resection of adjacent segment discs. If a cage is used, our strong preference is to use polyetheretherketone carbon fiber or a nonexpandable titanium mesh cage to minimize MRI

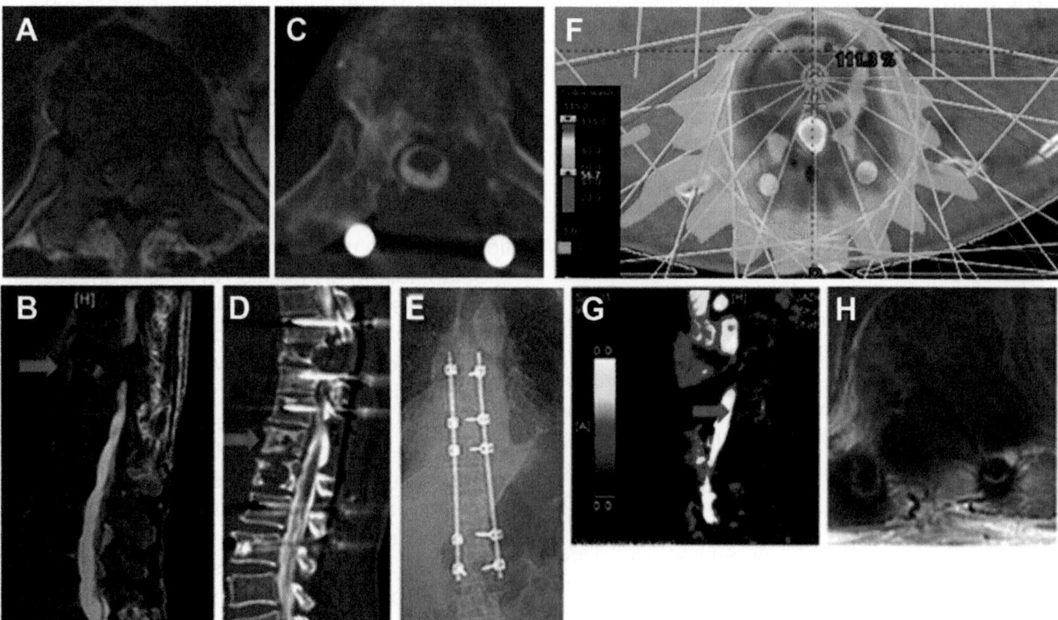

Fig. 1. A 64-year-old man with a history of non-small cell lung carcinoma presented with lower extremity weakness. (*A*) Axial T2-weighted image demonstrating high-grade ESCC T12. (*B*) Sagittal T2-weighted image demonstrating circumferential bone disease at T12 and a burst fracture at L1 (*arrow*). (*C*) After separation surgery myelogram-CT axial images showing reconstitution of the thecal sac and decompression of the spinal cord. (*D*) After separation surgery myelogram-CT sagittal images showing excellent T12 decompression (*arrow*). (*E*) Coronal plane radiographs demonstrating long posterior pedicle screw construct (*F*) Radiosurgery treatment plan color wash in the axial plane. (*G*) Dynamic contrast-enhanced MRI 12 months following stereotactic radiosurgery (SRS) showing a complete response (*arrow*). (*H*) Axial T1 post contrast MRI 12 months following SRS with no evidence of recurrence.

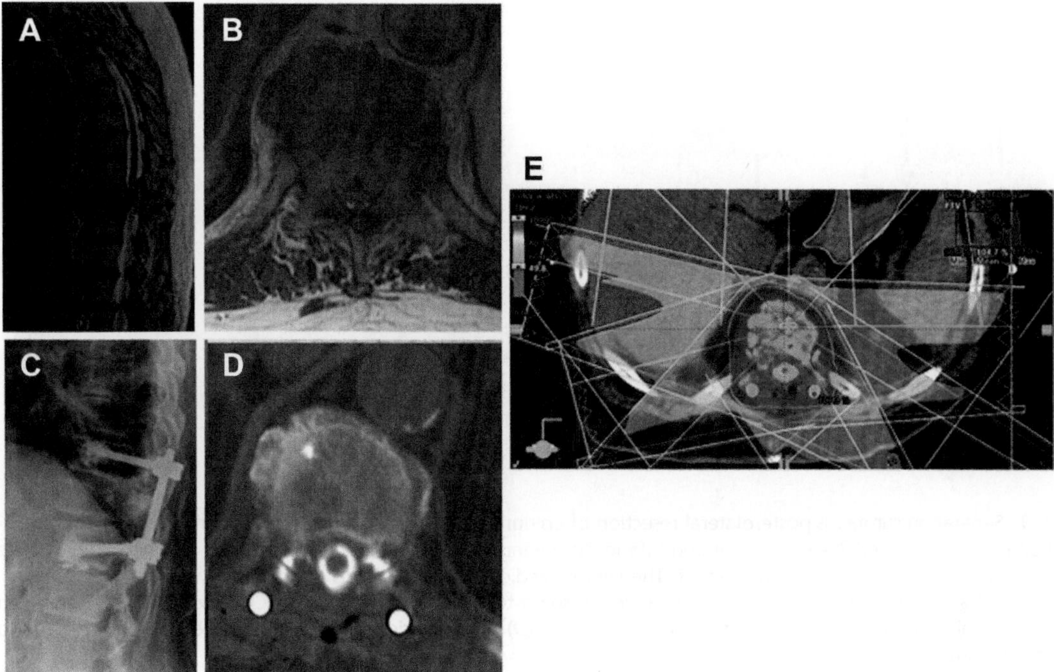

Fig. 2. A 77-year-old man with a history of melanoma presented with bilateral lower extremity weakness. (*A, B*) Sagittal and axial T2-weighed images show high-grade ESCC at T10. (*C*) Separation surgery with short segment pedicle screw fixation augmented by PMMA. (*D*) Postoperative myelogram demonstrating postoperative reconstitution of the thecal sac improving the target of SRS. (*E*) Radiosurgery treatment plan color wash in the axial plane.

artifact. Titanium expandable cages are typically avoided in tumor reconstruction due the inability to reliably image the spinal canal for recurrent epidural disease and a higher probability of subsidence. Importantly, aggressive or gross total resection of the vertebral body of paraspinal tumors are not required since postoperative SBRT will effectively treat these tumor components.

Spinal Cord Decompression

The 2 goals of decompression in separation surgery are recovery or maintenance of neurologic function and providing a sufficient margin to enable delivery of an ablative dose of SBRT within spinal cord constraints. In the setting of high-grade ESCC, it is crucial to avoid transmitting pressure to the spinal cord during decompression. This is most frequently achieved by using a 3-mm matchstick bur to carefully thin the bony elements to a shell before removal with a 15-blade or tenotomy scissors. To prevent inadvertent compression of the spinal cord, Kerrison punches should be avoided in cervical and thoracic decompression. Normal dural planes adjacent to the tumor are defined before excision to facilitate safe separation. Depending on tumor location, a surgical corridor to the ventral epidural space is created via unilateral or bilateral removal of the facet joint(s) and pedicle(s). To ensure that circumferential decompression is achieved, it is important to ensure adequate resection of the ventral epidural component of the tumor. The key to ventral tumor decompression is resection of the posterior longitudinal ligament (PLL). The PLL can be readily delineated with a Woodson dental tool and is cut sharply across the ventral dura with tenotomy scissors to facilitate release of Hoffmann's ligaments, which are fibrous connections from the ligament to the dura.[23] Blunt resection of the PLL should be avoided as it can create downward traction on the dura potentiating a spinal cord injury. Once a ventral cavity has been created, a dissector can be used to further separate the tumor from the dura and to ensure adequate ventral epidural decompression. Often, a partial vertebrectomy is performed to create a safe corridor for resection of the epidural disease (**Fig. 3**).[17]

To confirm ventral decompression, intraoperative ultrasonography can be a useful confirmatory adjunct, allowing visualization of reconstitution of ventral cerebrospinal fluid (CSF) space and decompression of the spinal cord.[24] Ultrasonography provides intraoperative confirmation of decompression that provides a margin for the safe delivery of postoperative SBRT.

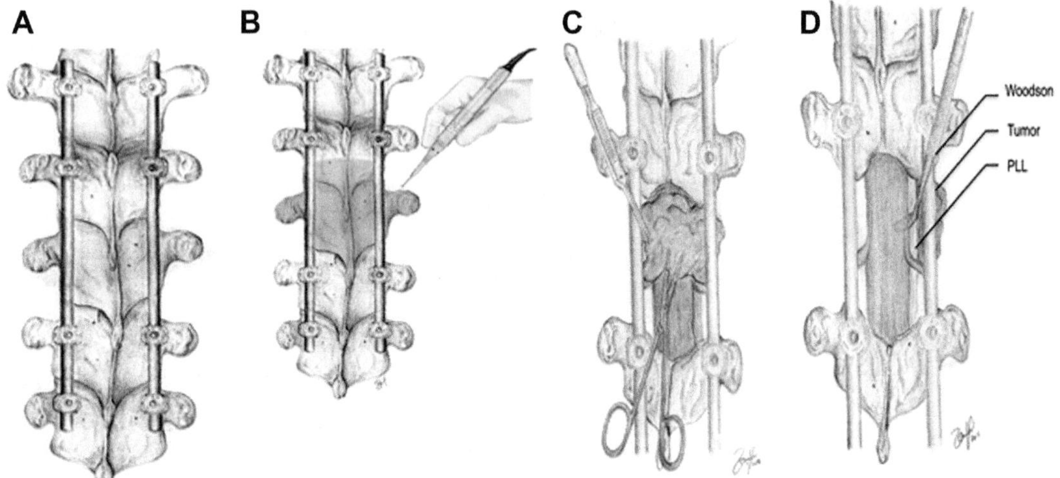

Fig. 3. Separation surgery is posterolateral resection of epidural tumor and instrumented fusion. (*A*) Spine instrumentation is typically placed 2-level superior and inferior to the index tumor level; however, PMMA-augmented screws are being explored to shorten the construct. (*B*) The lamina, pedicle, and facet joints are resected with a high-speed drill. The use of a Kerrison punch is avoided in the epidural space to avoid iatrogenic injury. (*C*) Tumor resection is initiated from normal dural planes typically with tenotomy scissors. (*D*) The posterior longitudinal ligament (PLL) is resected to affect a margin on the anterior dura.

Intraoperative Radiation Adjuvants

Delivery of a therapeutic radiation dose to the dural margin via intraoperative brachytherapy allows optimal postoperative dosimetry, particularly in the setting of circumferential tumor infiltration or previously irradiated targets.[25] Β-emitting radioisotopes, such as iridium-192, ytrium-90, and phosphorus-32, are ideal for epidural application as they have very high-dose delivery with a steep dose falloff. For example, a ^{32}P dural brachytherapy plaque can deliver 24 Gy to the surface of the dura within minutes with only 5% of the prescription dose being delivered at 3 mm, that is to the spinal cord. The dural plaque is comprised of ^{32}P impregnated in a thin, flexible silicon polymer and does not require shielding. The plaque is brought into the operating room, laid directly onto the targeted epidural space, and removed after a therapeutic dose has been delivered. In several series, ^{32}P brachytherapy has been demonstrated to provide local tumor control when used as an intraoperative surgical adjuvant following epidural decompression.[26]

Postoperative Stereotactic Body Radiotherapy

The second phase of hybrid therapy is the postoperative SBRT delivery. Circumferential decompression achieved via separation surgery allows for tumoricidal SBRT doses to be delivered to the entire tumor volume within the constraints of spinal cord tolerance.[27] Planning for SBRT can begin while the patient is still in the hospital and recovering from surgery.

Simulation

Simulation can be performed on postoperative days 2 to 3, with the goal of SBRT treatment approximately 2 weeks following separation surgery. Because MRI-related artifacts from hardware can limit radiosurgical treatment planning, computed tomography (CT) myelography is the preferred modality to better visualize the neural elements, surgical construct, and OARs.[28,29] Patients are immobilized during simulation in a reproducible manner using a patient-specific positioning frame. Preoperative MRI with and without contrast can be used to delineate the preoperative tumor volume and this volume is outlined on the postoperative CT myelogram simulation image for accurate delineation of tumor target, OARs, and for treatment planning.

TREATMENT

The Spine Radiosurgery Consensus Consortium contouring guidelines for spinal stereotactic radiosurgery and subsequent postoperative guidelines provide the basis for treatment planning.[4,29] Target volumes are defined according to the definitions set by the International Commission on Radiation Units and Measurements Report 50.[29,30] Gross tumor volume (GTV), being not only the residual tumor seen on imaging, but also the spinal and paraspinal regions involved before resection. Clinical target volume (CTV) includes the GTV and region of potential microscopic spread of tumor cells. The planning target volume (PTV) is a geometric construct that encompasses the CTV and adds an additional margin of tissue to ensure that the CTV receives the intended dose. This margin accounts for factors that create small deviations in delivery, such as patient positioning, motion during treatment, and physical distortions of the treatment machinery. In modern stereotactic spine radiosurgery, a typical PTV expansion on the CTV is 1 mm.

Treatment planning is ultimately a compromise between the prescribed dose and the allowable dose to surrounding normal structures (OARs). In general, for spine radiosurgery, dose uniformity within the target volume is sacrificed for steep dose gradients immediately outside the target volume to allow maximal sparing of OARs, such as the spinal cord or esophagus. Radiation "hotspots" over 130% of the prescribed dose are allowed. An ideal treatment plan would be able to cover at least 90% of the PTV with the prescribed dose, but better than 80% coverage of the PTV with the prescribed dose would be still considered acceptable. Because of the complexity of decision making in the setting of postoperative SBRT, it is helpful to use a multidisciplinary conference between radiation oncology and neurosurgery for treatment planning.

OUTCOMES

There is extensive level III evidence for use of hybrid therapy in the treatment of metastatic spinal disease. Laufer and colleagues[3] presented a series of 186 consecutive patients undergoing hybrid therapy for metastatic greater than 70% of patients were operated for high-grade ESCC with radioresistant tumor histologies and 50% had failed previous cEBRT. Three dose strategies were used: 24 Gy single fraction, 24 to 30 Gy in 3 fractions, or 30 Gy in 5 fractions. The 1-year cumulative incidence of recurrence was 16%, but the high-dose single or hypofractionated radiation regimens resulted in less than 10% 1-year incidence of recurrence. Local recurrence was not associated with radioresistant tumor histology, previous radiation, or the degree of preoperative epidural extension.

The study by Al-Omair and colleagues,[31] emphasizes the critical importance of epidural decompression and reconstitution of the thecal sac as the principle goal of separation surgery. They reported hybrid therapy outcomes in 80 patients undergoing postoperative SBRT at doses of 18 to 26 Gy in 1 to 2 fractions or 18 to 40 Gy in 3 to 5 fractions. The 1-year LC rate was 84%. The epidural space was the most common site of recurrence resulting in 66% of failures presenting as exclusively epidural. In multivariate analysis, delivery of 18 to 26 Gy as a single fraction and postoperative decompression resulting in no or minimal epidural impingement improved local tumor control. When looking at epidural failures, residual spinal cord compression postoperatively significantly decreased local disease control.

Compared with surgery followed by cEBRT, hybrid therapy has demonstrated significant improvement in quality of life based on patient-reported outcome (PRO) studies. Barzilai and colleagues,[32] showed improvement in multiple, validated PRO scales, including the Brief Pain Inventory and MD Anderson Symptom Inventory—Spine Tumor. A significant decrease in pain severity and symptom interference in activities of daily living were observed. In an international study by the AO Spine Knowledge Forum on Tumor, there was an improvement in multiple health-related quality of life PRO studies following hybrid therapy for spinal metastatic disease, regardless of the burden of spinal metastases.[33]

COMPLICATIONS

Immediate

Immediate complications after separation surgery are similar to those for all instrumented spinal surgery. In patients with highly vascular metastatic disease, such as renal cell carcinoma or hepatocellular carcinoma, there can be high rates of intraoperative blood loss with resultant postoperative anemia.[34] Intraoperative durotomy should be repaired primarily when feasible, or can be augmented with cadaveric allograft, muscle autograft, and/or fibrin glue. In cases of postoperative CSF leaks through the incision and pseudomeningocele formation, placement of a lumbar drain usually results in resolution of the leak. In cases of persistent leaks, plastic surgeons can help to provide extended coverage using local rotation or advancement muscle or omental flaps of the dural defect and soft-tissue reconstruction.

Patients with cancer are at increased risk of poor wound healing as a result of poor nutritional status, use of systemic therapy that impairs wound healing, and extensive use of radiation.[35] Keam and colleagues,[36] evaluated wound complication rates occurring in patients receiving cEBRT compared with radiosurgery before spine surgery and found no significant differences. Hence, preoperative SBRT is associated with clinically acceptable rates of wound morbidity and there is no need to delay surgical intervention for fear of wound breakdown following SBRT. Furthermore, this risk can be mitigated by preoperative identification of patients who might benefit from plastic surgery-assisted closure. Lau and colleagues,[37] examined 106 adult patients undergoing surgery for spinal metastatic disease and found that age greater than 65 years and presence of contiguous disease in 3 or more spinal levels were independent predictors of complications from surgery. Hence, high-risk patients, including those who have undergone recent cEBRT, reoperations, or cervicothoracic junction lesions may benefit from a prophylactic flap closure.

Delayed Complications

As patient survival improves with advances in systemic cancer therapies, a new set of delayed postoperative complications have emerged in the setting of separation surgery. The highly effective tumoricidal doses of SBRT can result in profound osteonecrosis of the vertebral body, resulting in delayed fracture progression and hardware failure.[38] Delayed vertebral body fracture can be treated with salvage vertebroplasty or kyphoplasty to avoid larger revision surgery in this high surgical risk population.[39] In addition, de novo disease in adjacent segments can be challenging to treat, especially if there is overlap with previous radiation treatment (ie, dose constraints). Given the low rates of solid arthrodesis, pseudoarthrosis and delayed instability can result in debilitating pain.[40] Interestingly, despite the high prevalence of poor bone quality in the metastatic cancer population, only 2.8% of patients required operative intervention for hardware failure in a large series of 318 patients who underwent separation surgery.[41] A recent evaluation of postoperative complications in long-term cancer survivors, evaluating patients who survived more than 2 years after surgery concluded that durable tumor control can be achieved in long-term cancer survivors surgically treated for symptomatic spinal metastases with limited complications. Complications observed after long-term follow-up include local tumor recurrence or progression, marginal tumor control failures, early or late hardware complications, late wound complications and progressive spinal instability or deformity.[42]

SUMMARY

Hybrid therapy for spinal metastatic disease-concomitant separation surgery and SBRT is an effective, tolerable, and reproducible treatment. Separation surgery provides rapid decompression, stabilization, and continuation of treatment, generally without a prolonged recovery period. Assuring adequate circumferential epidural decompression is crucial and allows for optimal SBRT dosing and durable local tumor control.

DISCLOSURE

Dr M.H. Bilsky receives consulting fees from DePuy/Synthes, Globus, and Brainla; Dr O. Barzilai: fellowship support to his institution from Globus for work performed outside of the current study; Dr D.M. Sciubba: Consultant for Baxter, DePuy-Synthes, Globus Medical, K2M, Medtronic, NuVasive. Unrelated grant funding from Baxter, North American Spine Society, Stryker. Drs R. Rothrock, Z. Pennington, J. Ehresman and N.J. Szerlip have nothing to dosclose.

REFERENCES

1. Yamada Y, Katsoulakis E, Laufer I, et al. The impact of histology and delivered dose on local control of spinal metastases treated with stereotactic radiosurgery. Neurosurg Focus 2017;42(1):E6.
2. Barzilai O, Laufer I, Yamada Y, et al. Integrating evidence-based medicine for treatment of spinal metastases into a decision framework: neurologic, oncologic, mechanicals stability, and systemic disease. J Clin Oncol 2017;35(21):2419–27.
3. Bilsky MH, Laufer I, Burch S. Shifting paradigms in the treatment of metastatic spine disease. Spine (Phila Pa 1976) 2009;34(22 Suppl):S101–7.
4. Redmond KJ, Lo SS, Fisher C, et al. Postoperative Stereotactic Body Radiation Therapy (SBRT) for spine metastases: a critical review to guide practice. Int J Radiat Oncol Biol Phys 2016;95(5):1414–28.
5. Patchell RA, Tibbs PA, Regine WF, et al. Direct decompressive surgical resection in the treatment of spinal cord compression caused by metastatic cancer: a randomised trial. Lancet 2005;366(9486):643–8.
6. Yamada Y, Bilsky MH, Lovelock DM, et al. High-dose, single-fraction image-guided intensity-modulated radiotherapy for metastatic spinal lesions. Int J Radiat Oncol Biol Phys 2008;71(2):484–90.
7. Ghia AJ, Guha-Thakurta N, Hess K, et al. Phase 1 study of spinal cord constraint relaxation with single session spine stereotactic radiosurgery in the primary management of patients with inoperable, previously unirradiated metastatic epidural spinal cord compression. Int J Radiat Oncol Biol Phys 2018;102(5):1481–8.
8. Lee I, Omodon M, Rock J, et al. Stereotactic radiosurgery for high-grade metastatic epidural cord compression. J Radiosurg SBRT 2014;3(1):51–8.
9. Lakomkin N, Zuckerman SL, Stannard B, et al. Preoperative risk stratification in spine tumor surgery: a comparison of the modified Charlson index, frailty index, and ASA score. Spine (Phila Pa 1976) 2019;44(13):E782–7.

10. Hopkins TJ, Raghunathan K, Barbeito A, et al. Associations between ASA Physical Status and postoperative mortality at 48 h: a contemporary dataset analysis compared to a historical cohort. Perioper Med (Lond) 2016;5:29.
11. Hackett NJ, De Oliveira GS, Jain UK, et al. ASA class is a reliable independent predictor of medical complications and mortality following surgery. Int J Surg 2015;18:184–90.
12. Ahmed AK, Goodwin CR, Heravi A, et al. Predicting survival for metastatic spine disease: a comparison of nine scoring systems. Spine J 2018;18(10): 1804–14.
13. Zacharia BE, Kahn S, Bander ED, et al. Incidence and risk factors for preoperative deep venous thrombosis in 314 consecutive patients undergoing surgery for spinal metastasis. J Neurosurg Spine 2017;27(2):189–97.
14. Khadem NR, Karimi S, Peck KK, et al. Characterizing hypervascular and hypovascular metastases and normal bone marrow of the spine using dynamic contrast-enhanced MR imaging. AJNR Am J Neuroradiol 2012;33(11):2178–85.
15. Nair S, Gobin YP, Leng LZ, et al. Preoperative embolization of hypervascular thoracic, lumbar, and sacral spinal column tumors: technique and outcomes from a single center. Interv Neuroradiol 2013;19(3):377–85.
16. Patsalides A, Leng LZ, Kimball D, et al. Preoperative catheter spinal angiography and embolization of cervical spinal tumors: outcomes from a single center. Interv Neuroradiol 2016;22(4):457–65.
17. Barzilai O, Laufer I, Robin A, et al. Hybrid therapy for metastatic epidural spinal cord compression: technique for separation surgery and spine radiosurgery. Oper Neurosurg (Hagerstown) 2019; 16(3):310–8.
18. Costa F, Dorelli G, Ortolina A, et al. Computed tomography-based image-guided system in spinal surgery: state of the art through 10 years of experience. Neurosurgery 2015;11(Suppl 2):59–67 [discussion: 67–8].
19. Frankel BM, Jones T, Wang C. Segmental polymethylmethacrylate-augmented pedicle screw fixation in patients with bone softening caused by osteoporosis and metastatic tumor involvement: a clinical evaluation. Neurosurgery 2007;61(3):531–7 [discussion: 537–8].
20. Barzilai O, McLaughlin L, Lis E, et al. Utility of cement augmentation via percutaneous fenestrated pedicle screws for stabilization of cancer-related spinal instability. Oper Neurosurg (Hagerstown) 2019;16(5):593–9.
21. Moussazadeh N, Rubin DG, McLaughlin L, et al. Short-segment percutaneous pedicle screw fixation with cement augmentation for tumor-induced spinal instability. Spine J 2015;15(7):1609–17.
22. Barzilai O, DiStefano N, Lis E, et al. Safety and utility of kyphoplasty prior to spine stereotactic radiosurgery for metastatic tumors: a clinical and dosimetric analysis. J Neurosurg Spine 2018;28(1):72–8.
23. Tardieu GG, Fisahn C, Loukas M, et al. The epidural ligaments (of Hofmann): a comprehensive review of the literature. Cureus 2016;8(9):e779.
24. Vasudeva VS, Abd-El-Barr M, Pompeu YA, et al. Use of intraoperative ultrasound during spinal surgery. Global Spine J 2017;7(7):648–56.
25. Folkert MR, Bilsky MH, Cohen GN, et al. Intraoperative ^{32}P high-dose rate brachytherapy of the dura for recurrent primary and metastatic intracranial and spinal tumors. Neurosurgery 2012;71(5):1003–10 [discussion: 1010–1].
26. Folkert MR, Bilsky MH, Cohen GN, et al. Local recurrence outcomes using the (3)(2)P intraoperative brachytherapy plaque in the management of malignant lesions of the spine involving the dura. Brachytherapy 2015;14(2):202–8.
27. Sahgal A, Roberge D, Schellenberg D, et al. The Canadian Association of Radiation Oncology scope of practice guidelines for lung, liver and spine stereotactic body radiotherapy. Clin Oncol (R Coll Radiol) 2012;24(9):629–39.
28. Sahgal A, et al. Stereotactic body radiotherapy for spinal metastases: current status, with a focus on its application in the postoperative patient. J Neurosurg Spine 2011;14(2):151–66.
29. Redmond KJ, et al. Consensus contouring guidelines for postoperative stereotactic body radiation therapy for metastatic solid tumor malignancies to the spine. Int J Radiat Oncol Biol Phys 2017;97(1):64–74.
30. Available at: https://icru.org/home/reports/prescribing-recording-and-reporting-photon-beam-therapy-report-50. Accessed January 8, 2019.
31. Al-Omair A, et al. Surgical resection of epidural disease improves local control following postoperative spine stereotactic body radiotherapy. Neuro Oncol 2013;15(10):1413–9.
32. Barzilai O, et al. Hybrid surgery-radiosurgery therapy for metastatic epidural spinal cord compression: a prospective evaluation using patient-reported outcomes. Neurooncol Pract 2018;5(2): 104–13.
33. Barzilai O, et al. Survival, local control, and health-related quality of life in patients with oligometastatic and polymetastatic spinal tumors: a multicenter, international study. Cancer 2019;125(5):770–8.
34. Quraishi NA, et al. Outcome of embolised vascular metastatic renal cell tumours causing spinal cord compression. Eur Spine J 2013;22(Suppl 1):S27–32.
35. Payne WG, et al. Wound healing in patients with cancer. Eplasty 2008;8:e9.
36. Keam J, et al. No association between excessive wound complications and preoperative high-dose, hypofractionated, image-guided radiation therapy

for spine metastasis. J Neurosurg Spine 2014;20(4): 411–20.

37. Lau D, et al. Independent predictors of complication following surgery for spinal metastasis. Eur Spine J 2013;22(6):1402–7.
38. Mantel F, Flentje M, Guckenberger M. Stereotactic body radiation therapy in the re-irradiation situation—a review. Radiat Oncol 2013;8:7.
39. Xu R, et al. Cement salvage of instrumentation-associated vertebral fractures. AJNR Am J Neuroradiol 2014;35(11):2197–201.
40. Zhang M, et al. Radiographic rate and clinical impact of pseudarthrosis in spine radiosurgery for metastatic spinal disease. Cureus 2018;10(11): e3631.
41. Amankulor NM, et al. The incidence and patterns of hardware failure after separation surgery in patients with spinal metastatic tumors. Spine J 2014;14(9): 1850–9.
42. Barzilai O, McLaughlin L, Lis E, et al. Outcome analysis of surgery for symptomatic spinal metastases in long-term cancer survivors. J Neurosurg Spine 2019;1–6.

Minimally Invasive Surgery Strategies

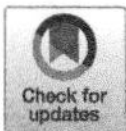

Changing the Treatment of Spine Tumors

Ori Barzilai, MD[a], Adam M. Robin, MS, MD[b], John E. O'Toole, MD, MS[c], Ilya Laufer, MS, MD[a,*]

KEYWORDS

• Minimal access surgery • Minimally invasive surgery (MIS) • Spinal tumor • Spinal metastases

KEY POINTS

- Innovation in surgical technique and contemporary spinal instrumentation paired with intraoperative navigation/imaging concepts allows for safer and less-invasive surgical approaches.
- The combination of stereotactic body radiotherapy, contemporary surgical adjuncts, and less-invasive techniques serves to minimize blood loss, soft tissue injury, and length of hospital stay without compromising surgical efficacy, potentially enabling patients to begin adjuvant treatment sooner.

INTRODUCTION

Minimally invasive surgical equipment and techniques have revolutionized spinal surgery. Although initially popularized in surgery for degenerative spinal disease and trauma, these techniques have also become widely applied in spinal tumor and deformity surgery. Among patients with malignant spinal tumors, minimizing the interruption or delay in systemic and radiation therapy plays a critical role in survival improvement. Utilization of minimally invasive techniques that facilitate postoperative recovery and decrease the risk of complications and systemic surgical stress may result in improved survival for patients with cancer and certainly plays a role in expediting their return to home and continuation of oncologic treatment.

The principal indications for surgery among patients with spinal tumors include tumor control, decompression of the spinal cord, and restoration of mechanical stability of the spinal column. Surgery for primary tumors may be undertaken with a curative intent, whereas metastatic tumor surgery is performed for symptom palliation. The key components of minimal access surgery include percutaneous spinal instrumentation, tubular and expandable retractors that facilitate transmuscular approaches, and neuronavigation. Endoscopic and robot-assisted surgery shows promise in further expanding the minimally invasive surgery (MIS) tumor surgery capabilities (**Figs. 1–3**).

MINIMALLY INVASIVE SPINAL TUMOR SURGERY TECHNIQUES

Spinal Stabilization

Vertebral cement augmentation provides reliable pain relief for patients with simple compression fractures without extensive cortical destruction or extension into the posterior elements. Kyphoplasty and vertebroplasty can be performed in the outpatient setting, representing the most enduring and the least-invasive spinal stabilization technique. The cement is injected into the

[a] Department of Neurosurgery, Memorial Sloan Kettering Cancer Center, Weill Cornell Medical College, 1275 York Avenue, New York, NY 10065, USA; [b] Department of Neurosurgery, Henry Ford Hospital, 2799 West Grand Boulevard, Detroit, MI, USA; [c] Department of Neurosurgery, Rush University Medical Center, 1653 West Congress Parkway, Chicago, IL 60612, USA
* Corresponding author.
E-mail address: lauferi@mskcc.org

Neurosurg Clin N Am 31 (2020) 201–209
https://doi.org/10.1016/j.nec.2019.11.003
1042-3680/20/

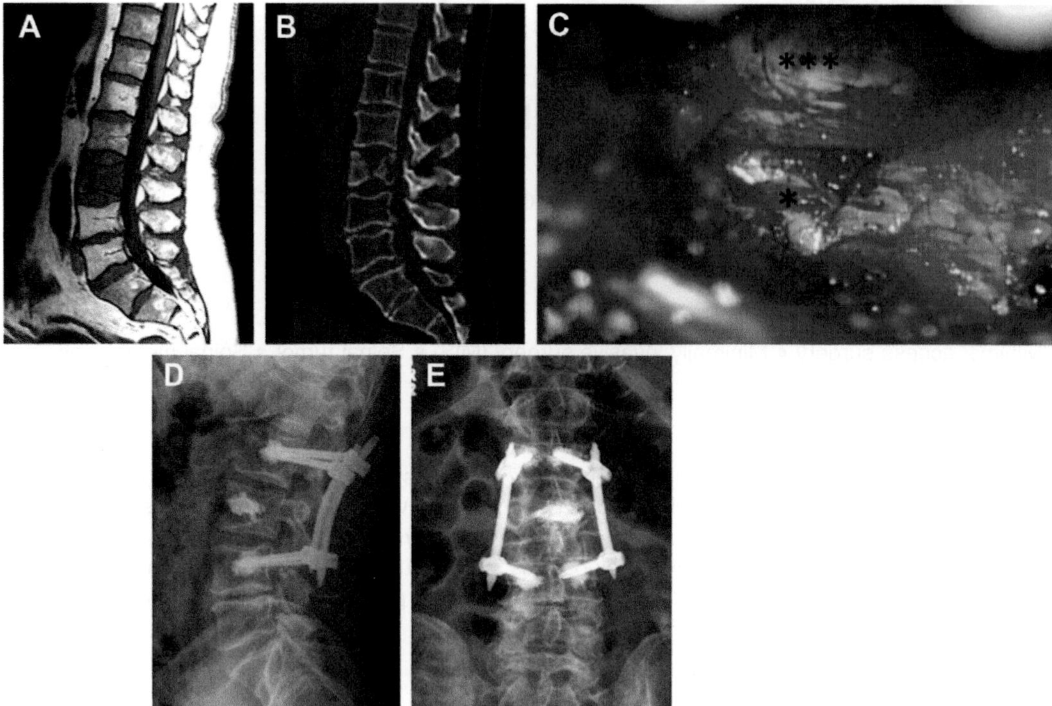

Fig. 1. A 61-year-old man with widely metastatic urothelial carcinoma treated with Pembrolizumab and concomitant radiation. He underwent SBRT to L3 vertebral body metastases with no significant compression fracture and no epidural disease (*A*). Several weeks after radiation, he experienced severe lower back pain and left-sided mechanical radiculopathy. CT scan showed progression of his L3 fracture with a fragment compressing the exiting nerve root (*B*). He underwent L2-L4 percutaneous stabilization with cement augmentation, L3 kyphoplasty, and left L3-4 minimally invasive facetectomy. Intraoperative image demonstrating the decompressed thecal sac (*triple asterisk*) and exiting nerve root (*asterisk*) (*C*). Postoperatively, his pain significantly improved, and he was discharged home on postoperative day 2. Postoperative anteroposterior (AP) (*D*) and lateral (*E*) views demonstrate the stabilizing construct.

vertebral body through a percutaneously placed needle and can be injected directly into the cancellous bone in vertebroplasty or into a cavity created with an inflatable balloon in kyphoplasty. In cases of epidural tumor extension, injection of cement into the vertebral body can displace the epidural tumor further into the canal and should be done with caution and avoided in cases of high-grade epidural disease.[1]

Percutaneous pedicle screw instrumentation (PPSI) permits minimally invasive stabilization of pathologic fractures that are not amenable to stand-alone percutaneous cement augmentation. The technique requires minimal approach-associated soft tissue disruption compared with open posterior instrumentation placement, avoiding muscle necrosis, devascularization, and denervation, and minimizing blood loss. Various techniques for radiographic or navigation guidance for PPSI placement have been described.

The use of cement augmentation can be used to provide additional spinal stability for patients requiring PPSI. Patients with cancer frequently suffer from impaired bone density, placing the patients at high risk for screw pull-out. Augmentation of osseous screw purchase with cement has been demonstrated to be an effective technique in overcoming this challenge. Fenestrated screws permit cement injection through the screw directly into the surrounding bone in the vertebral body.[2] Although traditionally, open pedicle screw instrumentation is placed at least 2 levels above and below the tumor in order to diminish the risk of screw pull-out, the use of fenestrated screws permits the use of short constructs with screws placed 1 level above and below the tumor.[2,3] In cases of significant lytic destruction of the vertebral body, cement augmentation of the tumor level can provide additional stability of the anterior column.[4]

Tumor Excision and Decompression

Among patients with primary tumors, surgical excision might be undertaken with curative intent. However, patients with metastatic tumors undergo

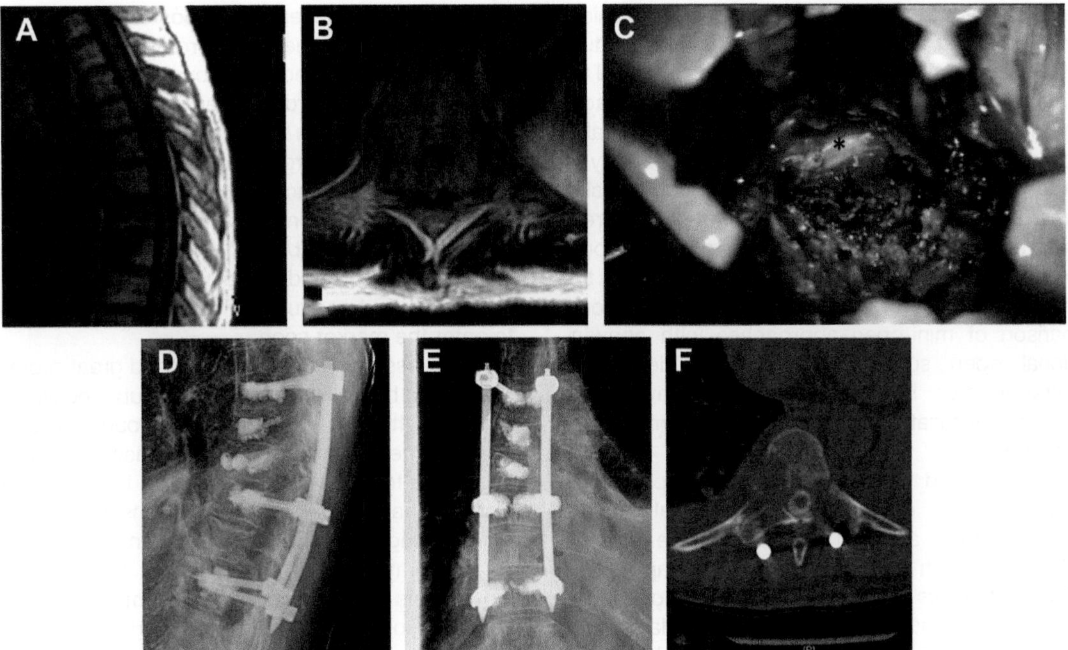

Fig. 2. A 66-year-old woman with no previous history of cancer, presented with severe movement-related back pain and imaging suggestive of metastatic lung cancer involving spine, liver, lung, lymph nodes, and left pleura. Her MRI scan was significant for multiple pathologic fractures (*A*) and multilevel epidural disease, notably high-grade compression with bilateral pedicle and joint involvement at the level of T10 (*B*). Given her mechanical instability and high-grade cord compression, she underwent T6-T10 percutaneous stabilization, T7 and T8 kyphoplasty, and a left-sided T10 minimally invasive decompression. The left caudal screw incision was extended, and decompression was performed via an expandable retractor (*C*; *asterisk*, thecal sac). Postoperative AP (*D*) and lateral (*E*) radiographs demonstrate the stabilizing construct, and postoperative CT myelogram (*F*) demonstrates the left-sided pediculectomy, partial facetectomy, and reconstitution of the thecal sac at the level of T10.

surgery for the purpose of symptom palliation. In both patient populations, the goals of excisional surgery include meaningful local control and decompression of the spinal cord and nerve roots.

The mini-open approach combines PPSI with conventional midline or anterior approaches for tumor excision and spinal cord decompression. This approach generally requires a 1- or 2-level midline

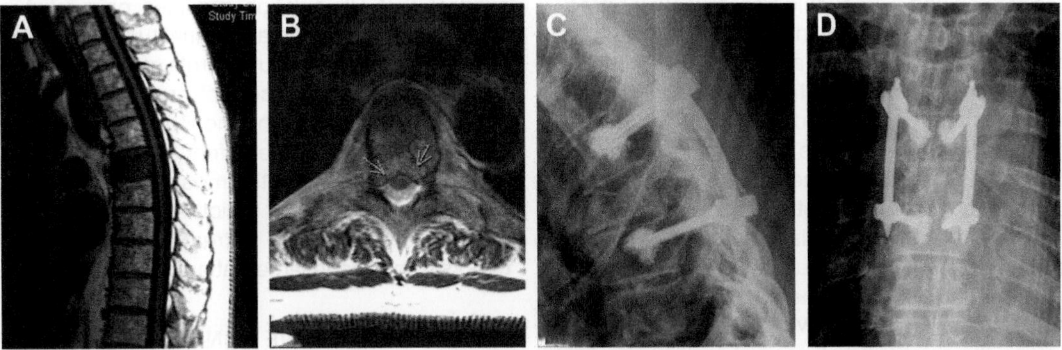

Fig. 3. A 67-year-old man with metastatic renal cell carcinoma to lungs, thoracic lymph nodes, adrenal glands, and T6 vertebra presenting with subacute movement-related back pain radiating to the bilateral chest wall, found to have a T6 metastasis (*A*) with epidural spinal cord compression 1C cord compression (*B*). Kyphoplasty was not performed because of the posterior vertebral body involvement extending into the canal. Patient underwent T5-T7 percutaneous stabilization with cement augmentation followed by adjuvant SBRT. Postoperative AP (*C*) and lateral (*D*) radiographs demonstrate the stabilization construct. At 1-year follow-up, the patient remains pain free with durable local tumor control.

approach for tumor exposure and decompression, while sparing the rest of the midline musculature that would have been dissected and retracted for the purpose of posterior instrumentation placement. Anterior mini-open approaches have also been described, largely using the thoracotomy or retroperitoneal approaches while limiting the skin and muscle dissection. The extent of decompression and tumor excision range from laminectomy to en bloc corpectomy and can be tailored to the oncologic goals of the operation. Matched comparison of mini-open approaches with conventional open surgery demonstrated decreased intraoperative blood loss, postoperative pain, and hospitalization duration after the mini-open approach.[5,6]

Tubular and expandable retractors provide a transmuscular exposure through serial muscle dilation, thus allowing greater muscle sparing compared with the midline mini-open approach. Such retractors have been used to remove intradural and extradural tumors. Fixed tubular retractors come in a range of diameters and lengths, allowing retractor selection specific to the patient's anatomy and surgical plan. Expandable retractors provide a wider surgical field and have mobile retractor blades that can be adjusted as the surgery progresses. These retractors can be placed through the incisions used for PPSI at a trajectory that allows targeted decompression or through a separate incision. Retractor trajectory is critical in providing adequate exposure and safe conditions for tumor removal. These retractors are placed over serial dilator tubes that are docked on the lamina. In patients with tumors causing lytic destruction of the lamina, serial dilation must be performed with great caution in order to avoid unintended entry in the spinal canal. The use of fixed and expandable transmuscular retractors has been described in a wide range of tumor operations from limited laminectomy to intralesional corpectomy for extradural tumors as well as for the removal of intradural tumors.

Endoscopy represents the next step in decreasing the invasiveness of spinal surgery. Current endoscopic systems provide a subcentimeter channel for visualization and single-port dissection. The popularity of such systems for the treatment of degenerative spinal problems has dramatically grown, with excellent data supporting the safety and efficacy of endoscopic spinal surgery. The use of thoracoscopy for anterior-approach corpectomy has been described in several case series and technical notes.[7,8] On the other hand, the use of endoscopic systems for posterior-approach spinal tumor work has been limited, described in only a few case reports.[9–12] However, the posterior-approach endoscopic technique holds promise for targeted tumor excision and bone removal for decompression of the spinal cord and nerve roots, and these applications will gain prominence as the technology improves and surgeons continue to gain experience with spinal endoscopy. Currently available endoscopic instruments have very limited capacity to control tumor bleeding, thus significantly limiting the role of endoscopy in tumor work; however, improved coagulation devices are expected to enter the market soon.

Robot-assisted surgery has gained great prominence in a broad range of surgical subspecialties, including thoracic, colorectal, genitourinary, and head and neck surgery. Most robot-assisted operations use transcavitary approaches that permit a working space for several robotic arms and a camera, allowing outstanding visualization of the surgical anatomy as well as controlled and precise movements of surgical instruments in small spaces. Robot-assisted spinal surgery has not been performed for posterior-approach spinal surgery; however, several reports describe its use in the removal of paraspinal thoracic and presacral tumors.[13–17]

Various ablation techniques have also been used in order to obtain local tumor control. The use of radiofrequency (RF), laser, microwave ablation, and cryoablation for the treatment of benign osseous spinal tumors has been described.[18–21] Ablation is often performed in combination with vertebral cement augmentation and radiotherapy. Proximity of tumors to nerve roots and vascular structures limits the utilization of percutaneous ablation; however, various organ displacement techniques and improved neuromonitoring might allow broader application. Multiple case series suggest that RF ablation provides pain relief in the treatment of metastatic spinal tumors; however, convincing data about the role of RF ablation in providing local tumor control are lacking. Laser ablation permits real-time monitoring of the ablation zone, improving the safety of the procedure. Spinal laser interstitial thermoablation combined with stereotactic body radiotherapy (SBRT) has been successfully used to treat spinal metastatic tumors, reported in large patient series.[22,23]

MINIMALLY INVASIVE SPINAL TUMOR INDICATIONS

Benign Epidural Tumors of the Spinal Column

Surgical treatment of benign osseous spinal tumors is indicated in cases of symptomatic or growing tumors and is generally undertaken with curative intent. Multiple reports describe curative treatment of osteoid osteomas and osteoblastomas using computed tomographic (CT)-guided percutaneous ablation techniques.[18] These series report complete pain relief with durable follow-up of up to 5 years without periprocedural complications or evidence of tumor recurrence. Because these lesions are frequently located in the posterior elements, including the pedicle and articular processes, open surgical excision may be associated with iatrogenic instability and the need for spinal stabilization. Percutaneous ablation avoids instability. Although proximity of these tumors to the spinal cord, nerve roots, and the vertebral artery may limit the use of ablation, modern neurologic monitoring techniques generally provide accurate information about the safety of the ablation.[21,24]

Although typical and atypical vertebral hemangiomas generally do not require treatment, they may occasionally cause pain, epidural venous congestion, and fractures. Most symptomatic hemangiomas can be treated with percutaneous cement injection.[25] Occasionally, the cement injection is performed in combination with alcohol ablation or transarterial embolization.[26]

Transtubular or endoscopic tumors excision provides another minimally invasive alternative to percutaneous ablation. Tubular retractors have been used to excise anterior cervical benign tumors using the anterior approach to C2 and the subaxial cervical spine, along with the posterior approach to thoracic and lumbar posterior element tumors.[27] Thoracoscopy has also been used for the removal of anteriorly located thoracic osteoid osteomas.[28]

Intradural Tumors

Similarly to benign osseous tumors, benign intradural intramedullary and extramedullary tumors are excised when they grow or cause symptoms. Surgery is undertaken with the goal of safe gross total excision and usually results in cure. Surgery for spinal astrocytomas may be limited to biopsy in cases of higher-grade tumors. The most commonly described minimal access approach to the intradural compartment involves a paramedian incision with sequential muscle dilation and the placement of a fixed tubular or expandable retractor. A hemilaminectomy with undercutting of the spinous process is performed. The intradural dissection is performed according to conventional microsurgical technique. Several techniques for dural closure through a tubular dilator have been described. Numerous case series and technical reports describe excellent outcomes after minimal access excision of intradural schwannomas, meningiomas, ependymomas, hemangioblastomas, and cavernous malformations.[29–34]

Metastatic Tumors

Instability

The diagnosis of spinal mechanical instability among patients with spinal metastatic tumors is facilitated using the Spinal Instability Neoplastic Score.[35] Generally, patients with pathologic fractures causing pain that is exacerbated by movement benefit from spinal stabilization. A prospective randomized trial demonstrated that balloon-assisted kyphoplasty provides superior pain relief and functional restoration compared with patients treated using noninterventional methods.[36] Cement augmentation works well among patients with simple pathologic compression fractures limited to the vertebral body.

Patients with thoracolumbar fractures, significant epidural tumor extension, fracture fragment retropulsion, fracture extension into the posterior elements, or severe lytic cortical destruction generally require instrumented stabilization because adequate cement fill may not be feasible. PPSI provides an excellent alternative to stand-alone cement augmentation, through stabilizing the anterior and posterior spinal elements. The small incisions and minimal muscle disruption required for PPSI lead to very low risk of wound complications and rapid postoperative recovery. The efficacy and safety of PPSI in stabilization of tumor-associated fractures have been reported by multiple investigators. Short-segment PPSI stabilization of painful pathologic fractures provides excellent pain relief when used as stand-alone or with fracture and screw cement augmentation.[3,37,38] Cement augmentation of the screw-bone interface using fenestrated screws has been shown to provide durable construct stability, with very low complication risk.[2] In addition to the use of cement for screw augmentation, cement stabilization of the fractured level may be performed using kyphoplasty or vertebroplasty technique in combination with PPSI in order to provide additional support to the anterior column.[3,4]

Various MIS pedicle screw placement strategies have been reported in the cancer literature. Most commonly, separate small skin incisions are made for each screw. However, in cases of multilevel constructs or decompressive surgery, some investigators advocate for a midline skin incision and transfacial transmuscular placement of the screws.[5,6] If a common midline incision is selected, a subcutaneous drain is usually required.

Metastatic epidural spinal cord compression and radiculopathy

Patients with symptomatic spinal cord compression benefit from surgical decompression. Furthermore, patients with fractures causing mechanical radiculopathy require nerve root decompression in order to attain pain relief.[39] Decompression strategies range from limited laminectomy or facetectomy to corpectomy, and all have been performed using various MIS techniques.

The midline mini-open approach has been used in order to perform tumor excision for circumferential spinal cord decompression in combination with posterior spinal instrumentation. Chou and Lu[40] used the mini-open approach to perform a transpedicular corpectomy with expandable cage and transfascial pedicle screw stabilization. They subsequently demonstrated that patients who underwent mini-open surgery had lower blood loss and shorter hospital stay compared with patients who underwent open corpectomy.[6] Similar comparison by Saadeh and colleagues[5] confirmed the reduction in blood loss, hospitalization duration, and postoperative pain.

Tubular retractors have been used in order to provide a posterior approach for the purpose of transpedicular vertebrectomy. Deutsch and colleagues[41] described transpedicular thoracic vertebrectomy using a 22-mm tubular retractor. Massicotte[42] has reported a series of patients who underwent thoracic and lumbar PPSI placement and corpectomies via an 18-mm tubular retractor in the outpatient setting.

Expandable retractors provide a wider and more flexible working corridor compared with fixed tubular retractors and have been used for posterior, posterolateral, and lateral approaches to spinal tumors. Taghva and colleagues[43] used dual expandable retractors to perform a bilateral T4 and T5 decompression, with a transpedicular approach on 1 side and a costotransversectomy approach on the contralateral side. A series of extracavitary corpectomies through an expandable retractor with short segment PPSI was also reported by Smith and colleagues.[44] The use of expandable retractors for facetectomy or transpedicular corpectomy with cage reconstruction in the lumbar spine has also been reported by several investigators.[45–47] Expandable retractors have also been used in transthoracic, transplural, and retroperitoneal approaches to the thoracic and lumbar spine in order to perform anterior corpectomy and cage reconstruction.[48,49] Thoracoscopy has also been used in order to perform anterior thoracic corpectomy.[7]

Finally, with popularization of SBRT, separation surgery, involving circumferential epidural decompression without corpectomy, has become a commonly performed operation for patients with metastatic epidural spinal cord compression. Because SBRT provides reliable tumor control without the need for extensive tumor excision, the goal of separation surgery is to create favorable conditions for SBRT by providing a separation between the tumor and the spinal cord.[50,51] The use of fixed tubular and expandable retractors in separation surgery has been described, followed by SBRT.[52,53] Tatsui and colleagues[54] have used LITT in order to perform focused ablation of epidural tumor in order to provide the separation necessary for successful SBRT. LITT is described in detail in a dedicated article in the current issue and provides a promising alternative to surgical tumor excision.

Algorithm for Minimally Invasive Surgery Strategy Selection in Patients with Metastatic Tumors

Clearly, surgeons use myriad MIS options in the treatment of spinal metastatic tumors. The choice of technique is dictated by the surgical indication, tumor location and morphology, hemorrhagic potential, prior surgery, and the degree of spinal cord compression. Not every tumor is amenable to safe and effective minimally invasive treatment. For example, a patient with renal cell carcinoma metastasis causing multilevel spinal cord compression might be better treated with open surgery after tumor embolization. On the other hand, focal tumors with low vascularity represent ideal targets for MIS decompression. The surgeon's experience with the MIS technique plays a critical role in the approach selection.

The authors have developed a treatment algorithm that considers the extent of epidural tumor extension, symptoms, tumor histology, and fracture morphology in order to facilitate and clarify MIS strategy selection.[47] They treat patients with solid tumors causing symptomatic spinal cord compression with PPSI and decompression through midline mini-open or transmuscular approach using an expandable retractor. Patients with lumbar tumors causing mechanical radiculopathy are treated with PPSI and facetectomy through a tubular or expandable retractor. Patients with mechanical instability caused by radiosensitive tumors with high-grade epidural extension are treated with PPSI with screw cement augmentation. In the absence of high-grade epidural extension, mechanically unstable fractures with extension into the posterior elements are treated with PPSI with screw and fracture cement augmentation. Finally, simple compression fractures can be treated with kyphoplasty.

SUMMARY

MIS presents clear advantages for patients with spinal tumors. For patients with benign osseous tumors, the minimal disruption of muscle and osseous structural elements may avoid iatrogenic instability and the need for fusion and diminish the risk of chronic pain. Patients with metastatic tumors usually require postoperative radiation and systemic therapy. The minimal soft tissue disruption with the use of MIS techniques facilitates healing and allows the patients to proceed to postoperative therapy with minimal delay. Finally, MIS diminishes the systemic surgical stress and facilitates postoperative recovery, thereby providing surgical options to patients at risk for priopative complications after open surgery and expediting their return to home. The use of MIS techniques will continue to expand in spine tumor surgery, and new techniques, such as endoscopy and robot-assisted surgery, will only improve outcomes and patient access to surgery.

DISCLOSURE

Dr I. Laufer is Consultant for SpineWave, Depuy/Synthes, Medtronic, Globus, and Brainlab. Dr Bilsky Royalties from Globus and Depuy, Brainlab and Varian speaker's bureau. Dr J.E. O'Toole Globus - Consulting/royalties, RTI Surgical - Royalties, Theracell: stock ownership.

REFERENCES

1. Lis E, Laufer I, Barzilai O, et al. Change in the cross-sectional area of the thecal sac following balloon kyphoplasty for pathological vertebral compression fractures prior to spine stereotactic radiosurgery. J Neurosurg Spine 2018;30(1):111–8.
2. Barzilai O, McLaughlin L, Lis E, et al. Utility of cement augmentation via percutaneous fenestrated pedicle screws for stabilization of cancer related spinal instability. Oper Neurosurg (Hagerstown) 2018;16(5):593–9.
3. Moussazadeh N, Rubin DG, McLaughlin L, et al. Short-segment percutaneous pedicle screw fixation with cement augmentation for tumor-induced spinal instability. Spine J 2015;15(7):1609–17.
4. Chang CW, Fu TS, Lin DY, et al. Percutaneous balloon kyphoplasty and short instrumentation compared with traditional long instrumentation for thoracolumbar metastatic spinal cord compression. World Neurosurg 2019;130:e640–7.
5. Saadeh YS, Elswick CM, Fateh JA, et al. Analysis of outcomes between traditional open versus mini-open approach in surgical treatment of spinal metastasis. World Neurosurg 2019;130:e467–74.
6. Lau D, Chou D. Posterior thoracic corpectomy with cage reconstruction for metastatic spinal tumors: comparing the mini-open approach to the open approach. J Neurosurg Spine 2015;23(2):217–27.
7. Ray WZ, Schmidt MH. Thoracoscopic vertebrectomy for thoracolumbar junction fractures and tumors: surgical technique and evaluation of the learning curve. Clin Spine Surg 2016;29(7): E344–50.
8. Ragel BT, Amini A, Schmidt MH. Thoracoscopic vertebral body replacement with an expandable cage after ventral spinal canal decompression. Neurosurgery 2007;61(5 Suppl 2):317–22 [discussion 322–3].
9. Archavlis E, Schwandt E, Kosterhon M, et al. A modified microsurgical endoscopic-assisted transpedicular corpectomy of the thoracic spine based on virtual 3-dimensional planning. World Neurosurg 2016;91:424–33.
10. Dhandapani S, Karthigeyan M. "Microendoscopic" versus "pure endoscopic" surgery for spinal intradural mass lesions: a comparative study and review. Spine J 2018;18(9):1592–602.
11. Telfeian AE, Choi DB, Aghion DM. Transforaminal endoscopic surgery under local analgesia for ventral epidural thoracic spinal tumor: case report. Clin Neurol Neurosurg 2015;134:1–3.
12. Xie T, Xiu P, Song Y, et al. Percutaneous endoscopic excision and ablation of osteoid osteoma of the lumbar spine and sacrum: a technical note and outcomes. World Neurosurg 2019;133:121–6.
13. Yin J, Wu H, Tu J, et al. Robot-assisted sacral tumor resection: a preliminary study. BMC Musculoskelet Disord 2018;19(1):186.
14. Perez-Cruet MJ, Welsh RJ, Hussain NS, et al. Use of the da Vinci minimally invasive robotic system for resection of a complicated paraspinal schwannoma with thoracic extension: case report. Neurosurgery 2012;71(1 Suppl Operative):209–14.
15. Chinder PS, Hindiskere S, Doddarangappa S, et al. Robotic surgery assisted staged en-bloc sacrectomy for sacral chordoma: a case report. JBJS Case Connect 2019;9(2):e0240.
16. Bederman SS, Lopez G, Ji T, et al. Robotic guidance for en bloc sacrectomy: a case report. Spine 2014; 39(23):E1398–401.
17. Finley D, Sherman JH, Avila E, et al. Thorascopic resection of an apical paraspinal schwannoma using the da Vinci surgical system. J Neurol Surg A Cent Eur Neurosurg 2014;75(1):58–63.
18. Faddoul J, Faddoul Y, Kobaiter-Maarrawi S, et al. Radiofrequency ablation of spinal osteoid osteoma: a prospective study. J Neurosurg Spine 2017; 26(3):313–8.
19. Gazis AN, Beuing O, Franke J, et al. Bipolar radiofrequency ablation of spinal tumors: predictability, safety and outcome. Spine J 2014;14(4):604–8.

20. Tomasian A, Wallace A, Northrup B, et al. Spine cryoablation: pain palliation and local tumor control for vertebral metastases. AJNR Am J Neuroradiol 2016;37(1):189–95.
21. Tomasian A, Wallace AN, Jennings JW. Benign spine lesions: advances in techniques for minimally invasive percutaneous treatment. AJNR Am J Neuroradiol 2017;38(5):852–61.
22. Ghia AJ, Rebueno NC, Li J, et al. The use of image guided laser interstitial thermotherapy to supplement spine stereotactic radiosurgery to manage metastatic epidural spinal cord compression: proof of concept and dosimetric analysis. Pract Radiat Oncol 2016;6(2):e35–8.
23. Tatsui CE, Lee SH, Amini B, et al. Spinal laser interstitial thermal therapy: a novel alternative to surgery for metastatic epidural spinal cord compression. Neurosurgery 2016;79(Suppl 1):S73–82.
24. Noel MA, Segura MJ, Sierre S, et al. Neurophysiological monitoring in radiofrequency ablation of spinal osteoid osteoma with a progressive time and temperature protocol in children. Spine Deform 2017;5(5):351–9.
25. Hadjipavlou A, Tosounidis T, Gaitanis I, et al. Balloon kyphoplasty as a single or as an adjunct procedure for the management of symptomatic vertebral haemangiomas. J Bone Joint Surg Br 2007;89(4): 495–502.
26. Premat K, Clarencon F, Cormier E, et al. Long-term outcome of percutaneous alcohol embolization combined with percutaneous vertebroplasty in aggressive vertebral hemangiomas with epidural extension. Eur Radiol 2017;27(7):2860–7.
27. Amendola L, Cappuccio M, Boriani L, et al. Endoscopic excision of C2 osteoid osteoma: a technical case report. Eur Spine J 2013;22(Suppl 3):S357–62.
28. Campos WK, Gasbarrini A, Boriani S. Case report: curetting osteoid osteoma of the spine using combined video-assisted thoracoscopic surgery and navigation. Clin Orthop Relat Res 2013;471(2): 680–5.
29. Kruger MT, Steiert C, Glasker S, et al. Minimally invasive resection of spinal hemangioblastoma: feasibility and clinical results in a series of 18 patients. J Neurosurg Spine 2019;1–10.
30. Afathi M, Peltier E, Adetchessi T, et al. Minimally invasive transmuscular approach for the treatment of benign intradural extramedullary spinal cord tumours: technical note and results. Neurochirurgie 2015;61(5):333–8.
31. Formo M, Halvorsen CM, Dahlberg D, et al. Minimally invasive microsurgical resection of primary, intradural spinal tumors is feasible and safe: a consecutive series of 83 patients. Neurosurgery 2018;82(3):365–71.
32. Ogden AT, Fessler RG. Minimally invasive resection of intramedullary ependymoma: case report. Neurosurgery 2009;65(6):E1203–4 [discussion: E1204].
33. Winkler EA, Lu A, Rutledge WC, et al. A mini-open transspinous approach for resection of intramedullary spinal cavernous malformations. J Clin Neurosci 2018;58:210–2.
34. Tredway TL. Minimally invasive approaches for the treatment of intramedullary spinal tumors. Neurosurg Clin N Am 2014;25(2):327–36.
35. Fisher CG, DiPaola CP, Ryken TC, et al. A novel classification system for spinal instability in neoplastic disease: an evidence-based approach and expert consensus from the Spine Oncology Study Group. Spine 2010;35(22):E1221–9.
36. Berenson J, Pflugmacher R, Jarzem P, et al. Balloon kyphoplasty versus non-surgical fracture management for treatment of painful vertebral body compression fractures in patients with cancer: a multicentre, randomised controlled trial. Lancet Oncol 2011;12(3):225–35.
37. Schwab JH, Gasbarrini A, Cappuccio M, et al. Minimally invasive posterior stabilization improved ambulation and pain scores in patients with plasmacytomas and/or metastases of the spine. Int J Surg Oncol 2011;2011:239230.
38. Hamad A, Vachtsevanos L, Cattell A, et al. Minimally invasive spinal surgery for the management of symptomatic spinal metastasis. Br J Neurosurg 2017;31(5):526–30.
39. Moliterno J, Veselis CA, Hershey MA, et al. Improvement in pain after lumbar surgery in cancer patients with mechanical radiculopathy. Spine J 2014;14(10): 2434–9.
40. Chou D, Lu DC. Mini-open transpedicular corpectomies with expandable cage reconstruction. Technical note. J Neurosurg Spine 2011;14(1):71–7.
41. Deutsch H, Boco T, Lobel J. Minimally invasive transpedicular vertebrectomy for metastatic disease to the thoracic spine. J Spinal Disord Tech 2008; 21(2):101–5.
42. Massicotte E. Minimal access spine surgery (MASS) for decompression and stabilization performed as an out-patient procedure for metastatic spinal tumours followed by spine stereotactic body radiotherapy (SBRT): first report of technique and preliminary outcomes. Technol Cancer Res Treat 2012;11(1):15–25.
43. Taghva A, Li KW, Liu JC, et al. Minimally invasive circumferential spinal decompression and stabilization for symptomatic metastatic spine tumor: technical case report. Neurosurgery 2010;66(3):E620–2.
44. Smith ZA, Li Z, Chen NF, et al. Minimally invasive lateral extracavitary corpectomy: cadaveric evaluation model and report of 3 clinical cases. J Neurosurg Spine 2012;16(5):463–70.
45. Donnelly DJ, Abd-El-Barr MM, Lu Y. Minimally invasive muscle sparing posterior-only approach for

lumbar circumferential decompression and stabilization to treat spine metastasis–technical report. World Neurosurg 2015;84(5):1484–90.

46. Venkatesh R, Tandon V, Patel N, et al. Solitary plasmacytoma of L3 vertebral body treated by minimal access surgery: common problem different solution! J Clin Orthop Trauma 2015; 6(4):259–64.
47. Barzilai O, McLaughlin L, Amato MK, et al. Minimal access surgery for spinal metastases: prospective evaluation of a treatment algorithm using patient-reported outcomes. World Neurosurg 2018;120: e889–901.
48. Uribe JS, Dakwar E, Le TV, et al. Minimally invasive surgery treatment for thoracic spine tumor removal: a mini-open, lateral approach. Spine 2010;35(26 Suppl):S347–54.
49. Serak J, Vanni S, Levi AD. The extreme lateral approach for treatment of thoracic and lumbar vertebral body metastases. J Neurosurg Sci 2019;63(4): 473–8.
50. Wang J, Boland P, Mitra N, et al. Single-stage posterolateral transpedicular approach for resection of epidural metastatic spine tumors involving the vertebral body with circumferential reconstruction: results in 140 patients. Invited submission from the Joint Section Meeting on Disorders of the Spine and Peripheral Nerves, March 2004. J Neurosurg Spine 2004;1(3):287–98.
51. Laufer I, Iorgulescu JB, Chapman T, et al. Local disease control for spinal metastases following "separation surgery" and adjuvant hypofractionated or high-dose single-fraction stereotactic radiosurgery: outcome analysis in 186 patients. J Neurosurg Spine 2013;18(3):207–14.
52. Nasser R, Nakhla J, Echt M, et al. Minimally invasive separation surgery with intraoperative stereotactic guidance: a feasibility study. World Neurosurg 2018;109:68–76.
53. Turel MK, Kerolus MG, O'Toole JE. Minimally invasive "separation surgery" plus adjuvant stereotactic radiotherapy in the management of spinal epidural metastases. J Craniovertebr Junction Spine 2017; 8(2):119–26.
54. Tatsui CE, Stafford RJ, Li J, et al. Utilization of laser interstitial thermotherapy guided by real-time thermal MRI as an alternative to separation surgery in the management of spinal metastasis. J Neurosurg Spine 2015;23(4):400–11.

Percutaneous Hybrid Therapy for Spinal Metastatic Disease

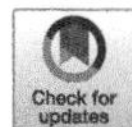

Laser Interstitial Thermal Therapy and Spinal Stereotactic Radiosurgery

Rafael A. Vega, MD, PhD[a], Amol J. Ghia, MD[b], Claudio E. Tatsui, MD[c,*]

KEYWORDS

• Image guidance • LITT • Magnetic resonance imaging • Metastatic spine tumors • Oncology • Minimally invasive spine surgery • Separation surgery • Spinal laser interstitial thermotherapy

KEY POINTS

- Spinal stereotactic radiosurgery (SSRS) is a form of radiation therapy by which advanced treatment delivery techniques (eg, intensity-modulated radiotherapy) are combined with image guidance and rigid immobilization to deliver a high dose of conformal radiation to the target while minimizing dose to nearby critical structures, such as the spinal cord. SSRS offers durable local control and pain relief, for carefully selected patients.
- Patients with metastatic epidural disease continue to pose a clinical treatment challenge.
- The ability for SSRS to deliver an ablative dose of radiation to the metastatic disease has changed treatment paradigms when used as definitive therapy or as a postoperative adjuvant.
- Based on improved responses to SSRS, surgery has largely transitioned from an aggressive gross-total or en bloc resection to a less aggressive approach aimed at spinal cord decompression in order to allow clearance for treatment with tumoricidal doses of radiation to the residual disease, while respecting the radiation constraints of the spinal cord.
- Spinal laser interstitial thermal therapy (SLITT) has been developed as a minimally invasive percutaneous alternative to open surgery. SLITT can be performed in select cases of epidural metastatic spinal cord compression in combination with SSRS.

INTRODUCTION

Spinal stereotactic radiosurgery (SSRS) is a form of radiation therapy by which advanced treatment delivery techniques (eg, intensity modulated radiotherapy) are combined with image guidance and rigid immobilization to deliver a high dose of conformal radiation to the target while minimizing dose to nearby critical structures, such as the spinal cord. SSRS offers durable local control and pain relief, for carefully selected patients.[1,2] However, patients with metastatic epidural disease continue to pose a clinical treatment challenge.

The ability for SSRS to deliver an ablative dose of radiation to the metastatic disease has changed

[a] Division of Neurosurgery, Beth Israel Deaconess Medical Center, Harvard Medical School, 110 Francis Street, Suite 3B, Boston, MA 02215, USA; [b] Department of Radiation Oncology, The University of Texas MD Anderson Cancer Center, 1515 Holcombe Boulevard, Houston, TX 77030, USA; [c] Department of Neurosurgery, The University of Texas MD Anderson Cancer Center, 1400 Holcombe Boulevard, Room FC7.2000, Unit 442, Houston, TX 77030, USA
* Corresponding author.
E-mail address: cetatsui@mdanderson.org

Neurosurg Clin N Am 31 (2020) 211–219
https://doi.org/10.1016/j.nec.2019.11.006

treatment paradigms when used as definitive therapy or as a postoperative adjuvant. Based on improved responses to SSRS, surgery has largely transitioned from an aggressive gross-total or en bloc resection to a less aggressive approach aimed at spinal cord decompression in order to allow clearance for treatment with tumoricidal doses of radiation to the residual disease, while respecting the radiation constraints of the spinal cord.[3–6]

SPINAL LASER INTERSTITIAL THERMAL THERAPY

Spinal laser interstitial thermal therapy (SLITT) uses laser energy to perform thermal ablation of soft tissue in the vertebral body and epidural space. The temperature and heat diffusion is monitored in real time by MRI thermography, allowing a visual feedback of the heat distribution and enabling precise interruption of the treatment when a preset temperature threshold occurs at the junction of the tumor and the thecal sac.[7–9] The goal is destruction of the epidural tumor, verified by an immediate postprocedure MRI, whereby the coagulative necrosis is identified by lack of contrast enhancement.

The rationale to add SLITT to SSRS is similar to the concept of separation surgery put forth by Bilsky and Smith[3] and consolidated by Laufer et al.[4,10] The authors' goal is to ablate the epidural tumor, allowing safe delivery of tumoricidal doses of stereotactic radiation to the residual disease. They typically perform the SSRS plan based on the preoperative MRI, prescribing 18 to 24 Gy to the gross tumor volume (GTV) and 16 Gy to the clinical target volume (CTV), using simultaneous integrated boost technique in a single fraction for radiation-naïve cases. The maximum dose to the spinal cord is restricted to 10 to 12 Gy, while aiming to deliver a minimum dose to the GTV of 14 Gy. The authors time the delivery of SSRS to be done within 5 days of the SLITT in order to optimize return to the oncologic treatment.

Operative Approach

SLITT is performed using intraoperative MRI (iMRI) (Brainlab Inc, Feldkirchen, Germany) with the patient under general anesthesia in the prone position. The operative workflow is illustrated in **Figs. 1–10**. A special trolley is used to transfer the patient in and out of the MRI magnet, because laser catheter placement uses ferromagnetic instruments and has to be performed outside of the high-power magnetic field. Skin fiducials (Izi Medical Products, Owing Mills, MD, USA) are placed over the region of interest in a unique pattern that distinguishes right from left and rostral from caudal. The patient is brought into the iMRI for acquisition of T2-weighted sequence of the region of interest, which is uploaded to a standard spinal navigation system (Stealth; Medtronic Inc, Minneapolis, MN, USA). The authors have demonstrated that surface matching of the skin fiducials allows image guidance registration with submillimeter accuracy.[11] Inline views of the reconstructed T2 images allow very clear identification of the tumor and its relationship to the surrounding neural elements for trajectory planning and safe insertion of the laser fibers.

The Weinstein-Boriani-Biagini tumor classification diagram[12] is used to select the ideal trajectory to ablate the epidural tumor. The oblique transpedicular and transforaminal approach is used to treat tumors in the ventral and lateral aspect of the spinal canal, whereas a contralateral translaminar trajectory is used for tumors located in the dorsal elements.[13] The optimal laser fiber placement should be approximately 5 to 6 mm from the thecal sac, and each catheter consistently achieves a 10-mm diameter of thermal injury. If the fiber is more than 8 mm away from the dura, the zone of ablation may not include the entire epidural tumor, increasing the chances of treatment failure. Depending on the extent of disease in the rostral-caudal plane, additional catheters are placed in tandem within a 10- to 12-mm distance of each other to ensure that there are no untreated segments in between successive ablations. Similarly, bilateral trajectories have been needed to completely treat wide ventral or lateral epidural disease. Of note, the authors have used up to 9 trajectories in a single patient to achieve adequate ablation.

Once all access cannulas have been placed, the surgical field is covered in a sterile fashion; the MRI coil is reapplied over the first layer of sterile drapes, allowing manipulation of all access cannulas, and covered with a second layer of sterile drapes. The laser catheters are secured to the sterile drapes over the MRI coil and introduced through each access cannulas. Finally, the patient is transferred back to the iMRI to obtain exact coplanar T2-weighted images of each catheter in preparation for the ablation.

The authors use the Visualase system (Medtronic Inc), which consists of a 980-nm diode encased within a 1.3-mm silica catheter, connected to a 15-W power source. MR thermography, based on gradient-echo acquisition, is used throughout the procedure to monitor the heat generated within the tissue.[14] The laser is deactivated when one of the 2 set temperature thresholds is reached. The authors identify the boundary between the dura and tumor and set an upper temperature limit of 48°C, whereas a

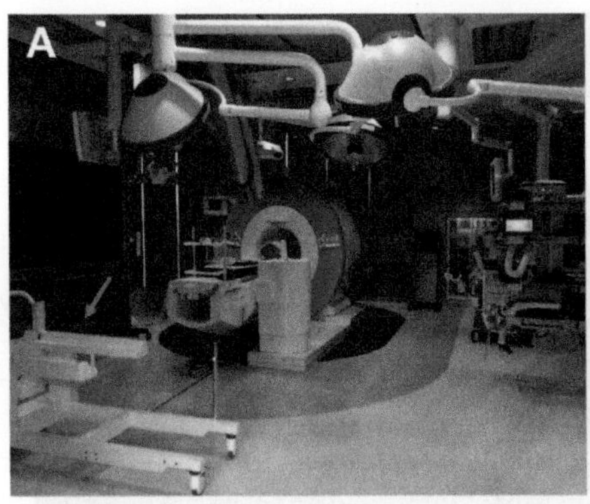

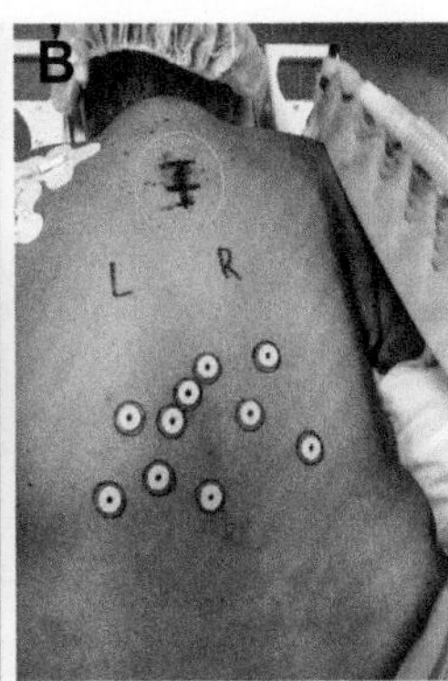

Fig. 1. Intraoperative workflow: Positioning. (*A*) The procedure is performed in the intraoperative MRI suite, and the patient is transported in and out of the MRI magnet by a special trolley (*arrow*). (*B*) The patient is intubated and positioned prone in the MRI transfer board. Skin fiducials are applied in a configuration that is easy to identify: superior/inferior and left/right over the area of interest. A skin incision overlying a spinous process is marked for placement of an MRI compatible navigation clamp (*circle*).

second threshold within the tissue adjacent to the laser fiber is set to 90°C, thereby preventing excessive heating and local tissue carbonization. MR thermography is significantly degraded with respiratory motion, requiring interruption of ventilation during the ablation cycles, which typically last up to 120 seconds and are closely monitored with pulse oximetry and capnography.

At the end of the procedure, final imaging analysis is performed by obtaining precontrast and postcontrast T1-weighted images. The coagulative necrosis induced by the laser ablation can be appreciated as a lack contrast enhancement. Postoperative image control is performed with MRI repeated every 8 to 12 weeks to monitor treatment response.

When required, spinal stabilization can be performed after SLITT, under the same anesthetic conditions or as a separate staged surgery. If performed the same day, the percutaneous posterior segmental instrumentation can be inserted inside the iMRI room after the patient is repositioned to a safe distance from the high magnetic field.[15,16] In such cases, a postoperative computed tomography (CT) myelogram is used for radiosurgery planning.

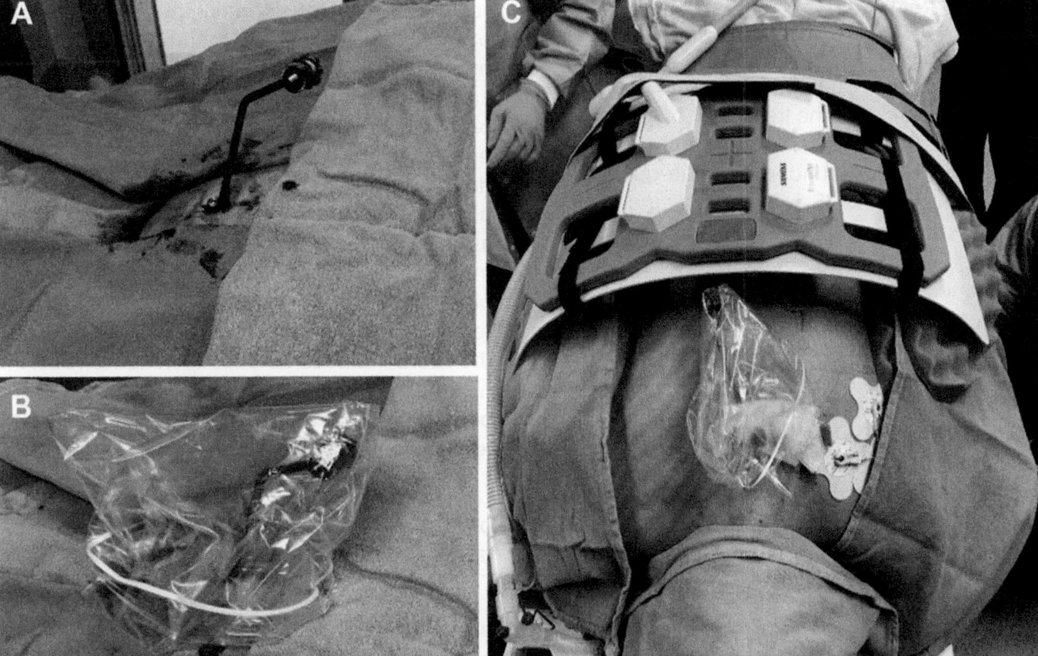

Fig. 2. Intraoperative workflow: Preparation for image guidance. (*A*) An MRI-compatible spinous process clamp is applied and (*B*) covered with a sterile plastic bag. (*C*) The MRI coil is placed over the fiducials supported by a plastic cradle to avoid contact with the skin and displacement of the fiducial markers. The patient is transferred to the MRI magnet for acquisition of T2 sequence of the region of interest overlying the fiducial markers.

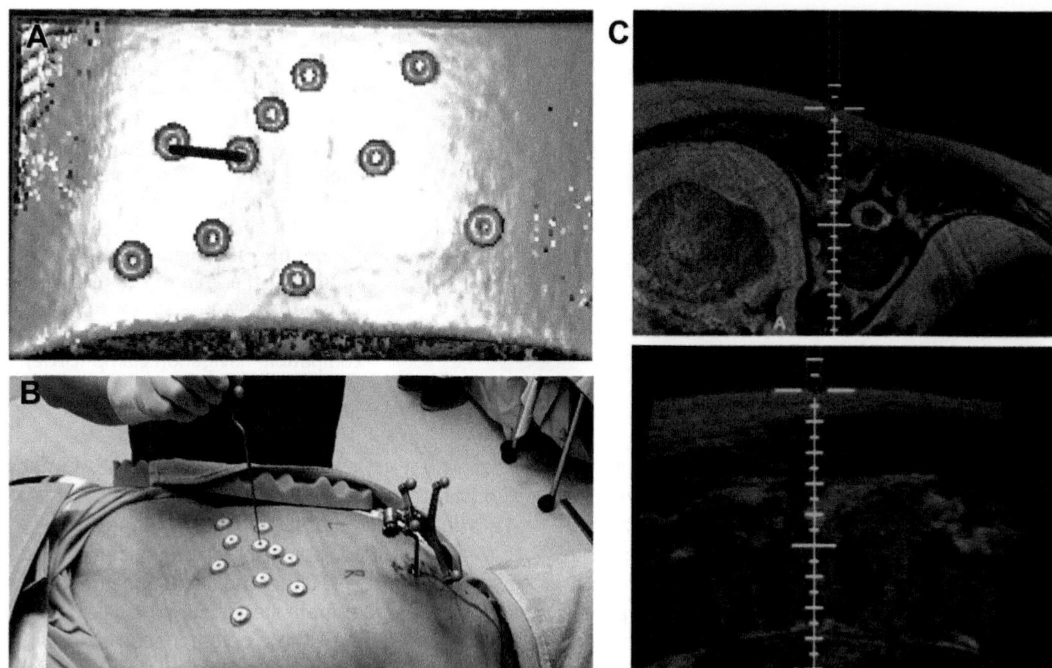

Fig. 3. Intraoperative workflow: Registration of image guidance. (*A*) A 3-dimensional model is reconstructed in the navigation software. (*B*) The reference array is attached to the spinous process clamp with sterile technique, and surface matching of the fiducial markers is performed. (*C*) Image guidance accuracy is confirmed and subsequently used for planning the trajectories to reach the tumor.

SPINAL STEREOTACTIC RADIOSURGERY

SSRS provides histology-independent, durable local tumor control constituting one of the most significant advances in the treatment of metastatic vertebral disease.[1,2,5,6,17,18] In the authors' practice, patients typically undergo image-guided intensity-modulated SSRS with CT guidance using a stereotactic linear accelerator delivery system with a cone-beam CT in addition to ExacTrac image guidance (Brainlab, Munich, Germany). In the radiation-naïve setting, single-fraction SSRS is used with the GTV receiving 18 to 24 Gy depending on histology with the CTV receiving 16 Gy. In the reirradiation setting, the authors use 3-fraction SSRS with the GTV receiving 27 Gy and CTV receiving 21 to 24 Gy. The maximum dose to the spinal cord is set to 10 to 12 Gy/1 fx for radiation-naïve cases and 10 Gy/3 fx for reirradiation cases. As is the authors' practice, planning target volumes are not used. The laser interstitial thermal therapy (LITT) procedure does not significantly alter the principal field design despite destroying the epidural component of disease.

RESULTS

SLITT is an emerging and minimally invasive method to treat spine metastases. The technology is still early in its development, and the authors do not advocate its use as a stand-alone therapy. They believe its use in conjunction with SSRS can provide an alternative to open surgical resection with effective local tumor control. Additional benefits over open surgery include shorter hospital admission, improved immediate postoperative pain control, and minimal blood loss. Furthermore, vascular tumors do not require preoperative embolization, and patients with significant medical comorbidities or in need for continued systemic therapy can safely be treated. Compared with other percutaneous ablative techniques, SLITT is unique in offering real-time monitoring of thermal coagulation, which allows safe treatment of tumors in close proximity to the spinal cord.

Spinal Laser Interstitial Thermal Therapy + Spinal Stereotactic Radiosurgery

In the authors' experience, the utilization of SLITT before SSRS is synergistic and can provide effective and durable local control with minimal morbidity.[9] SSRS was indicated in these subjects for oncologic control, but considering the degree of thecal sac compression, the dose prescribed to the epidural component has been restricted to respect the radiation toxicity constraints of the

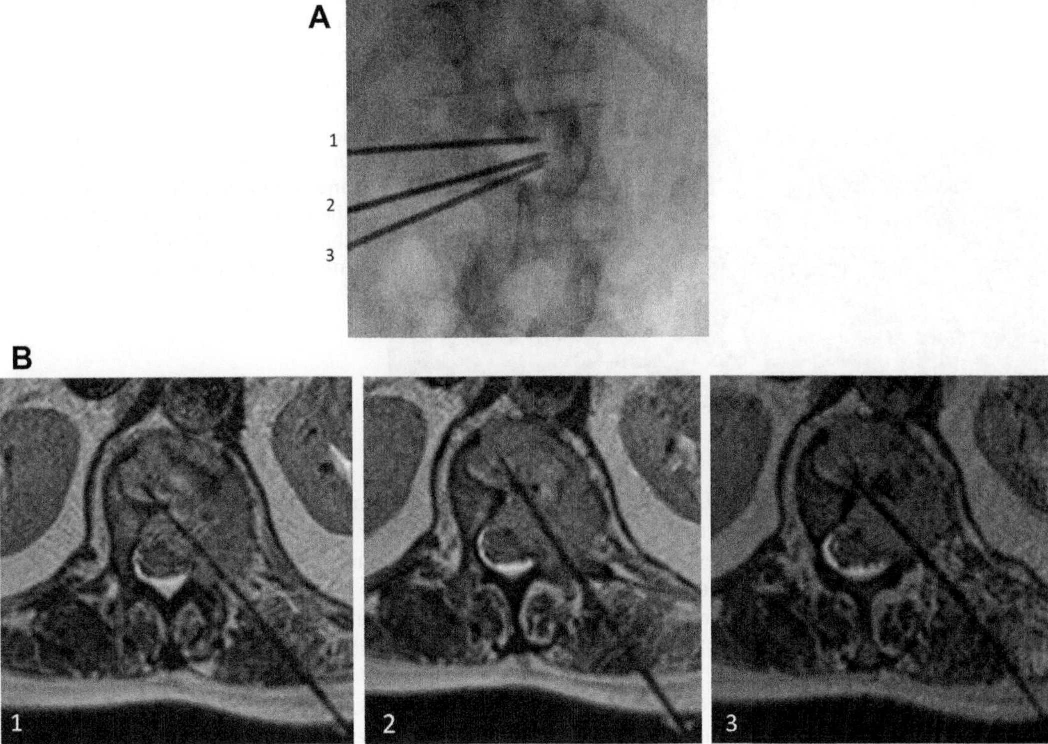

Fig. 4. Intraoperative workflow: Verification of catheter placement. (*A*) Intraoperative fluoroscopy demonstrating the final positioning of 3 access cannulas used to treat a metastatic renal cell carcinoma at the right T12 level. (*B*) Intraoperative sequences to localize the exact axial plane of each access catheter labeled in craniocaudal order.

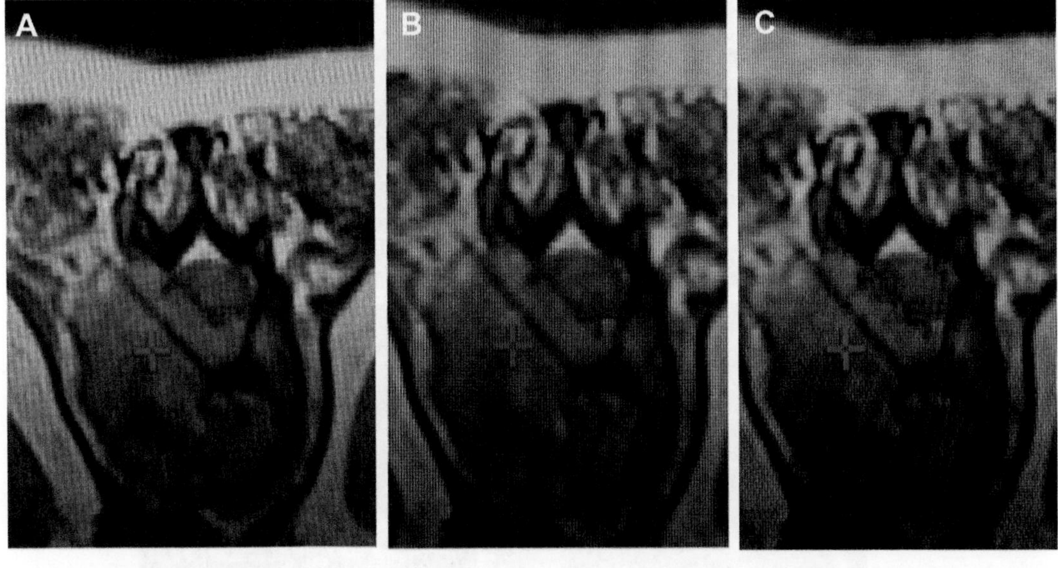

Fig. 5. Intraoperative workflow: Setting the MRI thermometry. (*A*) A point lateral to the laser fiber is selected to be a high temperature limit to avoid tissue carbonization. (*B*, *C*) Safety limits are applied in the junction of the tumor and the dura mater to avoid temperature damage of the spinal cord. The system will automatically shut off if these temperature thresholds are encountered during the procedure.

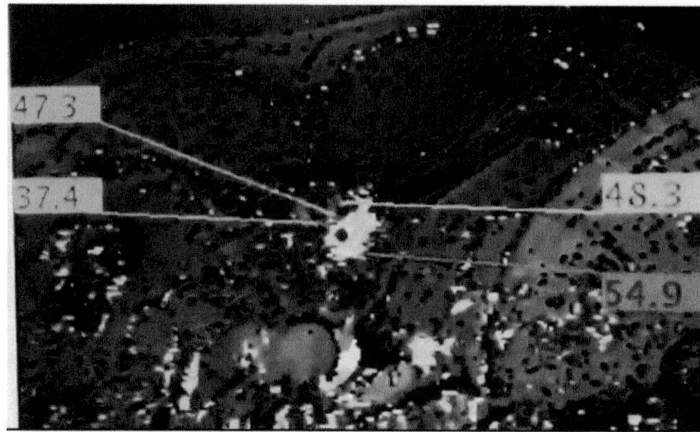

Fig. 6. Intraoperative workflow: MRI thermometry. During the laser ablation, MRI thermometry provides real-time feedback of temperature spread. The green boxes are monitoring the safety limits (displayed in Celsius degrees) in the junction of the tumor and the dura mater; in this example, the maximum temperature exceeded the limit of 48°C and the system automatically deactivated.

spinal cord.[19] In these settings, SLITT was used and provided a percutaneous alternative to open surgery with the benefit of an abbreviated hospital stay (median of 2 days) and durable local control. Progression was documented in only 2 of the 19 patients at 16 and 33 weeks and was ultimately re-treated with a subsequent SLITT.[9] Furthermore, there was a statistically significant reduction in the dimensions of epidural tumor seen at 2 months and improvement in the degree of epidural compression. Pain scores (Visual Analog Scale) were also significantly improved following SLITT.[9] Complications in the authors' initial series included a transient monoparesis in 1 patient, wound dehiscence requiring reoperation, and a delayed compression fracture.

To date, more than 125 cases of SLITT have been performed over the past 5 years to treat a

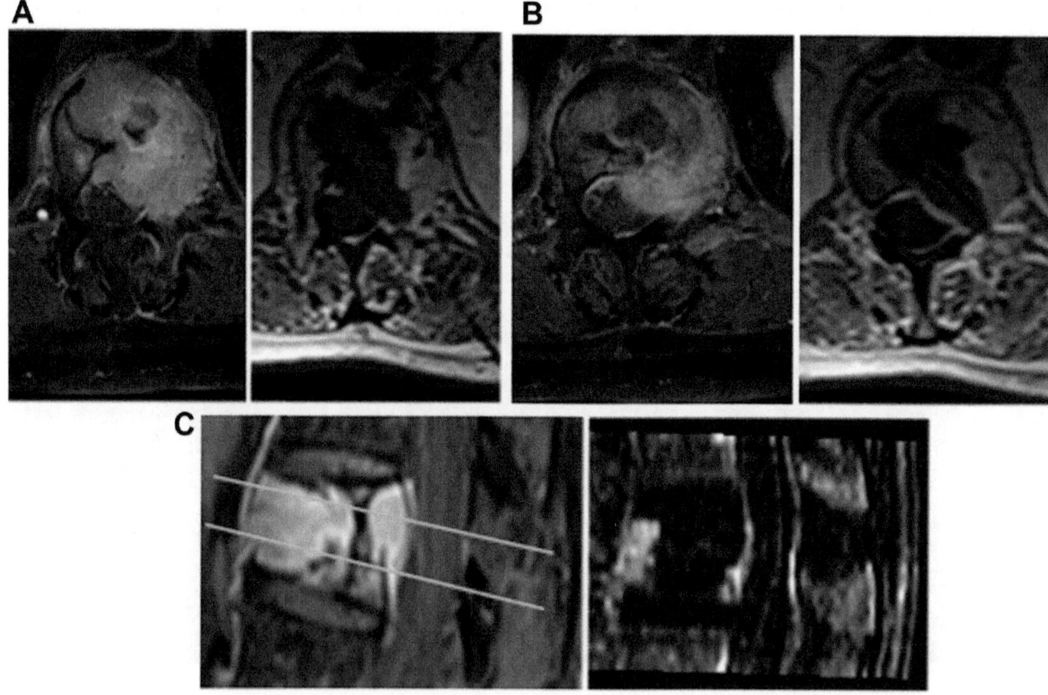

Fig. 7. Intraoperative workflow: Immediate results. (*A, B*) Axial images comparing the preablation and immediately postablation contrast MRI demonstrating the coagulative necrosis as a lack of contrast enhancement in the epidural space. (*C*) Sagittal reconstruction of the preablation and postablation MRI demonstrating complete ablation from upper and lower endplates. The yellow lines represent the axial planes of the postablation images depicted in panels *A* and *B*.

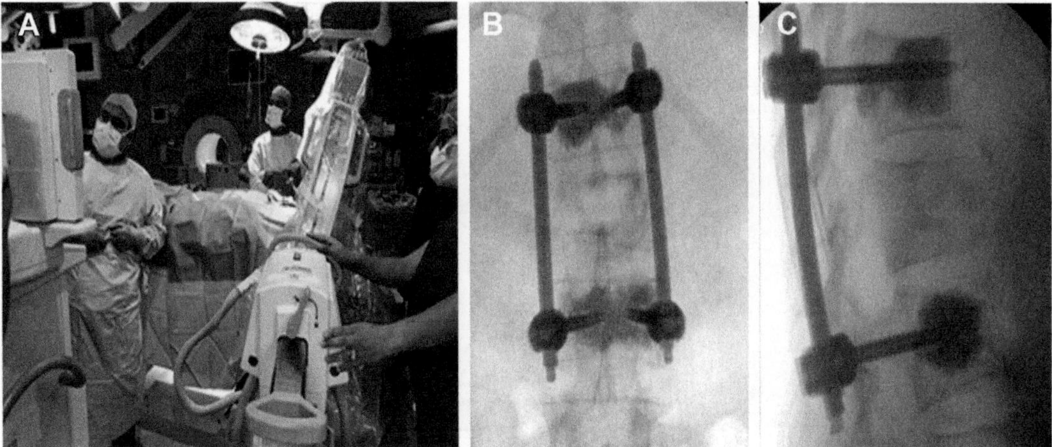

Fig. 8. Intraoperative workflow: Posterior segmental stabilization. (*A*) After completion of the laser ablation, the patient is positioned away from the high-powered magnetic field, and percutaneous stabilization can be performed with standard technique. (*B, C*) Anteroposterior and lateral fluoroscopy images demonstrating placement of percutaneous pedicle screws with cement augmentation.

wide variety of tumor histologies. In the authors' unpublished total series analysis, local tumor progression has been found to be at a total of 17 treated sites, 15 of which were in-field, whereas 2 were at the treatment margins of the SSRS field. Median follow-up was 35 weeks for the entire cohort, with time to recurrence measuring a mean of 26 weeks. Approximately one-third of patients also underwent a concomitant spinal stabilization procedure.

Spinal Laser Interstitial Thermal Therapy Lessons

From this larger experience of more than 125 cases, several lessons have emerged. The ideal candidate for SLITT is a patient with intact neurologic examination, with the spinal lesion arising from the vertebral body contained by the posterior longitudinal ligament, which acts like a capsule, preventing swelling of the tumor and

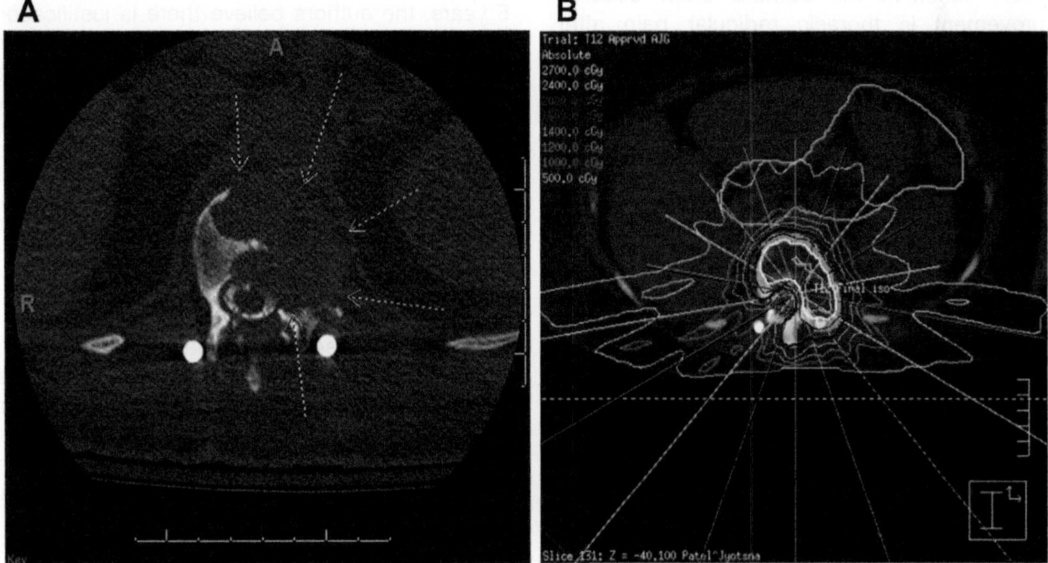

Fig. 9. SSRS planning. (*A*) CT myelogram obtained after SLITT demonstrating the presence of mild improvement in the mass effect in the epidural space and persistence of the large tumor destroying the left side of the vertebral body (*arrows*). In this case, the SSRS planning was performed after the ablation because of the need for placement of pedicle screws for spinal stabilization. (*B*) SSRS dosimetry plan in order to deliver 24 Gy in single fraction to the CTV and 16 Gy to the GTV.

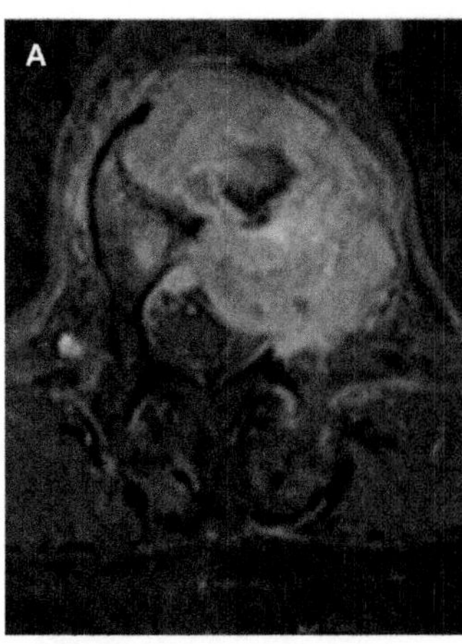

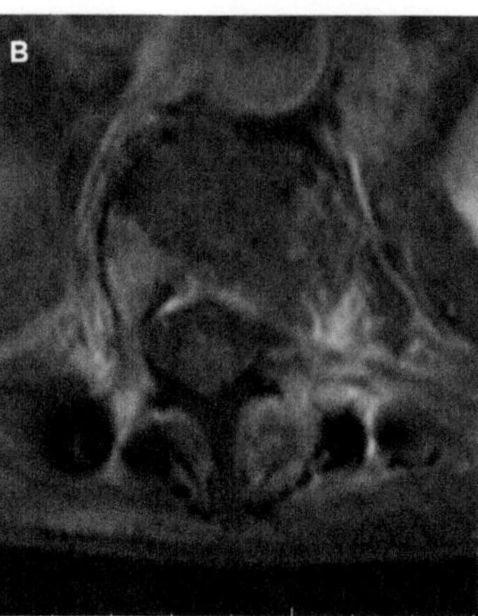

Fig. 10. Comparison of pre-LITT + SSRS and post-LITT + SSRS. (*A*) Preoperative MRI demonstrating the large tumor mass compressing the left T12 nerve root. (*B*) Postoperative contrast-enhanced MRI demonstrating complete resolution of the mass effect and regression of the tumor mass 18 months after treatment. The patient has durable local control; however, the patient presented systemic progression and had to change systemic treatment in the follow-up period.

worsening of the cord compression. Epidural disease free in the epidural space (ie, chest wall disease entering the epidural space in multiple neuroforamen) is a poor target for ablation because the extent of epidural extension is not well delineated, and a complete ablation is seldom achieved. The authors limit treatment to lesions within the thoracic spine located between T2 and T12 to avoid injury to the cervical or lumbosacral plexus. Initial efforts to treat lesions in the upper lumbar spine were complicated by injury to motor roots at the corresponding level. Because the thoracic nerve roots have mostly sensory function, the authors often observe improvement in thoracic radicular pain after ablating the tumor in combination with the nerve root in the intervertebral foramens.

The authors do not recommend this technique for patients presenting with neurologic deficits. The decompression achieved with SLITT takes approximately 2 to 3 weeks to occur, and patients with acute neurologic dysfunction owing to malignant spinal cord compression are better served with an open surgical decompression.

Although the zone of thermal injury typically measures 10 mm in diameter per laser catheter, the ablation is not universally homogenous. Regions of tumor that are adjacent to spinal fluid, large vessels, or cystic areas are more difficult to treat because these structures function as a heat-sink. Similarly, vascular tumors, such as renal cell carcinoma, may require longer treatment times and multiple trajectories to adequate ablate the tumor at risk. Osteoblastic tumors present additional challenges, because highly calcified tissue have low MRI signal, which negatively affects the quality of temperature monitoring by MR thermography.

FUTURE DIRECTIONS

The authors currently perform contouring, dosimetry planning, and treatment delivery of SSRS independently from the SLITT. Up until now, this strategy has proven to be successful, with local control similar to conventional open surgery. The concept of adaptive surgery could be implemented to couple both techniques by performing the SSRS based on the post-SLITT result, where the contouring and dosimetry plans would be adapted to cover eventual areas of suboptimal ablation, potentially improving the local control.

Given the success of SLITT over the past 5 years, the authors believe there is justification for a prospective randomized study to compare open surgical decompression and SLITT followed by SSRS in the management of epidural spinal cord compression (ESCC).

SUMMARY

The authors have been using SLITT as an alternative to open surgery in select cases of epidural spinal cord compression secondary to radioresistant metastatic disease before treatment with SSRS. Laser fibers are placed under MRI-based image guidance, and the epidural tumor is ablated while temperature in the junction of tumor with the dura-mater is monitored in real time and kept to safe levels. SLITT can be performed with minimal surgical morbidity given the correct patient selection and allows fast recovery, avoiding the traditional 2- to 3-week interval of convalescence after a standard open spinal decompression and stabilization. In the authors' experience, comparison between equivalent cases treated with SLITT or open surgery has shown no difference with respect to local tumor control. Last, patients undergo SSRS with minimal delay following thermal ablation with minimal disruption in the oncologic management of the systemic metastatic disease.

DISCLOSURE

Drs R.A. Vega and A.J. Ghia have nothing to disclose. Dr C.E. Tatsui receives research support from Medtronic inc.

REFERENCES

1. Garg AK, Shiu AS, Yang J, et al. Phase 1/2 trial of single-session stereotactic body radiotherapy for previously unirradiated spinal metastases. Cancer 2012;118(20):5069–77.
2. Nguyen QN, SHiu AS, Rhines LD, et al. Management of spinal metastases from renal cell carcinoma using stereotactic body radiotherapy. Int J Radiat Oncol Biol Phys 2010;76(4):1185–92.
3. Bilsky M, Smith M. Surgical approach to epidural spinal cord compression. Hematol Oncol Clin North Am 2006;20(6):1307–17.
4. Laufer I, Iorgulescu JB, Chapman T, et al. Local disease control for spinal metastases following "separation surgery" and adjuvant hypofractionated or high-dose single-fraction stereotactic radiosurgery: outcome analysis in 186 patients. J Neurosurg Spine 2013;18(3):207–14.
5. Gerszten PC, Burton SA, Ozhasoglu C, et al. Radiosurgery for spinal metastases: clinical experience in 500 cases from a single institution. Spine (Phila Pa 1976) 2007;32(2):193–9.
6. Gerszten PC, Mendel E, Yamada Y. Radiotherapy and radiosurgery for metastatic spine disease: what are the options, indications, and outcomes? Spine (Phila Pa 1976) 2009;34(22 Suppl):S78–92.
7. Tatsui CE, Stafford RJ, Li J, et al. Utilization of laser interstitial thermotherapy guided by real-time thermal MRI as an alternative to separation surgery in the management of spinal metastasis. J Neurosurg Spine 2015;23(4):400–11.
8. Tatsui CE, Belsuzarri TA, Oro M, et al. Percutaneous surgery for treatment of epidural spinal cord compression and spinal instability: technical note. Neurosurg Focus 2016;41(4):E2.
9. Tatsui CE, Lee SH, Amini B, et al. Spinal laser interstitial thermal therapy: a novel alternative to surgery for metastatic epidural spinal cord compression. Neurosurgery 2016;79(Suppl 1):S73–82.
10. Laufer I, Rubin DG, Lis E, et al. The NOMS framework: approach to the treatment of spinal metastatic tumors. Oncologist 2013;18(6):744–51.
11. Tatsui CE, Nascimento CNG, Suki D, et al. Image guidance based on MRI for spinal interstitial laser thermotherapy: technical aspects and accuracy. J Neurosurg Spine 2017;26(5):605–12.
12. Boriani S, Weinstein JN, Biagini R. Primary bone tumors of the spine. Terminology and surgical staging. Spine (Phila Pa 1976) 1997;22(9):1036–44.
13. Thomas JG, Al-Holou WN, de Almeida Bastos DC, et al. A novel use of the intraoperative MRI for metastatic spine tumors: laser interstitial thermal therapy for percutaneous treatment of epidural metastatic spine disease. Neurosurg Clin N Am 2017;28(4):513–24.
14. Ahrar K, Stafford RJ. Magnetic resonance imaging-guided laser ablation of bone tumors. Tech Vasc Interv Radiol 2011;14(3):177–82.
15. Rao PJ, Thayaparan GK, Fairhall JM, et al. Minimally invasive percutaneous fixation techniques for metastatic spinal disease. Orthop Surg 2014;6(3):187–95.
16. Moussazadeh N, Rubin DG, McLaughlin L, et al. Short-segment percutaneous pedicle screw fixation with cement augmentation for tumor-induced spinal instability. Spine J 2015;15(7):1609–17.
17. Sahgal A, Larson DA, Chang EL. Stereotactic body radiosurgery for spinal metastases: a critical review. Int J Radiat Oncol Biol Phys 2008;71(3):652–65.
18. Yamada Y, Bilsky MH, Lovelock DM, et al. High-dose, single-fraction image-guided intensity-modulated radiotherapy for metastatic spinal lesions. Int J Radiat Oncol Biol Phys 2008;71(2):484–90.
19. Ghia AJ, Rebueno NC, Li J, et al. The use of image guided laser interstitial thermotherapy to supplement spine stereotactic radiosurgery to manage metastatic epidural spinal cord compression: proof of concept and dosimetric analysis. Pract Radiat Oncol 2016;6(2):e35–8.

Benign Intradural and Paraspinal Nerve Sheath Tumors: Advanced Surgical Techniques

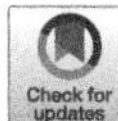

Ziev B. Moses, MD[a], Ori Barzilai, MD[b], John E. O'Toole, MD, MS[c,*]

KEYWORDS

• Peripheral nerve sheath tumor • Schwannoma • Neurofibroma • Minimally invasive spine surgery

KEY POINTS

- Most benign nerve sheath tumors are located in a dorsolateral location and are accessed via a posterior approach using minimally invasive tubular retractors.
- In the thoracic spine, select dumbbell, extraforaminal, and paraspinal tumors are accessed via thoracoscopic approaches combined with a posterior limited laminectomy, avoiding the need for spinal fusion and the morbidity of open thoracotomy.
- Robotic-assisted and full endoscopic surgery are two areas of innovation with promising initial early results for the resection of benign nerve sheath tumors.

INTRODUCTION

Benign nerve sheath tumors are the second most common primary spinal cord tumors in adults, predominantly consisting of schwannomas and neurofibromas.[1,2] They can either be intradural, extradural, or have a dumbbell configuration with intradural and extradural components. Nerve sheath tumors occur throughout the spine with fairly equal distributions, with one recent large series of 221 cases reporting a distribution of 38% cervical, 28% thoracic, and 33% lumbosacral.[3] This same series also reported that 59% were intradural, 12% extradural, and 24% with a dumbbell configuration. Most schwannomas arise from the dorsal nerve root, whereas neurofibromas tend to originate in the ventral nerve root. Surgery is often curative and remains the mainstay of treatment. This article reviews the surgical techniques used to manage these tumors in light of contemporary surgical innovations.

NERVE SHEATH ANATOMY

The nerve sheath is comprised of three component layers: (1) the endoneurium, (2) the perineum, and (3) the epineurium. Whereas the endoneurium individually envelops each axon traveling within a nerve bundle known as a fascicle, the perineurium is the supportive structure surrounding the fascicle itself and forms the blood-nerve barrier. The component fascicles make up the peripheral nerve, which is itself enveloped by an outermost denser connective tissue layer known as the epineurium. The epineurium is a continuation of the dura that envelops the spinal nerve as it exits the intervertebral foramen. Historically, peripheral nerve sheath tumors have been thought to arise from the dorsal root entry zone, a narrow region where myelin production shifts from oligodendrocytes to Schwann cells. Some have called into question this site of origin, especially with regards to cranial vestibular schwannomas.[4]

[a] Department of Neurosurgery, Rush University Medical Center, Chicago, IL 60612, USA; [b] Department of Neurosurgery, Memorial Sloan Kettering Cancer Center, New York, NY 10065, USA; [c] Department of Neurosurgery, Coleman Foundation Comprehensive Spine Tumor Clinic, Rush University Medical Center, 1725 West Harrison Street, Suite 855, Chicago, IL 60612, USA
* Corresponding author.
E-mail address: JOHN_OTOOLE@rush.edu

Neurosurg Clin N Am 31 (2020) 221–229
https://doi.org/10.1016/j.nec.2019.11.002
1042-3680/20/

NERVE SHEATH TUMOR CLASSIFICATION

The most recent World Health Organization classification of central nervous system tumors organizes cranial and paraspinal nerve tumors into the following categories: schwannoma, neurofibroma, perineurioma, and malignant peripheral nerve sheath tumors.[5,6]

Schwannomas

Schwannomas are typically benign encapsulated tumors composed of differentiated Schwann cells. They have a predilection for the vestibular division of the eighth cranial nerve and when intraspinal they tend to arise from the sensory nerve roots with much rarer involvement of motor nerves. Most schwannomas are solitary and sporadic, but they are seen in genetic conditions, such as schwannomatosis, Carney complex, and neurofibromatosis type 2. Their microscopic appearance is characterized by compact cellular areas with a nuclear palisading growth pattern (ie, Verocay bodies) known as Antoni A and loose, paucicellular regions known as Antoni B. On immunohistochemistry, the tumor cells diffusely express S-100 protein, with variable degrees of staining for Leu-7 and calretinin. Other variants include cellular schwannoma, melanotic schwannoma, and ancient schwannoma.

Neurofibromas

Neurofibromas are often benign intraneural or diffusely infiltrating tumors comprised of a mixture of fibroblasts, perineurial cells, and Schwann cells. Most are solitary and sporadic without relation to a syndrome; however, multiple neurofibromas and plexiform neurofibromas are often seen in neurofibromatosis type 1. Most neurofibromas are localized to the skin; however, less often they occur in a peripheral nerve or as diffuse plexiform expansions of a major nerve trunk or plexus. They occasionally involve a spinal nerve root and do not have as much of a discrete plane separating them from the nerve fascicles. Often, the nerve is nonfunctional and must be sacrificed to ensure a total resection. Identifying axons within the tumor on microscopy helps distinguish them from schwannomas. In addition, on immunohistochemistry, the spindle cells often are only moderately positive for S-100 and Leu-7.

SURGICAL INDICATIONS

Indications

Given the slow-growing and generally benign nature of peripheral nerve sheath tumors, surgery remains the mainstay of treatment. Even in nonsyndromic patients with no symptoms but large and/or growing lesions, surgery continues to be indicated given the positive safety profile with experienced neurosurgeons.

Alternatives to Surgery: Conservative and Radiation Management

Patients who are asymptomatic or poor surgical candidates in the setting of neurofibromatosis may be managed conservatively with surveillance imaging. Radiation and chemotherapy have traditionally had no role in benign peripheral nerve sheath tumors. Stereotactic radiation has been used in older patients and those with significant comorbidities, in addition to patients with residual disease after surgery.[7] In patients with symptoms/signs or radiographic evidence to suggest the possibility of malignant peripheral nerve sheath tumor, a biopsy should first be considered before proceeding with definitive surgery, because there is evidence that neoadjuvant treatment may improve disease-specific survival.[8]

SURGICAL APPROACHES

Cervical

Posterior/posterolateral

Most spinal schwannomas are positioned eccentrically in a dorsolateral position given their common origin from the dorsal roots. Therefore, they can often be approached via a traditional midline trajectory with posterior cervical laminectomy over the involved segments. Awake fiberoptic intubation is used in cases with significant cord compression and all patients undergoing surgical removal of these tumors should be monitored with neurophysiology including somatosensory evoked potentials (SSEPs) and motor evoked potentials (MEPs). A Mayfield skull clamp is used during the prone position and allows for a neutral head position in the case a fusion is planned and as a way to keep pressure of the eyes.

A midline vertical incision is planned using fluoroscopy and a laminectomy is performed in standard fashion using a combination of rongeurs and a high-speed drill. A subperiosteal dissection and removal of the laminae laterally to the facet joints is performed. It is important to ensure the laminectomy provides adequate exposure of the inferior and superior edges of the tumor. Intraoperative ultrasound is helpful to ensure the tumor is well-exposed before opening the dura. The operating microscope is then brought into the field, and the dura is then opened in the midline and tacked up to the paraspinal muscles using a 4-0 Nurolon suture. Microsurgical resection is then performed using standard technique (see section on special considerations by tumor type for microsurgical nuances). The dura is then closed using a running 4–0 Nurolon and the wound is closed in layers. The decision for posterior instrumentation is left to the surgeon but in general if less than half the facet is violated a fusion can be avoided.

In cases where the tumor is ventral or ventrolateral, a posterior approach may still be attempted. In cases with a large ventral tumor producing lateral displacement of the spinal cord, internal debulking can lead to improved visualization of the remaining tumor and the possibility of safe total removal. Otherwise, the traditional approach can be modified to allow for more ventral access by removing bone, such as the facet, pedicle, and/or posterior vertebral body. Additionally, sectioning the dentate ligament and gently rotating the spinal cord can allow for further access.[9] This has also been described for intramedullary lesions.[10]

Ventral

In cases where tumors arise in a purely ventral location and/or with bilateral ventral tumor extension, a ventral approach to the spine may be required.[11,12] In a series of 28 intradural extramedullary mass lesions, four patients had ventral subaxial cervical tumors.[11] Of these, three underwent an anterior approach including a corpectomy, structural allograft, and anterior cervical plate. One patient developed a cerebrospinal fluid leak that resolved with spinal drainage and another patient developed temporary swallowing difficulty because of sustained retraction of the ventral soft tissue. In another large study series of 140 patients with intradural extramedullary ventral tumors, 57 patients had cervical region tumors, and the ventrolateral approach was used in 9 (15.8%) of these patients.[13] The authors described their approach to dumbbell tumors by first removing the extravertebral part followed by widening the intervertebral foramen with Kerrison rongeurs, removing the foraminal component, and then opening the dural ring of the nerve root to debulk the remainder of the tumor. Total removal was possible in 65% of cases using the ventrolateral approach.

Minimal access approaches

Minimal access approaches for cervical nerve sheath tumors are especially important because traditional laminectomy in the posterior cervical spine may result in delayed spinal deformity given the importance of the posterior elements in maintaining stability in this region.[14,15] In addition, although a traditional posterior cervical laminectomy typically provides enough exposure for removal of an intradural lesion, dumbbell lesions with extraforaminal extension may require facetectomy, thus requiring spinal fusion. A Japanese group described the use of a modified cervical hemilaminoplasty using a thread wire saw as a way to provide the requisite exposure for dumbbell tumors while allowing for restoration of the normal anatomy after their removal.[16] This involved making cuts such that half the lamina, inferior articular process, and half the spinous process is removed as one mass. In their series of 10 patients with cervical spinal schwannomas, all were successfully resected including seven dumbbell-shaped tumors. No patients required a posterior cervical fusion or had evidence of instability on postoperative radiographs. In another series of 16 patients with cervical schwannomas, a variety of minimal access approaches including hemilaminectomy, subtotal hemilaminectomy, interlaminar fenestration, and osteoplastic hemilaminotomy were used.[17] The wider space between the C1 and C2 vertebrae allowed for an interlaminar fenestration to be used for two C2 schwannomas. A tubular approach for removal of cervical peripheral nerve sheath tumors is an alternative to cervical hemilaminoplasty and interlaminar approaches. Proposed benefits of tubular approaches include reduced blood loss and avoiding the need for muscle dissection. In a retrospective review of open surgery compared with a tubular minimally invasive approach for intradural-extramedullary tumors, the cerebrospinal fluid leak rate, mean hospital stay, and mean estimated blood loss (EBL) were all improved with an minimally invasive surgery (MIS) approach.[18]

Thoracic

Posterior/posterolateral

A large proportion of intradural extramedullary masses in the spine (eg, schwannomas) arise from the dorsal nerve roots and thus a traditional midline subperiosteal dissection and laminectomy is appropriate for these lesions as described previously. However, given the ventral thoracic spine is obstructed by the spinal cord posteriorly, thoracic cage laterally, and mediastinum anteriorly, there are several modified approaches to accessing thoracic tumors that have ventrolateral deviation or extraforaminal extension. Some authors have advocated that tumors with a paravertebral component greater than 3 cm across require more than a standard laminectomy and foraminotomy.[19] These include transpedicular, costotransversectomy, and lateral extracavitary approaches, the primary difference between the latter two being the amount of underlying rib removed and more lateral trajectory with the extracavitary approach.[20] In a series of six patients with myelopathy and ventral intradural extramedullary thoracic tumors, the lateral extracavitary and a modification of it for higher thoracic lesions named the lateral parascapular extrapleural approach were used to resect these masses.[21] This involves resection of the facet and pedicle, in addition to dorsally removing the rib from its posterior bend to the costotransverse and costovertebral articulations. These steps allow for almost complete access to the ventral thoracic spine. For dumbbell thoracic tumors, several authors have described their experience with single-stage posterolateral approaches.[22–25] In a series of 16 patients, a costotransversectomy allowed for a single-stage removal of large dumbbell tumors in the thoracic spine with a mean extraforaminal tumor extension of 5.3 cm.[22] The authors used spinal instrumentation in all patients. In a Chinese series of 14 patients with dumbbell thoracic tumors, a modified single-stage approach using an arc incision to allow for more lateral exposure resulted in a total resection in 13 patients and no instrumentation was used. The need for stabilization following costotransversectomy remains controversial.[26,27] Advantages of a single-stage posterolateral approach include the need for only one incision, better familiarity of all the steps to the neurosurgeon, and avoiding a chest tube.

Minimally invasive alternative posterolateral approaches for thoracic nerve sheath tumors have also been described.[28–31] In a series of two patients, the authors described the use of an expandable tubular retractor to remove dumbbell-shaped tumors.[29] First, they placed unilateral pedicle screws at the adjacent segments, followed by gross total resection, and then placement of an interbody cage. They used the criteria that the medial border of the spinal component be near the midline of the canal and for the pedicles to be intact on computed tomography before proceeding with their approach. Another group described the use of a minimally invasive lateral extrapleural approach to treat a purely extradural foraminal nerve sheath tumor.[31] The authors used the Nuvasive (NuVasive, Inc., San Diego, CA) table-mounted expandable tube to resect an extradural 3.1 × 3 cm neurofibroma in the lower thoracic spine. Importantly, the authors did not need to stabilize the spine afterward; however, this approach is limited in treating intradural tumors or those located medial to the facet.

Open thoracotomy

Masses that are not able to be fully resected from a posterolateral approach, such as those with a large extraforaminal component or components anterior to the vertebral body, attachments to vascular structures, or an inability to make an accurate preoperative diagnosis, may require a combined approach with a second-stage thoracotomy.[32] Others advocate for a single-stage combined neurosurgical and thoracic approach, either via a single incision[33–35] or separate incisions.[36,37] In one series, in most cases the laminectomy was performed after the thoracotomy.[35] The authors reported that in six patients the tumor was able to be completely removed from the thoracic approach avoiding a laminectomy. They described a complete resection in all 16 patients and advocate for a single-stage procedure instead of a second stage to minimize complications. The largest tumor in their series was 10 cm. Some authors have described tumor size as the criterion for choosing whether to use a single posterolateral approach or a combined posterior and transthoracic approach, with a combined approach being more appropriate for larger tumors, particularly in the anteroposterior direction.[38,39]

Thoracoscopic approaches

Thoracoscopy is an alternative to open thoracotomy for resection of tumors extending into or limited to the mediastinum. The best tumors for this approach include those that are peripherally located within the intercostal nerves or extend into the chest cavity from the neural foramina. This approach has been associated with less postoperative pain, shorter hospitalization, and fewer complications than open thoracotomy.[40] The procedure involves placing several triangulated ports along the posterior and anterior axillary lines with an additional portal for diaphragm retraction.[41] Combined with a limited laminectomy, dumbbell tumors of the thoracic spine are resected without the need to violate the facet and necessitate fusion. Performing the laminectomy first to remove the intracanalicular portion avoids traction on the spinal cord during thoracoscopic resection and allows for a watertight dural closure. In one series of five patients, total gross resection was achieved in all patients with no evidence of recurrent tumor for at least a minimum of 3 years.[42] Complications were limited to one hemothorax.

Lumbosacral

Posterior/posterolateral

Similar principles as described previously in the posterior approach for cervical nerve sheath tumors are incorporated for dorsal nerve sheath tumors in the lumbosacral region, including the use of neurophysiologic monitoring. Patients are positioned on a Wilson frame or an open Jackson table. All dependent areas are padded. A midline incision is made and a subperiosteal dissection is carried out to the lamina, with special care not to violate the facet capsule, unless a fusion is to be performed. Laminectomies over the intended area are carried out using rongeurs and a high-speed drill. A dural opening is made in the midline over the tumor. Depending on the tumor size, either a piecemeal resection is carried out or a circumferential dissection followed by an *en bloc* removal. Hemostasis is obtained and normal saline irrigation is used to ensure the subarachnoid space is clear of blood products. The dura is then closed in a watertight fashion and a dural sealant is applied to the suture line. The wound is then closed in layers, or if a laminoplasty was performed, the posterior elements are then plated and replaced before closing.

Lateral

Extradural foraminal schwannomas of the lumbar spine are much rarer than their cervical and thoracic counterparts, with a rate of 4.2% in one series.[43] A traditional posterior approach requires aggressive facetectomies resulting in iatrogenic instability and the need for posterior stabilization. More recently, the lateral retroperitoneal approach has gained increasing popularity as a minimally invasive method for treating degenerative lumbar spine disease.[44] By directly approaching the foramen from a lateral approach, its use has also been described as a fusion-sparing approach to extradural foraminal nerve sheath tumors.[31] In two patients with lumbar neurofibromas at L1-2 and L3-4, with tumors ranging in size from 3.4 to 4 cm, an expandable tube retractor was used to resection these masses without complication. The authors note that tumors located below L4-5 are not easily accessed given the iliac crest. For tumors below L4-5, a standard anterior retroperitoneal approach for tumor resection has been described.[45] The authors describe that by taking an anterior approach, a patient with an L5-S1 foraminal schwannoma did not have to go undergo fusion because initially they had been booked for a posterior approach with total facetectomy and pedicle screw fixation at another institution. For lesions further lateral than the foramen and in the lumbar plexus, a similar direct retroperitoneal lateral approach using an expandable tubular retractor has been described. In one case report, the authors used a well-known lateral retractor system (MaXcess System, NuVasive, Inc, San Diego, CA) to traverse the psoas and dock onto the L4-5 disk, where they were able to identify the tumor and remove it using standard microsurgical technique.[46] Critical to all these lateral approaches is the use of continuous and directional electromyography monitoring to identify traversing nerves and avoid injury.

Minimal access approaches

With the increasing use of minimally invasive approaches to treat degenerative pathology, their application to removal of nerve sheath tumors has also expanded. Several series describing the use of minimally invasive tubular systems for removing nerve sheath tumors have been published.[28,30,47,48] Although no randomized control studies comparing open with minimally invasive approaches for nerve sheath tumor exists, case series comparing these approaches have shown decreased blood loss and shorter hospital stays to be associated with minimally invasive techniques.[18,49] Please see **Fig. 1** for an example of a tubular access approach to removal of a concomitant L4-5 disc herniation and nerve sheath tumor. In one study comparing costs between open and minimally invasive removal of intradural extramedullary tumors, in patients undergoing the latter approach, the costs of treatment were significantly lower.[50] This was attributed to the lower rate of requiring fusion and the shorter intensive care unit and overall hospitals stays. Apart from tubular approaches, one group has described their interlaminar approach in the lumbar spine for removal of intradural extramedullary tumors.[51,52] This technique takes advantage of the larger interlaminar space in the lumbar spine. The authors describe its use in 18 patients with postoperative imaging confirming total removal of these lesions and no evidence of bony removal. In three cases given the smaller relative interlaminar window, an endoscope was used to assist in the resection of these tumors.

Special Surgical Considerations

Neurofibroma

Neurofibromas typically appear as an enlargement of a sensory nerve and are typically intimately involved with the dorsal root. Many times, total removal of a neurofibroma requires sacrifice of the nerve root. It is important to use intraoperative stimulation to assess whether the nerve root can be sacrificed. If the nerve shows motor function at 0.5 to 1 mA then every effort is made to save the root, especially in the cervical and lumbar regions.

Schwannoma

Schwannomas typically arise from one or more dorsal rootlets. Typically, there is a plane between the tumor and the rootlets that can be developed using Rhoton microsurgical instruments. Whereas smaller tumors can typically be removed *en bloc*, larger tumors often require internal debulking and piecemeal removal. The ultrasonic aspirator allows for internal decompression with minimal stress on the surrounding neural structures.

FUTURE DIRECTIONS

Robotic-Assisted Tumor Resection

The use of robotic surgery has a strong basis in robot-assisted video-assisted thoracic surgery for various procedures, including pulmonary lobectomy, and has been shown to be superior to open thoracotomy with improvements in postoperative morbidity, length of stay, and cost-effectiveness.[53] Given this rationale, it has been used to treat posterior mediastinal schwannomas, often in the midthoracic region.[54,55] Often these tumors are foraminal or paravertebral with no intraspinal component. In one series of two patients, the use of the da Vinci Xi robot (Intuitive Surgical Inc., Sunnyvale, CA) was extended to the superior and inferior margins of the thoracic cavity to treat paravertebral schwannomas with complete resections and favorable postoperative courses.[56] These were single-stage surgeries without the need for separate spinal access. In addition, the use of the robot has been extended for retroperitoneal tumors. In one patient with a large retroperitoneal schwannoma arising from the left L4 nerve root, a robotic-assisted resection was performed after splitting the psoas major.[57] There were no complications and the postoperative MRI revealed a complete resection. Please see **Fig 2** for an example of a combined neurosurgery and thoracic surgery approach to a T4 dumbbell schwannoma.

Endoscopic-Assisted Tumor Resection

Minimally invasive approaches using tubular retractors have been shown to be a successful strategy for removal of peripheral nerve sheath tumors. The principles of avoiding prolonged retraction, minimizing soft tissue damage and muscle denervation, and reducing bony resection have all motivated the ongoing evolution of minimally invasive surgery. The next frontier of this endeavor is full endoscopic spine surgery, which represents a shift from the use of the endoscope as a visual tool, which was supplanted by the use of microscope to see down the shaft of the tubular retractor, to the primary working and visual channel.[58] Although the full endoscopic technique has been described in interlaminar and transforaminal surgery for degenerative pathologies, its use in the removal of nerve sheath tumors has been somewhat limited. In the lumbar spine its use was limited to assisting in cases with small interlaminar windows.[51] In a case series using the Destandau endoscopic technique, 18 patients with intradural extramedullary tumors underwent surgery.[59] The authors did not have to perform complete facetectomies or perform a stabilization in any patients. Dural repair was performed bimanually using the endoscope for visualization. Other studies have shown the use of the endoscope to be critical in evaluating an intramedullary tumor cavity in the cervical spine of a pediatric patient, where it

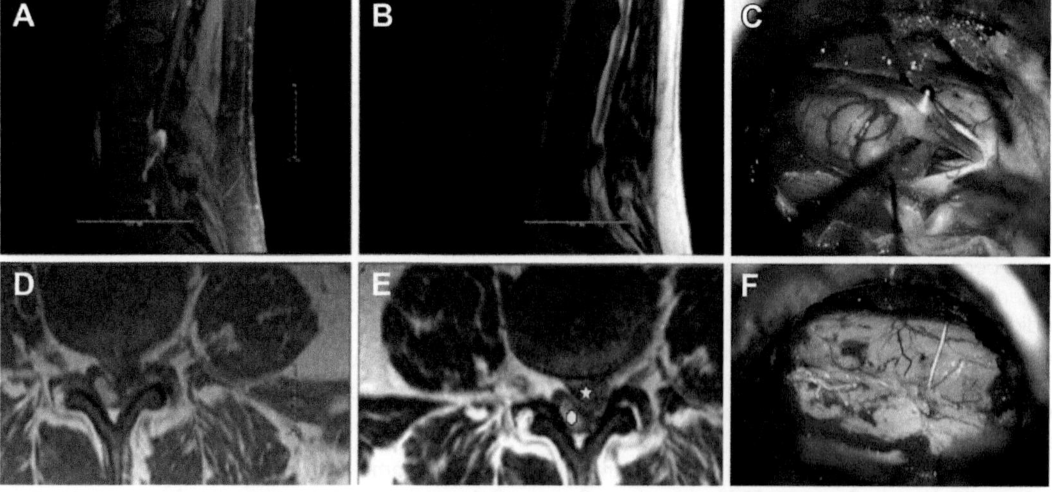

Fig. 1. (*A*) Sagittal T1 and (*D*) axial T1 postcontrast, (*B*) sagittal T2 and (*E*) axial T2 lumbar MRI revealing an L4-5 disk herniation (*asterisk*) and concomitant nerve sheath tumor (*cross*). An MIS tubular left L4-5 microdiscectomy was performed followed by a dural opening and removal of the schwannoma. (*C*) The dorsal rootlet did not stimulate and was sacrificed for a total removal of the tumor. (*F*) The dura was closed primarily using specialized tubular microequipment. MIS, minimally invasive surgery.

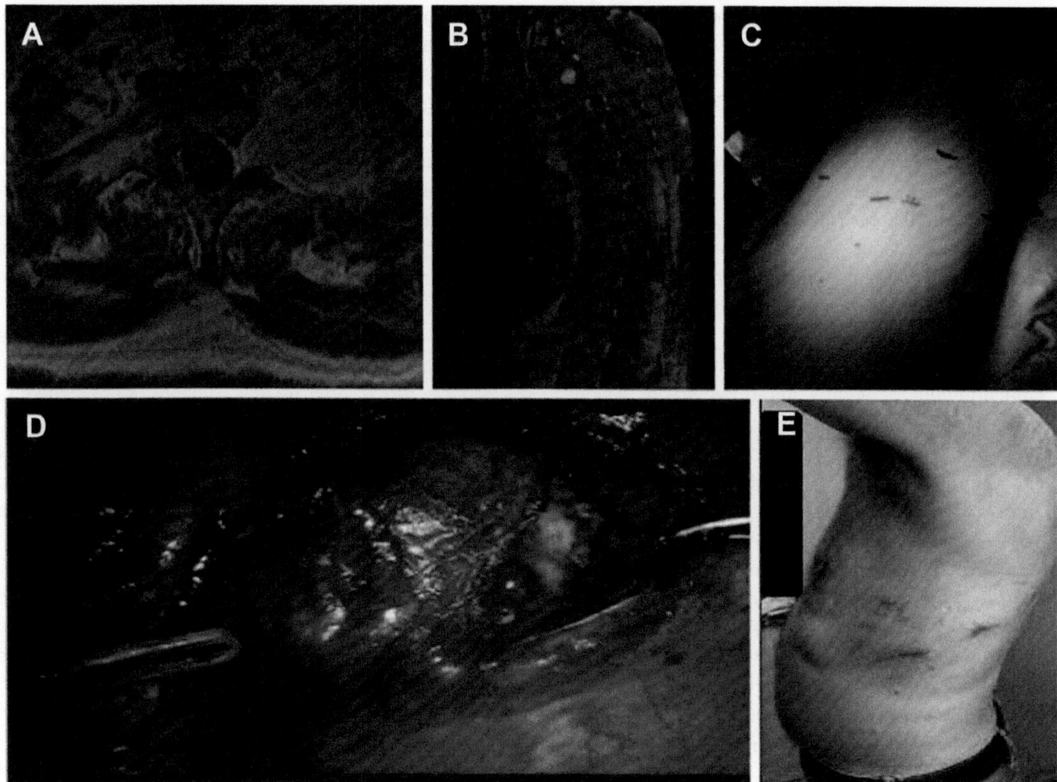

Fig. 2. (*A*) Axial and (*B*) sagittal T1 postcontrast thoracic spine MRI reveals a left T2 dumbbell schwannoma. After performing an MIS tubular left T2-3 hemilaminectomy with ligation of the left T2 nerve root and tumor release, (*C*) the patient was positioned in a lateral decubitus position for robotic-assisted thoracic resection. (*D*) The tumor was resected using a robotic surgical system requiring ligation of one large feeding vessel from the superior intercostal artery using a locking polymer clip. (*E*) The small access incisions were well healed at his first follow-up visit. MIS, minimally invasive surgery.

discovered abnormal tissue that was subsequently removed with endoscopic bipolar cautery and suction.[60] In another case report, it was used to biopsy and partially resect a recurrent ventral extradural thoracic spine mass in an awake patient.[61] Several limitations of the approach are the poor visualization in the context of tumor bleeding and the availability of proper working channel tools to resect these lesions. It is anticipated as improvements in these areas are made, endoscopy may have a more prominent role in the removal of peripheral nerve sheath tumors.

DISCLOSURE

The authors have nothing to disclose.

REFERENCES

1. Duong LM, McCarthy BJ, McLendon RE, et al. Descriptive epidemiology of malignant and nonmalignant primary spinal cord, spinal meninges, and cauda equina tumors, United States, 2004-2007. Cancer 2012;118(17):4220–7.
2. Dolecek TA, Propp JM, Stroup NE, et al. CBTRUS statistical report: primary brain and central nervous system tumors diagnosed in the United States in 2005-2009. Neuro Oncol 2012;14(Suppl 5):v1–49.
3. Safaee MM, Lyon R, Barbaro NM, et al. Neurological outcomes and surgical complications in 221 spinal nerve sheath tumors. J Neurosurg Spine 2017;26(1):103–11.
4. Xenellis JE, Linthicum FH Jr. On the myth of the glial/Schwann junction (Obersteiner-Redlich zone): origin of vestibular nerve schwannomas. Otol Neurotol 2003;24(1):1.
5. Louis DN, Perry A, Reifenberger G, et al. The 2016 World Health Organization classification of tumors of the central nervous system: a summary. Acta Neuropathol 2016;131(6):803–20.
6. Enzinger FM, Weiss SW. Malignant tumours of perpheral nerves, vol. 31. St Louis (MO): CV Mosby Company; 2001.
7. Purvis TE, Goodwin CR, Lubelski D, et al. Review of stereotactic radiosurgery for intradural spine tumors. CNS Oncol 2017;6(2):131–8.
8. Shurell-Linehan E, DiPardo BJ, Elliott IA, et al. Pathologic response to neoadjuvant therapy is associated

with improved long-term survival in high-risk primary localized malignant peripheral nerve sheath tumors. Am J Clin Oncol 2019;42(5):426–31.
9. Sorenson TJ, Lanzino G, Rangel Castilla L. Surgical resection of cervical meningioma: 3-dimensional operative video. Oper Neurosurg (Hagerstown) 2019;16(6):768.
10. Martin NA, Khanna RK, Batzdorf U. Posterolateral cervical or thoracic approach with spinal cord rotation for vascular malformations or tumors of the ventrolateral spinal cord. J Neurosurg 1995;83(2): 254–61.
11. Angevine PD, Kellner C, Haque RM, et al. Surgical management of ventral intradural spinal lesions. J Neurosurg Spine 2011;15(1):28–37.
12. O'Toole JE, McCormick PC. Midline ventral intradural schwannoma of the cervical spinal cord resected via anterior corpectomy with reconstruction: technical case report and review of the literature. Neurosurgery 2003;52(6):1482–5 [discussion: 1485–6].
13. Slin'ko EI, Al-Qashqish II. Intradural ventral and ventrolateral tumors of the spinal cord: surgical treatment and results. Neurosurg Focus 2004; 17(1):ECP2.
14. Deutsch H, Haid RW, Rodts GE, et al. Postlaminectomy cervical deformity. Neurosurg Focus 2003; 15(3):E5.
15. Fassett DR, Clark R, Brockmeyer DL, et al. Cervical spine deformity associated with resection of spinal cord tumors. Neurosurg Focus 2006;20(2):E2.
16. Kato Y, Kaneko K, Kataoka H, et al. Cervical hemilaminoplasty: technical note. J Spinal Disord Tech 2007;20(4):296–301.
17. Raysi Dehcordi S, Marzi S, Ricci A, et al. Less invasive approaches for the treatment of cervical schwannomas: our experience. Eur Spine J 2012; 21(5):887–96.
18. Wong AP, Lall RR, Dahdaleh NS, et al. Comparison of open and minimally invasive surgery for intradural-extramedullary spine tumors. Neurosurg Focus 2015;39(2):E11.
19. Thorat JD, Rajendra T, Thirugnanam A, et al. Single-stage posterior midline approach for dumbbell tumors of the thoracic spine, with intraoperative CT guidance. Surg Neurol Int 2011;2:31.
20. Lubelski D, Abdullah KG, Steinmetz MP, et al. Lateral extracavitary, costotransversectomy, and transthoracic thoracotomy approaches to the thoracic spine: review of techniques and complications. J Spinal Disord Tech 2013;26(4):222–32.
21. Steck JC, Dietze DD, Fessler RG. Posterolateral approach to intradural extramedullary thoracic tumors. J Neurosurg 1994;81(2):202–5.
22. Ando K, Imagama S, Ito Z, et al. Removal of thoracic dumbbell tumors through a single-stage posterior approach: its usefulness and limitations. J Orthop Sci 2013;18(3):380–7.
23. Rong HT, Fan YS, Li SP, et al. Management of dumbbell and paraspinal tumors of the thoracic spine using a single-stage posterolateral approach: case series. Orthop Surg 2018;10(4):343–9.
24. Marhx Bracho A, Munoz Montoya JE, Pena Rosas NP, et al. Costotransversectomy plus hemilaminectomy as alternative surgical approach for extramedullary intradural thoracic schwannoma resection with and without extradural extension in pediatric population three cases and literature review. J Spine Surg 2019;5(2):285–90.
25. Valle-Giler EP, Garces J, Smith RD, et al. One-stage resection of giant invasive thoracic schwannoma: case report and review of literature. Ochsner J 2014;14(1):135–40.
26. Oda I, Abumi K, Lu D, et al. Biomechanical role of the posterior elements, costovertebral joints, and rib cage in the stability of the thoracic spine. Spine (Phila Pa 1976) 1996;21(12):1423–9.
27. Watkins Rt, Watkins R 3rd, Williams L, et al. Stability provided by the sternum and rib cage in the thoracic spine. Spine (Phila Pa 1976) 2005;30(11):1283–6.
28. Nzokou A, Weil AG, Shedid D. Minimally invasive removal of thoracic and lumbar spinal tumors using a nonexpandable tubular retractor. J Neurosurg Spine 2013;19(6):708–15.
29. Li C, Ye Y, Gu Y, et al. Minimally invasive resection of extradural dumbbell tumors of thoracic spine: surgical techniques and literature review. Eur Spine J 2016;25(12):4108–15.
30. Tredway TL, Santiago P, Hrubes MR, et al. Minimally invasive resection of intradural-extramedullary spinal neoplasms. Neurosurgery 2006;58(1 Suppl): ONS52–8 [discussion: ONS52–58].
31. Dakwar E, Smith WD, Malone KT, et al. Minimally invasive lateral extracavitary resection of foraminal neurofibromas. J Clin Neurosci 2011;18(11):1510–2.
32. Heltzer JM, Krasna MJ, Aldrich F, et al. Thoracoscopic excision of a posterior mediastinal "dumbbell" tumor using a combined approach. Ann Thorac Surg 1995;60(2):431–3.
33. Grillo HC, Ojemann RG, Scannell JG, et al. Combined approach to "dumbbell" intrathoracic and intraspinal neurogenic tumors. Ann Thorac Surg 1983;36(4):402–7.
34. Reeder LB. Neurogenic tumors of the mediastinum. Semin Thorac Cardiovasc Surg 2000; 12(4):261–7.
35. Shadmehr MB, Gaissert HA, Wain JC, et al. The surgical approach to "dumbbell tumors" of the mediastinum. Ann Thorac Surg 2003;76(5):1650–4.
36. Akwari OE, Payne WS, Onofrio BM, et al. Dumbbell neurogenic tumors of the mediastinum. Diagnosis and management. Mayo Clin Proc 1978;53(6):353–8.
37. Yuksel M, Pamir N, Ozer F, et al. The principles of surgical management in dumbbell tumors. Eur J Cardiothorac Surg 1996;10(7):569–73.

38. Payer M, Radovanovic I, Jost G. Resection of thoracic dumbbell neurinomas: single posterolateral approach or combined posterior and transthoracic approach? J Clin Neurosci 2006;13(6):690–3.
39. Miura J, Doita M, Miyata K, et al. Horner's syndrome caused by a thoracic dumbbell-shaped schwannoma: sympathetic chain reconstruction after a one-stage removal of the tumor. Spine (Phila Pa 1976) 2003;28(2):E33–6.
40. Dickman CA, Apfelbaum RI. Thoracoscopic microsurgical excision of a thoracic schwannoma. Case report. J Neurosurg 1998;88(5):898–902.
41. Dickman CA, Karahalios DG. Thoracoscopic spinal surgery. Clin Neurosurg 1996;43:392–422.
42. Konno S, Yabuki S, Kinoshita T, et al. Combined laminectomy and thoracoscopic resection of dumbbell-type thoracic cord tumor. Spine (Phila Pa 1976) 2001;26(6):E130–4.
43. Celli P, Trillo G, Ferrante L. Spinal extradural schwannoma. J Neurosurg Spine 2005;2(4):447–56.
44. Kwon B, Kim DH. Lateral lumbar interbody fusion: indications, outcomes, and complications. J Am Acad Orthop Surg 2016;24(2):96–105.
45. Phan K, Mobbs RJ. Anterior retroperitoneal approach for removal of L5-S1 foraminal nerve sheath tumor-case report. Spine J 2016;16(4):e283–6.
46. Benjamin CG, Oermann EK, Thomas JA, et al. Minimally invasive direct lateral transpsoas approach for the resection of a lumbar plexus schwannoma: technique report. Surg J (N Y) 2016;2(3):e66–9.
47. Haji FA, Cenic A, Crevier L, et al. Minimally invasive approach for the resection of spinal neoplasm. Spine (Phila Pa 1976) 2011;36(15):E1018–26.
48. Mannion RJ, Nowitzke AM, Efendy J, et al. Safety and efficacy of intradural extramedullary spinal tumor removal using a minimally invasive approach. Neurosurgery 2011;68(1 Suppl Operative):208–16 [discussion: 216].
49. Lee SE, Jahng TA, Kim HJ. Different surgical approaches for spinal schwannoma: a single surgeon's experience with 49 consecutive cases. World Neurosurg 2015;84(6):1894–902.
50. Fontes RB, Wewel JT, O'Toole JE. Perioperative cost analysis of minimally invasive vs open resection of intradural extramedullary spinal cord tumors. Neurosurgery 2016;78(4):531–9.
51. Zhu YJ, Ying GY, Chen AQ, et al. Minimally invasive removal of lumbar intradural extramedullary lesions using the interlaminar approach. Neurosurg Focus 2015;39(2):E10.
52. Anghileri M, Miceli R, Fiore M, et al. Malignant peripheral nerve sheath tumors: prognostic factors and survival in a series of patients treated at a single institution. Cancer 2006;107(5):1065–74.
53. Yang CF, Sun Z, Speicher PJ, et al. Use and outcomes of minimally invasive lobectomy for stage I non-small cell lung cancer in the national cancer data base. Ann Thorac Surg 2016;101(3):1037–42.
54. Ruurda JP, Hanlo PW, Hennipman A, et al. Robot-assisted thoracoscopic resection of a benign mediastinal neurogenic tumor: technical note. Neurosurgery 2003;52(2):462–4 [discussion: 464].
55. Cerfolio RJ, Bryant AS, Minnich DJ. Operative techniques in robotic thoracic surgery for inferior or posterior mediastinal pathology. J Thorac Cardiovasc Surg 2012;143(5):1138–43.
56. Pacchiarotti G, Wang MY, Kolcun JPG, et al. Robotic paravertebral schwannoma resection at extreme locations of the thoracic cavity. Neurosurg Focus 2017;42(5):E17.
57. Ragu R, Blanchard C, Meurette G. Robotic excision of large retroperitoneal schwannoma (with video). J Visc Surg 2017;154(4):297–9.
58. Hasan S, Hartl R, Hofstetter CP. The benefit zone of full-endoscopic spine surgery. J Spine Surg 2019;5(Suppl 1):S41–56.
59. Parihar VS, Yadav N, Yadav YR, et al. Endoscopic management of spinal intradural extramedullary tumors. J Neurol Surg A Cent Eur Neurosurg 2017;78(3):219–26.
60. Chern JJ, Gordon AS, Naftel RP, et al. Intradural spinal endoscopy in children. J Neurosurg Pediatr 2011;8(1):107–11.
61. Telfeian AE, Choi DB, Aghion DM. Transforaminal endoscopic surgery under local analgesia for ventral epidural thoracic spinal tumor: case report. Clin Neurol Neurosurg 2015;134:1–3.

Stereotactic Radiosurgery for Benign Spinal Tumors

Antonio Meola, MD, PhD[a], Scott Soltys, MD[b], Adam Schmitt, MD[c], Peter C. Gerszten, MD[d], Steven D. Chang, MD[a,*]

KEYWORDS

• Neurofibroma • Meningioma • Schwannoma • Stereotactic radiosurgery • Spine

KEY POINTS

- Surgery is the mainstay for treatment of benign spinal tumors.
- Schwannomas, meningiomas, and neurofibromas are the most common benign spinal tumors and are usually located in the intradural, extramedullary compartment.
- Spinal stereotactic radiosurgery is a safe and effective alternative in selected patients.

INTRODUCTION

Spinal tumors account for 4% of all central nervous system tumors.[1] Primary intradural tumors are usually extramedullary (80%), or, less commonly, intramedullary (20%). Extramedullary tumors include different histologic subtypes, such as meningiomas, schwannomas, and neurofibromas. Although these tumors are usually benign, they may be malignant in exceptional cases. Schwannomas are the most frequent intradural spinal tumors, followed by meningiomas and neurofibromas.[2]

From a clinical standpoint, spinal extramedullary tumors can present with a broad variety of symptoms including pain, radicular sensory impairment or loss, paresthesias, motor impairment, and bowel or bladder dysfunction.[3] The main treatment is open surgical resection; however, alternative treatment techniques, principally stereotactic radiosurgery (SRS), can be used in selected cases. Specifically, complete surgical resection is associated with an excellent prognosis with good functional outcome in greater than 90% of cases and a low risk of recurrence reported to be 1% to 6% after gross-total resection.[4] When subtotal resection is pursued, a second resection or adjuvant SRS can be performed in order to achieve local tumor control. Although the location, clinical presentation, and treatment workflow are common for schwannomas, meningiomas, and neurofibromas, each of these tumors has unique pathologic and radiological features.

Although meningiomas are more common in the intracranial cavity than in the spine, spinal meningiomas account for about one-fourth of spinal tumors.[5] Spinal meningiomas arise from arachnoid cap cells of the meninges and are graded by the World Health Organization (WHO) in a similar fashion as their intracranial counterparts. Most are benign tumors (World Health Organization [WHO] grade 1), belonging to the meningothelial or psammomatous variety.[6] Foci of calcification, known as psammoma bodies, are often found in spinal meningiomas. Prior radiation therapy and neurofibromatosis type 2 are risk factors for the development of these tumors.[7] Meningiomas are typically located in the thoracic spine and often arise from the ventral dural surface.[8,9] MR-images

[a] Department of Neurosurgery, Stanford University, 300 Pasteur Drive, Stanford, CA 94305, USA; [b] Department of Radiation Oncology, Stanford University, 875 Blake Wilbur Dr, Stanford, CA 94305, USA; [c] Department of Radiation Oncology, Memorial Sloan Kettering Cancer Center, 1275 York Avenue, New York, NY 10065, USA; [d] Department of Neurosurgery, University of Pittsburgh Medical Center, 200 Lothrop St, Pittsburgh, PA 15213, USA

* Corresponding author. Department of Neurosurgery, 300 Pasteur Drive, Room R-225, Stanford, CA 94305.
E-mail address: sdchang@stanford.edu

Neurosurg Clin N Am 31 (2020) 231–235
https://doi.org/10.1016/j.nec.2019.12.003
1042-3680/20/

are characteristically T1-isointense, T2-hyperintense, contrast-enhancing characteristic dural enhancing attachment (ie, dural tail).

Spinal schwannomas are the most common peripheral nerve sheath tumors arising from the Schwann cells of the spinal nerves.[1] Schwannomas do not have a marked gender or spinal location predilection. On MRI these lesions appear as T1-isointense, T2 hyperintense, gadolinium-enhancing ovoid-shaped lesions usually arising from the dorsal nerve roots.[10] As a consequence, these tumors tend to displace the spinal cord medially and ventrally within the spinal canal. This aspect makes them accessible via a traditional posterior laminectomy surgical approach.

Spinal neurofibromas also arise from the nerve sheath cells, although they rarely arise in the intradural space.[11] Spinal neurofibromas, especially when multiple, should raise the clinical suspicion of neurofibromatosis type 1, which requires a thorough radiological evaluation of the head and spine and periodic follow-up imaging. On MRI, neurofibromas appear as T1-isointense, T2-hyperintense, gadolinium-enhancing round tumors, which usually arise from the ventral spinal roots, mainly in the cervical section of the spine and importantly without an evident capsule. The absence of a capsule makes these tumors more adherent to the nerve fibers, and, as consequence, more challenging to resect, with potentially higher surgical morbidity.[12]

STEREOTACTIC RADIOSURGERY: TECHNIQUE, INDICATIONS, AND RISKS

Spinal stereotactic radiosurgery (SSRS) is associated with unique clinical challenges that impose high quality and technical standards in selected centers. SSRS consists of the delivery of a lethal dose to a target within the spine with submillimetric accuracy. This goal may be achieved by using different radiosurgery platforms. The treatment is planned and delivered by a multidisciplinary team including a neurosurgeon, radiation oncologist, medical physicist, and radiation oncologists. The radiosurgical planning is a critical part of the SSRS, and requires an accurate registration of multiple pretreatment image sets, typically thin-sliced MRI with and without contrast, contrast-enhanced computed tomography (CT), and selective myelogram-CT. The radiation target and the organs at risk (OARs), namely all the organs adjacent to the tumor itself that could suffer from the inadvertent radiation, should be contoured.[13] The OARs include the spinal cord, nerve roots, and other organs such as the esophagus, larynx, kidney, and bowel.. The spinal cord is one of the most sensitive OARs and requires special attention. CT myelogram and T2 MRI sequences can be registered in the radiosurgical plan in order to visualize the spinal cord during the tumor contouring and the subsequent dose planning (**Fig. 1**). Failure to protect the spinal cord can result in radiation-induced myelopathy (RIM).[3] Tolerable doses for the spinal cord are maximum 45 to 50 Gy at 1.8 to 2 Gy per fraction or up to 12 Gy delivered in a single fraction SSRS.[14–16] The risk for RIM depends upon the radiation dose, number of fractions, length of spinal cord exposed, and duration of treatment.[17] Another potential adverse effect of SSRS is secondary malignancy in the radiated field. However, this risk has been reported as null in a large (1836 patients) retrospective series of benign intracranial tumors treated with SRS.[18]

The mainstay of the treatment of benign spinal tumors is surgical resection. The indications for SSRS[3,19] are limited and include: medical comorbidities contraindicating general anesthesia; adjuvant treatment after subtotal resection or recurrent tumors; histologically-proven high-grade tumors (ie, WHO grade 2 and 3 meningiomas); special surgical challenges, such as tumors located ventrally to the spinal cord (especially where the spinal canal is narrower in the cervical and thoracic spin); and multiple growing tumors requiring treatment, such as in the case of neurofibromatosis type 1.

STEREOTACTIC RADIOSURGERY: OUTCOMES

There is relative paucity of studies assessing the use of SSRS for benign spinal lesions. The largest series[3,19–23] on the topic, including more than 30 patients, is summarized in **Table 1**. Across different studies, the delivered dose ranged between 12 and 30 Gy, in 1 to 5 fractions. The median follow-up of the studies ranged between 23 and 54 months. The tumor local control ranged between 76% and 100% of the cases. Comparisons between the studies are difficult because of their retrospective nature, different tumor histologies, different treatment protocols at each institution, and short length of follow-up. However, the outcome of SSRS for benign spinal tumors appears to be good, with excellent tumor-control rates. As an example, Gerszten and colleagues[23] presented a series including 35 schwannomas, 25 neurofibromas, and 13 meningiomas. Among these patients, SSRS was used as definitive treatment in 55 patients and as a postoperative adjuvant in 18patients. At the end of follow-up, none of the patients progressed, regardless of whether they received surgery before SRS.

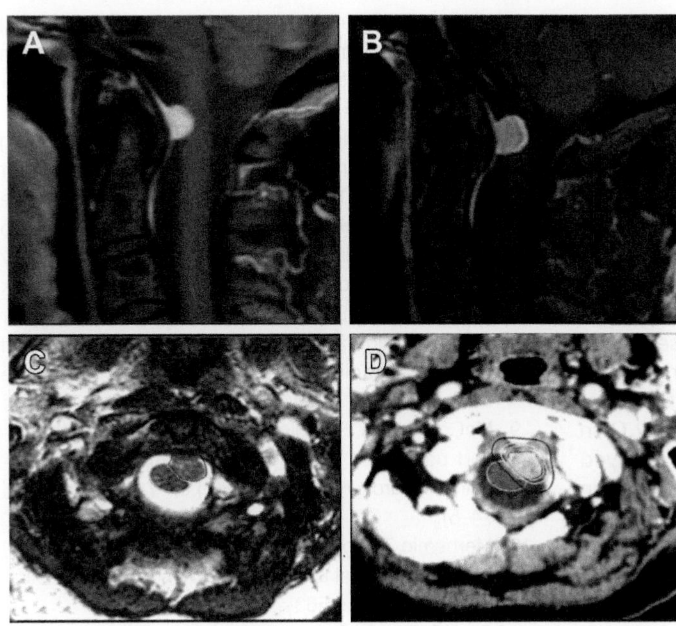

Fig. 1. 82-year-old woman with an asymptomatic tumor at C1, diagnosed as a meningioma by imaging (*A*). On observation, this tumor displayed slow growth over 4 years (*B*). She received stereotactic radiosurgery; the spinal cord (*cyan contour*) and tumor (*red contour*) were delineated on a FIESTA/CISS image (*C*) and confirmed on postcontrast images (*D*). The prescription dose was 24 Gy (*green isodose line in panel D*) in 3 fractions with 89% tumor coverage, 21 Gy (*yellow isodose line*) with 98% tumor coverage. The maximum spinal cord dose was 20 Gy.

Dodd and colleagues[3] treated 30 schwannomas, 16 meningiomas, and 9 neurofibromas with 16 to 30 Gy in up to 5 fractions. At a median follow-up of 36 months, all tumors were smaller (39%) or stable (61%). Importantly, 3 patients required intervention because of persisting or worsening symptoms. Importantly, in selected patients, SSRS can still be considered as an alternative to surgery, while the resection of the tumor is performed in patients with failed symptomatic

Table 1
Published studies (with more than 30 cases) on intraspinal meningioma, schwannomas, and neurofibroma

Publication	Tumor Types	Patients	Dose (Gy)	Fractionation	Median Follow-up (Months)	Outcome
Chin et al,[24] 2018	39 meningiomas 84 schwannomas 26 neurofibromas	120	12.0–22.0	1–5	49	Local control rates of 98%, 95%, and 88% at 3, 5, and 10 y, respectively
Kalash et al,[21] 2018	15 meningiomas 13 schwannomas	38	9.0–21.0	1–3	54	76% local control
Shin et al,[22] 2015	47 schwannomas	58	Median 13.0	1	44	95% local control
Gerszten et al,[19] 2012	10 meningiomas 16 schwannomas 14 neurofibromas	45	16.0	1–3	32	100% local control
Gerszten et al,[23] 2008	13 meningiomas 35 schwannomas 25 neurofibromas	73	15–25.0	1–3	37	100% local control
Dodd et al,[3] 2006	16 meningiomas 30 schwannomas 9 neurofibromas	51	16.0–30.0	1–5	23	95% local control

control by SSRS. In a recent series, Chin and colleagues[20] reported the outcomes of 120 patients with 149 benign spinal tumors (39 meningiomas, 26 neurofibromas, and 84 schwannomas) treated with 16 Gy in 1 fraction or 20 Gy in 2 fractions and with a median follow-up of 49 months. The local control rates were 98%, 95%, and 88% at 3, 5, and 10 years, respectively. The study reported that 9 patients experienced local failure. However, there was no statistically significant difference in the prescription dose or minimum dose between tumors that progressed with respect to the other tumors of the cohort. Importantly, SSRS can also be used for symptom control, including pain control. In the series by Chin and colleagues, local or radicular pain involved 55% of the tumors and, after SSRS, improved in 36% of tumors, remained stable in 53% of tumors, and worsened in 11% of tumors. Surgical resection can be performed after SRS when symptomatic or radiographic failure occurs.

SUMMARY

SSRS is a safe and effective therapeutic option for benign spinal tumors including meningiomas, schwannomas, and neurofibromas. Although surgery is the mainstay of treatment, SSRS can be performed as an alternative or as an adjuvant treatment to surgery in selected patients including, but not limited to, patients with severe medical comorbidities, high-grade tumors, residual or recurrent tumors, and tumors in locations difficult to access surgically. The radiosurgical planning requires accurate image registration and accurate contouring of the target and of the adjacent OARs. Radiation-induced myelopathy is a rare, yet potentially disabling complication that depends on total dose, fractionation schedule, length of radiated cord, and duration of treatment.

REFERENCES

1. Kufeld M, Wowra B, Muacevic A, et al. Radiosurgery of spinal meningiomas and schwannomas. Technol Cancer Res Treat 2012;11(1):27–34.
2. Mirimanoff RO, Dosoretz DE, Linggood RM, et al. Meningioma: analysis of recurrence and progression following neurosurgical resection. J Neurosurg 1985;62(1):18–24.
3. Dodd RL, Ryu MR, Kamnerdsupaphon P, et al. CyberKnife radiosurgery for benign intradural extramedullary spinal tumors. Neurosurgery 2006;58(4):674–85 [discussion: 674–5].
4. Klekamp J, Samii M. Surgical results for spinal meningiomas. Surg Neurol 1999;52(6):552–62.
5. Nabors LB, Portnow J, Ammirati M, et al. Central nervous system cancers, version 1.2015. J Natl Compr Canc Netw 2015;13(10):1191–202.
6. Louis DN, Perry A, Reifenberger G, et al. The 2016 World Health Organization classification of tumors of the central nervous system: a summary. Acta Neuropathol 2016;131(6):803–20.
7. Halliday AL, Sobel RA, Martuza RL. Benign spinal nerve sheath tumors: their occurrence sporadically and in neurofibromatosis types 1 and 2. J Neurosurg 1991;74(2):248–53.
8. Purvis TE, Goodwin CR, Lubelski D, et al. Review of stereotactic radiosurgery for intradural spine tumors. CNS Oncol 2017;6(2):131–8.
9. McCormick PC. Surgical management of dumbbell and paraspinal tumors of the thoracic and lumbar spine. Neurosurgery 1996;38(1):67–74 [discussion: 74–5].
10. Merhemic Z, Stosic-Opincal T, Thurnher MM. Neuroimaging of spinal tumors. Magn Reson Imaging Clin N Am 2016;24(3):563–79.
11. Conti P, Pansini G, Mouchaty H, et al. Spinal neurinomas: retrospective analysis and long-term outcome of 179 consecutively operated cases and review of the literature. Surg Neurol 2004;61(1):34–43 [discussion: 44].
12. Seppala MT, Haltia MJ, Sankila RJ, et al. Long-term outcome after removal of spinal neurofibroma. J Neurosurg 1995;82(4):572–7.
13. Sharma M, Bennett EE, Rahmathulla G, et al. Impact of cervicothoracic region stereotactic spine radiosurgery on adjacent organs at risk. Neurosurg Focus 2017;42(1):E14.
14. Isaacson SR. Radiation therapy and the management of intramedullary spinal cord tumors. J Neurooncol 2000;47(3):231–8.
15. Gibbs IC, Patil C, Gerszten PC, et al. Delayed radiation-induced myelopathy after spinal radiosurgery. Neurosurgery 2009;64(2 Suppl):A67–72.
16. Sahgal A, Chang JH, Ma L, et al. Spinal cord dose tolerance to stereotactic body radiotherapy. Int J Radiat Oncol Biol Phys 2019. [Epub ahead of print].
17. Ling DC, Flickinger JC, Burton SA, et al. Long-term outcomes after stereotactic radiosurgery for spine metastases: radiation dose-response for late toxicity. Int J Radiat Oncol Biol Phys 2018;101(3):602–9.
18. Pollock BE, Link MJ, Stafford SL, et al. The risk of radiation-induced tumors or malignant transformation after single-fraction intracranial radiosurgery: results based on a 25-year experience. Int J Radiat Oncol Biol Phys 2017;97(5):919–23.
19. Gerszten PC, Quader M, Novotny J Jr, et al. Radiosurgery for benign tumors of the spine: clinical experience and current trends. Technol Cancer Res Treat 2012;11(2):133–9.

20. Chin AL, Fujimoto D, Kumar KA, et al. Long-term update of stereotactic radiosurgery for benign spinal tumors. Neurosurgery 2019;85(5):708–16.
21. Kalash R, Glaser SM, Flickinger JC, et al. Stereotactic body radiation therapy for benign spine tumors: is dose de-escalation appropriate? J Neurosurg Spine 2018;29(2):220–5.
22. Shin DW, Sohn MJ, Kim HS, et al. Clinical analysis of spinal stereotactic radiosurgery in the treatment of neurogenic tumors. J Neurosurg Spine 2015;23(4):429–37.
23. Gerszten PC, Burton SA, Ozhasoglu C, et al. Radiosurgery for benign intradural spinal tumors. Neurosurgery 2008;62(4):887–95 [discussion: 895–6].
24. Chin AL, Fujimoto D, Kumar KA, et al. Long-Term Update of Stereotactic Radiosurgery for Benign Spinal Tumors. Neurosurgery 2019;85(5):708–16.

Surgical Management of Intramedullary Spinal Cord Tumors

Ibrahim Hussain, MD[a,b,*], Whitney E. Parker, MD, PhD[a,b], Ori Barzilai, MD[a], Mark H. Bilsky, MD[a,b]

KEYWORDS

• Intramedullary • Spinal cord tumor • Astrocytoma • Ependymoma • Hemangioblastoma

KEY POINTS

- Intramedullary spinal cord tumors (IMSCT) comprise are rare and can occur in all age groups with the most common types being astrocytoma, ependymoma, and hemangioblastoma.
- Presenting symptoms vary based on the region of the spinal cord involved and associated radiographic findings, such as peritumoral syrinx and reactive edema.
- Surgical approach, techniques, and goals vary based on tumor subtype and patient-specific factors, therefore an individualized and multi-disciplinary plan is paramount.
- Adjuncts such as preoperative embolization, ultrasonic aspirators, neurophysiologic monitoring, and image-guided radiation therapy and have improved surgical outcomes and survival.
- Targeted immunotherapies, advanced magnetic resonance-based imaging modalities, and intraoperative optical imaging agents are currently active of research for IMSCT.

INTRODUCTION

Intramedullary spinal cord tumors (IMSCTs) comprise a rare subset of central nervous system (CNS) tumors that can develop at any age and have distinct management strategies based on histopathology. Gliomas, including astrocytomas, ependymomas, and gangliogliomas, as well as nonglial tumors such as hemangioblastomas, are most common, with differences based on age at presentation, location within the spinal cord, and imaging characteristics. In pediatric patients, astrocytomas are the most common type of IMSCT, whereas ependymomas are more common in adults.[1] Other rare tumor types that can develop in the intramedullary compartment include lymphoma, primary CNS melanoma, primitive neuroectodermal tumors, and solid tumor metastases.[2–10]

Presenting symptoms vary based on the region of the spinal cord involved and associated radiographic findings, such as peritumoral syrinx and reactive edema. The most common presenting complaints include sensorimotor deficits, myelopathy, proprioceptive deficits, and localized neck or back pain. More aggressive tumors tend to become symptomatic in a shorter period of time. The Modified McCormick[11] and the Klekamp-Samii[12] clinical scoring systems are the most frequently cited tools used to assess neurologic function of preoperative and postoperative patients with IMSCTs. The Modified McCormick Scale comprises 5 grades ranging from neurologically normal (grade 1) with no ambulatory difficulty, to nonindependent, wheelchair-bound paraplegic and quadriplegic (grade 5). The Klekamp-Samii Scale ranges from 0 to 5 and

[a] Department of Neurological Surgery, Memorial Sloan Kettering Cancer Center, 1275 York Avenue, New York, NY 10065, USA; [b] Department of Neurological Surgery, Weill Cornell Medical College, 525 E. 68th St, New York, NY 10065, USA
* Corresponding author.
E-mail address: ibh9004@nyp.org

Neurosurg Clin N Am 31 (2020) 237–249
https://doi.org/10.1016/j.nec.2019.12.004

considers pain, sensory disturbance/dysesthesia, weakness, ataxia, and sphincter function. Grade 5 individuals have no symptoms, whereas grade 0 patients are plegic, incontinent, and functionally incapacitated.

Enormous progress has been made over the past 2 decades in imaging capabilities, microscopy, microsurgical techniques, neurophysiologic monitoring, and intraoperative devices (eg, ultrasonic aspirators, ultrasonography). Moreover, there have been increasing studies focused on determining optimal adjuvant therapy regimens involving radiation therapy, chemotherapy, and immunotherapy, which have opened promising new avenues for disease control. Nonetheless, these tumors represent a challenging and high-risk disorder to manage within the surgical neuro-oncology realm. This article discusses the classic characteristics of the most common IMSCTs and further focuses on perioperative management considerations germane to successful outcomes.

ASTROCYTOMA

As with their intracranial counterparts, spinal astrocytomas are classified according to progressive grades of aggressiveness, including pilocytic (grade 1), diffuse (grade II), anaplastic (grade III), and glioblastoma (grade IV). Most are low-grade tumors (grades I and II), with high-grade lesions seen more commonly in adults than in children. In adults presenting with spinal cord astrocytomas, the average age at diagnosis ranges from 36 to 52 years, whereas the average duration of symptoms before diagnosis is 15 months.[13–15]

On MRI, these tumors are typically T1 isointense to hypointense and T2 hyperintense. Most enhance with administration of gadolinium contrast, although up to 18% may be nonenhancing.[16] The enhancement pattern can vary, but most are heterogeneous or patchy (**Fig. 1**). Compared with ependymomas, which are classically midline, these tumors tend to be eccentric, given their origin from the parenchyma of the spinal cord. In this regard, exophytic portions of tumor can be observed. They tend to be more infiltrative than ependymomas and have a less discernible interface with normal cord parenchyma. Intratumoral or polar cysts are common features.[17–19]

Because of their more invasive qualities, gross total resection (GTR) of spinal cord astrocytomas is difficult without incurring significant neurologic morbidity. As such, GTR rates are reported between 16% and 30%.[14,20] Survival varies widely based on grade at presentation and preoperative functional status.[21,22] Pilocytic astrocytomas have 10-year survival rate of 78%.[20] However, outcomes in high-grade astrocytomas are dismal, with 5-year and 10-year survival rates of 32% and 0%, respectively.[15] The association of overall survival and progression-free survival (PFS) with extent of resection remains controversial in the literature.[15,23–25] Most investigators agree that overall survival is not improved by aggressive surgical resection in high-grade astrocytomas, and thus that the surgical goal should be safe resection or biopsy only without causing significant deficit.[20,26,27]

The benefit of adjuvant chemotherapy remains unclear, although agents such as temozolomide, cisplatin, carboplatin, bevacizumab, and irinotecan have been described to have some degree of efficacy.[28–31] Radiation therapy seems to show benefit in decreasing recurrence rates following subtotal resection, especially in cases of high-grade tumors.[32] In 1 study, 5-year survival rates following postoperative radiation have been reported to be as high as 79%[33]; however, other studies have failed to show efficacy regardless of extent of resection.[20,34] At present, for patients who undergo subtotal resection or experience relapse, even in the setting of low-grade histology (World Health Organization [WHO] grades I–II), adjuvant radiotherapy is recommended.[35]

Multiple studies have investigated targeted therapy and clinical efficacy of various agents in the treatment of intracranial astrocytoma, but data regarding the potential treatment of spinal astrocytomas remain scarce, likely because of the rarity of this condition. Common genetic mutations observed in cranial astrocytomas are also noted in spinal astrocytomas, including those in the *p16* gene, *PTEN*, *BRAF*, *p53*, and the replication independent histone 3 variant H3.3 gene. Spinal astrocytomas have also been found to harbor the *BRAF-KIAA1549* fusion gene and *BRAFV600E* mutation, which suggests potential targeted molecular treatment options, as has been shown in intracranial gliomas.[36,37] Downstream targets from *PTEN* have been identified, such as mammalian target of rapamycin (mTOR) and Akt, and several potential drugs are currently under clinical investigation for managing cranial astrocytoma, which may offer the possibility of expanding treatments to spinal astrocytoma.[38,39]

EPENDYMOMA

Ependymomas are the most common IMSCTs seen in adults and the second most common seen in children.[40] These tumors most commonly present in the fourth and fifth decades of life, and have a mean symptomatic duration of 21 to

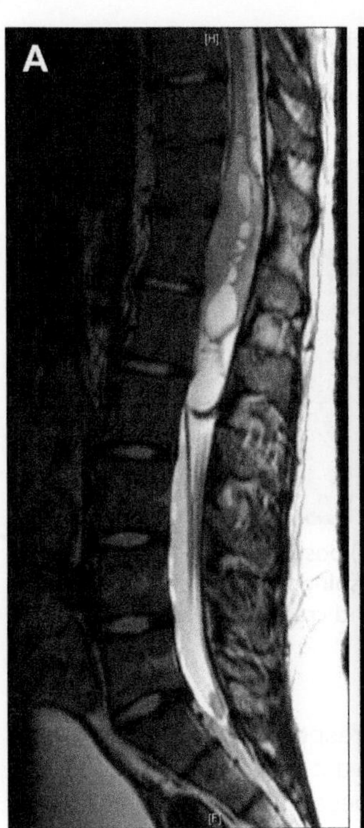

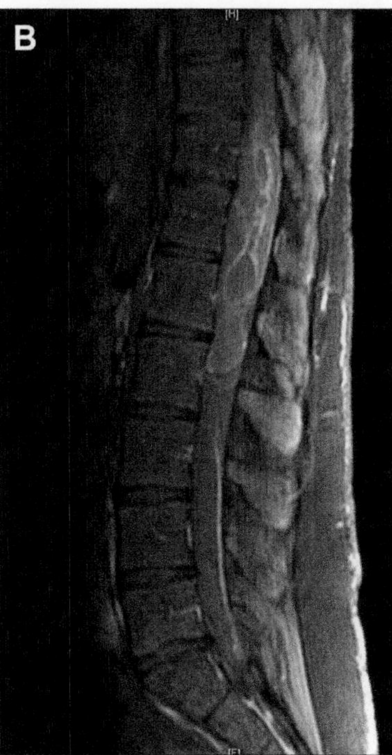

Fig. 1. Sagittal (*A*) T2 and (*B*) T1 postcontrast images of an intramedullary pilocytic astrocytoma at the level of the conus medullaris. The tumor is T2 isointense to hyperintense with an intratumoral cyst that enhances with gadolinium administration.

37 months before diagnosis.[1,11,41] Grade I variants are referred to as subependymomas, which are exceedingly rare, with about 105 pathology-confirmed cases reported in the literature.[42] Grade II tumors are the classic ependymomas and show perivascular rosettes (pseudorosettes) and encompass distinct histologic variants including cellular, papillary, clear cell, and tanycytic. Higher grade (anaplastic) variants are rare, typically invasive, less amenable to gross total excision, and carry a worse prognosis.[43] Compared with the general population, spinal ependymomas are more commonly observed in individuals with the inherited tumor predisposition syndrome neurofibromatosis type 2.[44] These patients may develop multiple lesions leading to a characteristic string-of-pearls sign on imaging.[45,46] Although still an active area of investigation, the vascular endothelial growth factor (VEGF) receptor inhibitor bevacizumab has shown some benefit with regard to improved symptoms and radiographic response in neurofibromatosis type 2–associated spinal ependymomas.[47,48]

Spinal ependymomas most commonly occur in the cervicothoracic region and span an average of 3 to 4 segments within the spinal cord.[1,49] These T1-hypointense, T2-hyperintense tumors heterogeneously enhance with administration of gadolinium contrast (**Fig. 2**), although in rare cases can be nonenhancing, confounding differentiation from astrocytoma.[50,51] In contrast with astrocytomas, ependymomas typically occupy a more central location within the spinal cord because they arise from the ependymal cells that line the central canal and cause symmetric expansion of the spinal cord. As with astrocytomas, osseous remodeling can be seen because of ependymomas' slow-growing nature. Scalloping of the posterior vertebral bodies, thinning of the laminae, erosion of the medial aspects of the pedicles, and reactive scoliosis can be seen in up to 11% of cases.[51] Intratumoral or satellite cysts and syringohydromyelia can be seen in up to 90% of tumors at the rostral and/or caudal ends.[49,52] Intratumoral cysts tend to contrast enhance, whereas satellite cysts do not.[52] A cap sign can be observed with these tumors, with a hypointense rim caused by hemosiderin deposition on T2-weighted imaging in up to one-third of cases.[17,18] Calcifications are not commonly observed with spinal ependymomas, as opposed to their intracranial counterparts.

A specific subtype of these tumors is myxopapillary ependymoma, which exclusively occurs in the region of conus medullaris and along the tract of the filum terminale (**Fig. 3**). Unlike nonmyxomatous ependymomas, these grade I tumors are more likely to be T1 hyperintense.[51] Overall, 10-year survival, PFS, and local control rates for these tumors are 97%, 62%, and 72%, respectively.[53] The role of adjuvant radiation is controversial, with conflicting findings on rates of recurrence, regardless of extent of resection.[53,54]

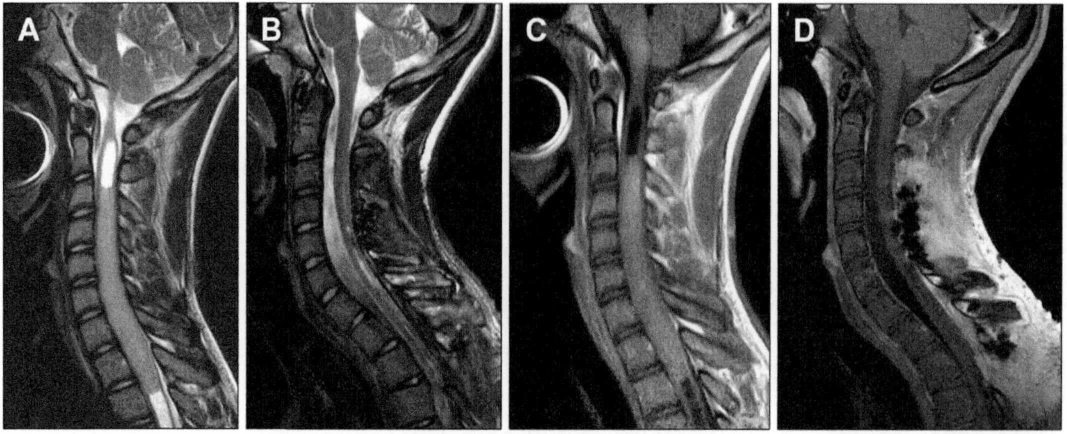

Fig. 2. (*A*) Preoperative and (*B*) postoperative T2 MRI and (*C*) preoperative and (*D*) postoperative T1 postcontrast MRI of an intramedullary ependymoma spanning the cervical and upper thoracic spine. The tumor symmetrically expands the spinal cord and heterogeneously contrast enhances. Satellite cysts and cranial and caudal poles are noted.

When safely feasible, GTR is the gold standard of surgical treatment of these tumors, with superior outcomes reported.[54–56] Although unencapsulated, these tumors usually have distinct borders and are not infiltrative.[49] They tend to have a red to brown tint, compared with the surrounding spinal cord parenchyma, making their margins more easily discernible than astrocytomas intraoperatively (see **Fig. 2**). Drop metastases can be seen with these tumors, most commonly described with myxopapillary ependymomas[57,58] or in individuals with intracranial posterior fossa ependymomas.[59,60] Drop metastases usually present in the low lumbar or sacral levels because of gravity-mediated effects.

The 5-year PFS for spinal ependymomas is 80%, with GTR being the most significant prognostic factor.[61] In children, PFS of 58 months has been described.[62] For myxopapillary ependymomas, the recurrence rate was 15.5% in patients treated by GTR and 32.6% in patients treated by subtotal resection, irrespective of whether or not they received adjuvant therapy. The role of chemotherapy for these tumors remains poorly defined. Small retrospective case series have shown some benefit with etoposide and temozolomide in the systemic management of residual or recurrent ependymomas.[29,63] Treatment of a spinal ependymoma with adjuvant radiation following subtotal resection has reported 5-year survival rates of 96% with improved PFS.[64,65] For patients with subtotally resected grade II or any grade III spinal ependymomas, adjuvant radiotherapy is recommended given the higher risk for disease relapse.[37] Adjuvant radiation therapy is generally discouraged after GTR of WHO II ependymomas because studies failed to show an additional benefit.[35,66]

Cranial and spinal ependymomas have been shown to be molecularly distinct.[67] Although studies have identified various potential molecular targets in ependymomas, including phosphatidylinositol 3

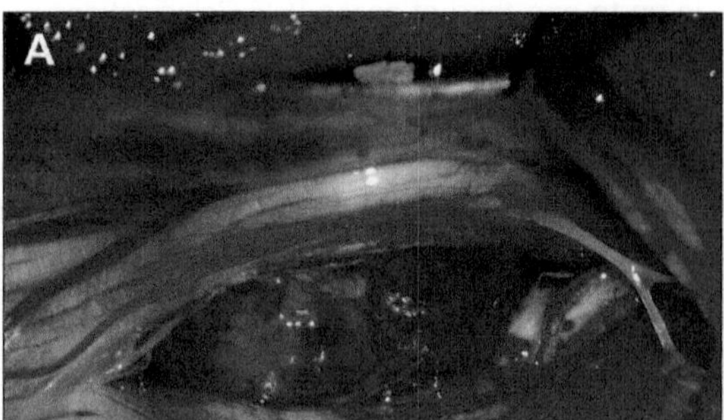

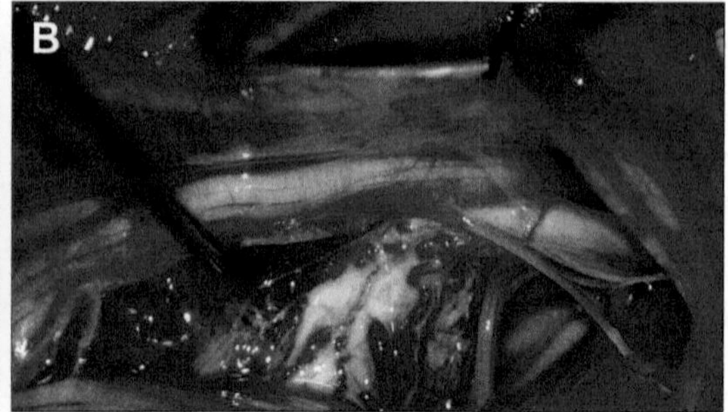

Fig. 3. A myxopapillary ependymoma at the level of the conus medullaris and cauda equina before (A) and after (B) near-total resection. Note the brownish coloration of the tumor and associated dense vascularity in this region.

kinase (PI3K) signaling pathway and epidermal growth factor receptor (EGFR), few clinical trials have explored the efficacy of treatments involving these targets and their efficacy remains unknown.[39] One report of a platelet-derived growth factor (PDGF)–expressing tumor that responded to treatment with imatinib suggests that this medication may have a potential for treating such tumors.[68]

HEMANGIOBLASTOMA

Hemangioblastomas are the third overall most common and the most common nonglial IMSCT, accounting for 2% to 6% of all cases. These WHO grade I tumors can be found throughout the CNS and, apart from the spinal cord, are most frequently encountered in the cerebellum.[69] Most of these tumors occur in the cervicothoracic spine.[70] The average age at presentation is approximately 47 years old. Unlike other IMSCTs, these vascular tumors rarely present with acute paresis caused by intramedullary hemorrhage, which requires urgent decompression to preserve neurologic function.[71–73] Up to 72% of patients with von Hippel-Lindau disease (VHL) develop 1 or more CNS hemangioblastomas.[74,75] Loss of the *VHL* gene promotes increased production of VEGF and erythropoietin. Patients with VHL often have new multiple, small, remote tumors.[76]

Macroscopically, these tumors appear as a cystic mass with a well-circumscribed mural nodule. Microscopically, they contain rich vascularity with tightly packed thin-walled capillary-type vessels separated by stromal cells.[69] Spinal hemangioblastomas can have varying appearances on T1-weighted imaging and are T2 isointense to hyperintense. Flow voids can be observed in larger lesions on T2 sequences, as well syringomyelia and cord edema, which may be secondary to venous hypertension.[75,77] With contrast administration, these tumors avidly and homogeneously enhance (**Fig. 4**).[18] They are almost exclusively found along the dorsal aspect of the spinal cord.[75]

Hemangioblastomas usually have a well-defined margin, compared with normal spinal cord parenchyma. Approximately 93% to 99% of tumors can achieve GTR, with an 86% rate of functional stability at 5 years postoperatively.[78,79] Recurrence rates following GTR in non–VHL-associated sporadic hemangioblastomas are less than 7%.[80] Patients with VHL-associated hemangioblastomas have poorer outcomes, mostly because of multifocal CNS or extra-CNS manifestations of disease.[78] Preoperative embolization has proved valuable for the surgical management of these tumors by reducing intraoperative blood loss and, anecdotally, by shrinking the tumor, and thus easing the ability to manipulate and resect it.[81] Hemangioblastomas typically show a prominent tumor blush on angiography and in many cases an early draining vein (see **Fig. 4**). However, given the predilection for their occurrence in the cervical spine, several hemangioblastomas may not be amenable to embolization, with feeding arteries in close proximity to the anterior spinal artery.[82] Complications related to vertebral artery and anterior spinal artery occlusion have been described, resulting in spinal cord and posterior fossa infarcts.[83]

Before the development of spinal radiosurgery, patients unable to undergo resection were treated with conventionally fractionated external beam radiotherapy to low doses with poor outcomes. Recent technological advancements have led to initial experience with radiosurgery for select patients who are unable to undergo resection, have VHL, or have multiple tumors. Initial series in select patients show promising results with high rates of local control and low complication rates.[84,85]

OTHER TUMORS

Primary intramedullary spinal cord lymphoma (PISCL) presents at an average age of 57 to 62 years, predominantly in white people.[2,86] Patients with human immunodeficiency virus or those who are immunosuppressed, as in the setting of organ transplant, are at greater risk for developing PISCL.[86,87] The most common subtype is diffuse B-cell type. Of note, follicular lymphomas are associated with accelerated failure time following treatment.[86] General cumulative survival percentages at 1 and 5 years after treatment are 73.8% and 63.1%, respectively.[86] Most patients present with multifocal, enhancing lesions on spinal MRI. Intravenous/intrathecal methotrexate and radiation therapy are treatment options once the diagnosis is confirmed, but aggressive surgical resection should not be undertaken, given the lack of added disease control and the incurring of significant neurologic morbidity.

Gangliogliomas are an exceedingly rare grade I class of intramedullary gliomas that are almost exclusively seen in the pediatric population. The median age of presentation is 14 years, and patients may possess BRAF V600E and H3 K27M mutations, as seen in histologically identical intracranial midline gliomas.[88–90] Astrocytomas and ependymomas share many similar features with ganglioglioma, including T2 hyperintensity, enhancement, tumoral cysts, and cord edema.[5] GTR is the optimal surgical treatment of intramedullary gangliogliomas, with 5-year and 10-year survival rates after treatment of 89% and 83%,

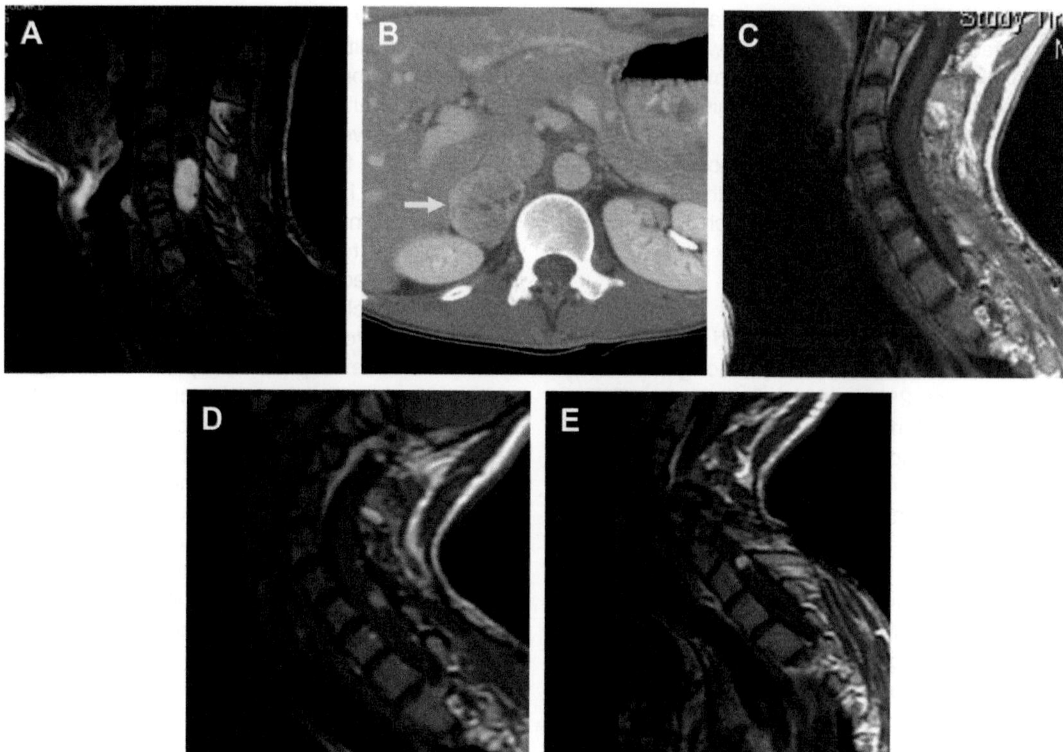

Fig. 4. Representative case showing the importance of VHL screening for hemangioblastoma. A 25-year-old musician presented with a 4-year history of neck pain with progressive right arm and hand weakness associated with dysesthetic pain. On examination, his right hand grip and triceps were graded as 3 out of 5 with normal proprioception. MRI showed a homogeneously enhancing intramedullary tumor (*A*) with polar cysts. He underwent cervical laminectomy and resection of the tumor. At surgery, the tumor was pial based and was circumferentially excised. In the recovery room, the patient had a hypertensive crisis, which was controlled with β-blockers. A computed tomography scan showed a right adrenal mass (*arrow*) compatible with pheochromocytoma (*B*). The patient was diagnosed with VHL and a pheochromocytoma was resected with resolution of hypertension off all medications. One-year postoperative image (*C*) shows no tumor recurrence. Nineteen-year follow-up MRI scans (*D, E*) show slowly progressive multiple cervical asymptomatic hemangioblastomas, which are followed radiographically with no need for surgical intervention.

respectively.[91] Given the predominance of children who present with these tumors, radiation therapy is not frequently used.[90]

Intramedullary metastases from solid tumor primary malignancies indicate late-stage systemic disease with a poor prognosis. The most frequent extra-CNS histologies reported to metastasize to the intramedullary compartment are non–small cell lung and breast cancers.[4] The mean interval from the time of the primary cancer diagnosis to the development of symptomatic intramedullary metastases is 38 months. The mean survival time after surgery for such metastases is 11.6 months even with aggressive surgical treatment and radiation, indicating that these are a late-stage event.[4]

PREOPERATIVE CONSIDERATIONS

Among the most controversial aspects in the management of IMSCT is the management of patients who present with classic radiographic findings but no symptoms or minimal pain-related symptoms without neurologic deficits. The decision-making algorithm in such cases accounts for the following considerations: (1) is tissue diagnosis required to guide further management? (2) Does intervention itself, even for biopsy, result in a worse clinical status than the patient's current preoperative state? (3) Does resectability of the tumor become more complicated by delaying treatment? Up to 10% of patients who present with no or minimal symptoms end up with worse neurologic status after surgical intervention.[41] Although philosophies vary from center to center, at our institution we have adopted the stance of close radiographic and clinical follow-up in patients with asymptomatic or incidentally discovered lesions. Surgical intervention is reserved for those who develop neurologic symptoms or for rapid growth observed on short-interval imaging.

OPERATIVE CONSIDERATIONS

Once the decision has been made to proceed with surgery, several adjuncts may be used to increase the likelihood of successful outcomes. The process begins with the anesthesiology team. With large tumors that occupy a significant portion of the spinal canal from tumor bulk and edema, spinal cord perfusion is of the utmost importance. All patients should have an arterial line placed for continuous and accurate mean arterial pressure (MAP) readings. Total intravenous anesthetics should be used and paralytics avoided to optimize intraoperative neurophysiologic monitoring. Initial induction with certain anesthetics (eg, propofol) can decrease systemic MAPs and result in spinal cord hypoperfusion, leading to ischemia and a potentially catastrophic infarct. This consequence can be potentiated in patients with concomitant peripheral vascular disease.[92]

Technique

After appropriate localization, a midline skin incision is created. The soft tissue dissection is carried down to the level of the spinous processes. A meticulous subperiosteal dissection is performed exposing the laminae. Care is taken not to expose or disrupt the joint capsules. A midline laminectomy is performed, again taking care to not injure the facet joints or pars interarticularis laterally. In most situations that involve 4 or fewer levels and do not cross the cervicothoracic or thoracolumbar junctions, instrumented stabilization is not required. However, case-by-case exceptions are often made, based on the number or levels requiring laminectomy, preoperative alignment, iatrogenic destabilization, and medical comorbidities. Following laminectomy, meticulous hemostasis is obtained, and all bone done dust should be irrigated out before dural opening, to prevent seepage into the intradural compartment, which can cause an aseptic meningitis. Intraoperative ultrasonography is a useful adjunct to determine whether the cranial and caudal extent of dural exposure is adequate.

For dural opening, the operative microscope is brought in and suction devices should be switched to finger-controlled suctions. A midline durotomy is performed and dural edges are tacked up to the adjacent paraspinal musculature for additional exposure and to prevent epidural bleeding from obscuring the field. Cottonoid patties should be placed along the epidural gutters for additional hemostasis. The arachnoid is opened and cerebrospinal fluid (CSF) is drained, presenting the dorsal aspect of the spinal cord. Based on tumor pathology, there may or may not be superficial color-related changes of the spinal cord to indicate the precise location of disorder. There are 2 main entry zones to the spinal cord: the midline raphe and the dorsal root entry zone. Typically, the midline myelotomy is preferred because of the lower rates of postoperative deficits. The midline dorsal raphe is identified and is usually determined based on where veins course toward the midline and then traverse into the parenchyma (**Fig. 5**). Sharp excision of the pia with an 11 blade is made by focused bipolar cauterization of the pia, and slow advancement of the myelotomy is accomplished with blunt dissection.

Once the tumor is encountered, the technique for resection is based on pathology and tumor anatomy. Most commonly, an intralesional tumor resection is accomplished using the CUSA (Integra, Plainsboro, NY). Ependymomas have a discernible interface with the spinal cord; thus, the tumor can be separated from normal parenchyma using blunt dissection and mild traction using microinstruments rendering a GTR. Care must be taken to coagulate the feeding vessels, which emanate from the anterior spinal artery. In contrast, most astrocytomas do not have discernible plane. As such, most astrocytomas are simply biopsied, although tumor debulking using an inside-out technique can be used to accomplish a safe maximal resection, which is terminated once a significant decrease in somatosensory or motor signal occurs during intraoperative monitoring.

Hemangioblastomas require a unique surgical approach, compared with glial IMSCTs. These tumors usually have a distinct tumor–spinal cord interface and are often unilateral and visualized

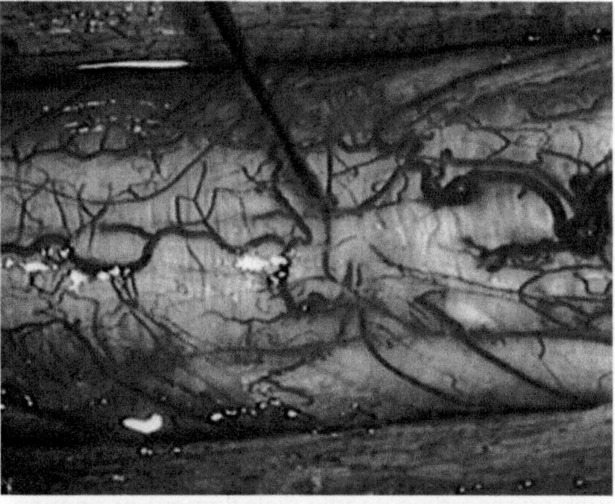

Fig. 5. The midline dorsal raphe. At this region, veins course toward the midline, then dive deep into the spinal cord parenchyma. This landmark serves as the entry point for resection of intramedullary tumors that are not apparent superficially by minimizing dorsal column dysfunction.

on the surface. The inside-out technique is not advised given their dense vascularity, even after successful embolization. Our group uses techniques that mirror those previously described by McCormick and Lonser.[93–95] The pial interface surrounding the tumor is sharply incised with an arachnoid knife or microscissors. Bipolar cautery is used to define this border circumferentially, shrink the tumor bulk, and ablate any large surface vessels. Once the tumor is circumferentially separated, the dissection is continued to define the ventral surface. Care must be taken, because draining veins may be present on the undersurface. Once completely detached ventrally, the tumor can be removed en bloc. In some situations in which only a small portion of the tumor is visible at the surface, longitudinal myelotomies at the poles may be required to define the circumferential borders.

At the conclusion of surgical resection, hemostasis is achieved with combination of thrombin-soaked gel foam, hemostatic matrix, and bipolar cautery. A watertight dural closure is performed, then meticulous multilayer deep tissue, fascial, and superficial tissue closure. The use of subfascial or suprafascial drains is usually at the discretion of the operating surgeon, with no high-quality evidence arguing for or against their use in these cases.

Neuromonitoring

The goal of intraoperative neurophysiologic monitoring (IONM) in IMSCT surgery is to monitor in real time the functional integrity of the motor and sensory systems and detect iatrogenic injury at early, reversible stages. The gold standard for IONM is a multimodality approach consisting of continuous electromyography, somatosensory evoked potentials (SSEPs), motor evoked potentials (MEPs), and transcranial MEPs (tcMEPs).[96] In addition to monitoring the integrity of the neural circuit, IONM can also be performed to delineate functional areas, such as mapping the spinal cord dorsal columns in order to delineate a physiologic midline or safe-entry zone, and localizing the corticospinal tract within the tumor cavity in order to delineate danger zones worth avoiding.

With any acute change in monitoring, a systematic approach for troubleshooting should be adopted. First, technical factors should be excluded, such as recording needle dislodgment or connectivity issues at any point from the patient to the neuromonitoring station. Second, the MAP should be assessed, because spinal cord hypoperfusion can affect signals. Increasing MAP and irrigation with warm saline to increase perfusion with a return of signals to baseline can confirm this suspicion. In addition, intravenous steroid bolus should be considered. Third, reversal correctable surgical maneuvers should be addressed, including removal of hemostatic material such as gel foam or cottonoid patties and release of pial tack-up sutures. When there is persistent reduction of signals despite these steps, a case-by-case decision must be made on whether to proceed with resection or to perform a wake-up test based on the degree of signal loss, volume of remaining tumor, and tumor pathology.

MEP recording has shown a sensitivity and specificity in detecting motor deficits of 95% and 98%, respectively.[97] tcMEP monitoring has a sensitivity and specificity for detecting motor deficits of 80% and 71.4%, respectively.[98] SSEP recording has a sensitivity and specificity of detecting postoperative sensory deficits of 94% and 97%, respectively.[97] Sala and colleagues[99] found better improvement in McCormick grade at 3 months postoperatively in patients who were monitored compared with historical controls. Quinones-Hinojosa and colleagues[100] found that a loss of tcMEP waveform in 12 patients correlated with worse motor deficits, compared with patients without loss of waveform. Mehta and colleagues[101] showed dorsal column dysfunction in only 9% of patients with dorsal column mapping, versus 50% of patients without.

An important limitation of MEP and SSEP monitoring is that there may be a few-second delay from the time an insult occurs to the time at which signal changes become evident. This brief delay can have significant impact, because potentially irreversible damage can occur in this short time as the surgeon continues to operate. D (direct)-wave monitoring provides faster, real-time feedback of the integrity of the corticospinal tracts during IMSCT surgery. Motor potentials are evoked transcranially to stimulate the motor cortex of the brain. Impulses travel through the spinal cord and are recorded caudal to the area of surgery by electrodes placed in the epidural or subdural space. Decreases in amplitude of D-wave recordings greater than 50% are associated with motor deficits that may be permanent.[102,103] Preservation of D-wave recordings predicts good motor outcome despite deterioration or loss of MEPs.[104] New techniques to allow continuous mapping of the spinal cord during resection of IMSCTs are currently under investigation.[96]

POSTOPERATIVE MANAGEMENT

Steroids and strict blood pressure control to avoid hypotension for the first 24 to 48 hours are paramount in the postoperative period. These measures can minimize spinal cord edema and optimize spinal cord perfusion. Hypertension conversely can lead to hemorrhage along the surgical corridor or in the intramedullary tumor cavity, resulting in high-grade compression, requiring emergent decompression to salvage neurologic function. Steroids are also effective in treating inflammation associated with aseptic meningitis that may occur from tumor proteins, blood, and bone dust that circulates within the CSF postoperatively, and should be tapered off slowly to prevent acute-onset symptoms. Patients are typically placed on bed rest and flat in bed for prevention of spinal headaches for a minimum of 24 hours after surgery. Even among patients for whom the intended surgical goal was achieved without adverse events intraoperatively, almost all have some degree of proprioceptive deficit caused by the myelotomy through the dorsal columns. Abnormalities in the sensation of joint location in space can be especially debilitating during the early ambulatory phase of recovery. Intense physical therapy usually helps to recover this deficit over a period of 12 months. Postoperative imaging is typically obtained before discharge, to assess the extent of resection and to serve as a new baseline for comparison with future scans.

FUTURE DIRECTIONS

Diffusion tensor imaging (DTI) tractography is a noninvasive MRI sequence that enables visualization of the white matter tracts.[105] Tractography can be used as an additional tool for suggesting diagnosis preoperatively, as well predicting the resectability of an IMSCT. Setzer and colleagues[105] used DTI tractography to divide IMSCTs into 3 categorical groups: (1) fibers were splayed around solid lesions; (2) fiber tracts were partially mixed but mostly splayed around solid lesions; and (3) more than 50% of fiber tracts were indistinguishable from the solid lesion. They were able to show substantial agreement between preoperative tractography and intraoperative findings using this technology. The utility of DTI in IMSCT treatment may also prove valuable in the preoperative counseling of patients on the likely outcomes of surgery.

5-Aminolevulinic acid (5-ALA) is a part of the heme biosynthetic pathway and, when metabolized, gets transformed through a series of reactions in the mitochondria into protoporphyrin IX, a fluorescent metabolite. This drug is able to penetrate the blood-brain barrier, most notably in areas with a high density of malignant cells. 5-ALA has been used in European centers for glioma surgery for more than a decade, showing more complete resections of high-grade gliomas compared with conventional techniques, but was only approved by the Food and Drug Administration (FDA) in the United States in 2017.[106] Small case series have reported that most intramedullary ependymomas show 5-ALA fluorescence, as do drop metastases and hemangiopericytomas.[107,108] This adjunct may also be especially useful in determining the amount of residual tumor left in intramedullary anaplastic astrocytomas and glioblastoma but may have limited benefit in low-grade astroctyomas.[107,109,110]

SUMMARY

Patients with IMSCT are best served by multidisciplinary management involving, but not limited to, neurosurgeons, neurologists, medical oncologists, radiation oncologists, physiatrists, and physical therapists. Preoperative neurologic status and maximally safe resection predict better outcomes. Microsurgical technique and acceptable operative aggressiveness are dictated by tumor pathology and grade. The benefit of chemotherapy, biologic therapy, and targeted therapies remains unclear, whereas there is increasing evidence that radiation therapy is beneficial, especially with recent advances in stereotactic body radiation therapy. Future clinical trials, better understanding of molecular pathogenesis, and technological advancements will serve to more precisely determine optimal treatment paradigms for IMSCT as the era of personalized medicine continues to evolve.

DISCLOSURE

M.H. Bilsky receives royalties from Globus and DePuy/Synthes and is on the Speaker's Bureau for Brainlab and Varian. The other authors have nothing to disclose.

REFERENCES

1. Klekamp J. Spinal ependymomas. Part 1: intramedullary ependymomas. Neurosurg Focus 2015; 39(2):E6.
2. Yang W, Garzon-Muvdi T, Braileanu M, et al. Primary intramedullary spinal cord lymphoma: a population-based study. Neuro Oncol 2017;19(3): 414–21.
3. Wuerdeman M, Douglass S, Abda RB, et al. A rare case of primary spinal cord melanoma. Radiol Case Rep 2018;13(2):424–6.
4. Payer S, Mende KC, Westphal M, et al. Intramedullary spinal cord metastases: an increasingly common diagnosis. Neurosurg Focus 2015;39(2):E15.

5. Oppenheimer DC, Johnson MD, Judkins AR. Ganglioglioma of the spinal cord. J Clin Imaging Sci 2015;5:53.
6. Niemeyer B, Marchiori E. Anaplastic ganglioglioma involving the entire length of the spinal cord. Eur Neurol 2018;79(3–4):125.
7. Murakami T, Koyanagi I, Kaneko T, et al. Intramedullary spinal cord ganglioglioma presenting as hyperhidrosis: unique symptoms and magnetic resonance imaging findings: case report. J Neurosurg Spine 2013;18(2):184–8.
8. Lotfinia I, Vahedi P. Intramedullary cervical spinal cord ganglioglioma, review of the literature and therapeutic controversies. Spinal Cord 2009; 47(1):87–90.
9. Deme S, Ang LC, Skaf G, et al. Primary intramedullary primitive neuroectodermal tumor of the spinal cord: case report and review of the literature. Neurosurgery 1997;41(6):1417–20.
10. Harbhajanka A, Jain M, Kapoor SK. Primary spinal intramedullary primitive neuroectodermal tumor. J Pediatr Neurosci 2012;7(1):67–9.
11. McCormick PC, Torres R, Post KD, et al. Intramedullary ependymoma of the spinal cord. J Neurosurg 1990;72(4):523–32.
12. Klekamp J, Samii M. Introduction of a score system for the clinical evaluation of patients with spinal processes. Acta Neurochir (Wien) 1993;123(3–4):221–3.
13. Rabadan AT, Hernandez D, Paz L. Extent of resection and postoperative functional declination of Klekamp's type A intramedullary tumors in adult patients. Surg Neurol Int 2016;7(Suppl 40):S976–9.
14. Hamilton KR, Lee SS, Urquhart JC, et al. A systematic review of outcome in intramedullary ependymoma and astrocytoma. J Clin Neurosci 2019;63:168–75.
15. Khalid S, Kelly R, Carlton A, et al. Adult intradural intramedullary astrocytomas: a multicenter analysis. J Spine Surg 2019;5(1):19–30.
16. Seo HS, Kim JH, Lee DH, et al. Nonenhancing intramedullary astrocytomas and other MR imaging features: a retrospective study and systematic review. AJNR Am J Neuroradiol 2010;31(3):498–503.
17. Nemoto Y, Inoue Y, Tashiro T, et al. Intramedullary spinal cord tumors: significance of associated hemorrhage at MR imaging. Radiology 1992; 182(3):793–6.
18. Koeller KK, Rosenblum RS, Morrison AL. Neoplasms of the spinal cord and filum terminale: radiologic-pathologic correlation. Radiographics 2000;20(6):1721–49.
19. Bansal S, Suri A, Borkar SA, et al. Management of intramedullary tumors in children: analysis of 82 operated cases. Childs Nerv Syst 2012;28(12): 2063–9.
20. Minehan KJ, Brown PD, Scheithauer BW, et al. Prognosis and treatment of spinal cord astrocytoma. Int J Radiat Oncol Biol Phys 2009; 73(3):727–33.
21. Cooper PR, Epstein F. Radical resection of intramedullary spinal cord tumors in adults. Recent experience in 29 patients. J Neurosurg 1985;63(4):492–9.
22. Innocenzi G, Raco A, Cantore G, et al. Intramedullary astrocytomas and ependymomas in the pediatric age group: a retrospective study. Childs Nerv Syst 1996;12(12):776–80.
23. Garces-Ambrossi GL, McGirt MJ, Mehta VA, et al. Factors associated with progression-free survival and long-term neurological outcome after resection of intramedullary spinal cord tumors: analysis of 101 consecutive cases. J Neurosurg Spine 2009; 11(5):591–9.
24. Bansal S, Ailawadhi P, Suri A, et al. Ten years' experience in the management of spinal intramedullary tumors in a single institution. J Clin Neurosci 2013;20(2):292–8.
25. Ahmed R, Menezes AH, Awe OO, et al. Long-term disease and neurological outcomes in patients with pediatric intramedullary spinal cord tumors. J Neurosurg Pediatr 2014;13(6):600–12.
26. Seki T, Hida K, Yano S, et al. Clinical factors for prognosis and treatment guidance of spinal cord astrocytoma. Asian Spine J 2016;10(4):748–54.
27. Cohen AR, Wisoff JH, Allen JC, et al. Malignant astrocytomas of the spinal cord. J Neurosurg 1989; 70(1):50–4.
28. Mora J, Cruz O, Gala S, et al. Successful treatment of childhood intramedullary spinal cord astrocytomas with irinotecan and cisplatin. Neuro Oncol 2007;9(1):39–46.
29. Chamberlain MC. Temozolomide for recurrent low-grade spinal cord gliomas in adults. Cancer 2008; 113(5):1019–24.
30. Hassall TE, Mitchell AE, Ashley DM. Carboplatin chemotherapy for progressive intramedullary spinal cord low-grade gliomas in children: three case studies and a review of the literature. Neuro Oncol 2001;3(4):251–7.
31. Gwak SJ, An SS, Yang MS, et al. Effect of combined bevacizumab and temozolomide treatment on intramedullary spinal cord tumor. Spine (Phila Pa 1976) 2014;39(2):E65–73.
32. Shrivastava RK, Epstein FJ, Perin NI, et al. Intramedullary spinal cord tumors in patients older than 50 years of age: management and outcome analysis. J Neurosurg Spine 2005;2(3):249–55.
33. Jyothirmayi R, Madhavan J, Nair MK, et al. Conservative surgery and radiotherapy in the treatment of spinal cord astrocytoma. J Neurooncol 1997;33(3):205–11.
34. Benes V 3rd, Barsa P, Benes V Jr, et al. Prognostic factors in intramedullary astrocytomas: a literature review. Eur Spine J 2009;18(10):1397–422.
35. Kotecha R, Mehta MP, Chang EL, et al. Updates in the management of intradural spinal cord tumors: a

radiation oncology focus. Neuro Oncol 2019;21(6): 707–18.
36. Zadnik PL, Gokaslan ZL, Burger PC, et al. Spinal cord tumours: advances in genetics and their implications for treatment. Nat Rev Neurol 2013;9(5): 257–66.
37. Del Bufalo F, Ceglie G, Cacchione A, et al. BRAF V600E inhibitor (Vemurafenib) for BRAF V600E mutated low grade gliomas. Front Oncol 2018;8:526.
38. Karsy M, Guan J, Sivakumar W, et al. The genetic basis of intradural spinal tumors and its impact on clinical treatment. Neurosurg Focus 2015; 39(2):E3.
39. Sami A, Karsy M. Targeting the PI3K/AKT/mTOR signaling pathway in glioblastoma: novel therapeutic agents and advances in understanding. Tumour Biol 2013;34(4):1991–2002.
40. Smith AB, Soderlund KA, Rushing EJ, et al. Radiologic-pathologic correlation of pediatric and adolescent spinal neoplasms: part 1, intramedullary spinal neoplasms. AJR Am J Roentgenol 2012;198(1):34–43.
41. Aghakhani N, David P, Parker F, et al. Intramedullary spinal ependymomas: analysis of a consecutive series of 82 adult cases with particular attention to patients with no preoperative neurological deficit. Neurosurgery 2008;62(6):1279–85 [discussion: 85-6].
42. Soleiman HA, Ironside J, Kealey S, et al. Spinal subependymoma surgery: do no harm. Little may be more! Neurosurg Rev 2019. https://doi.org/10.1007/s10143-019-01128-x.
43. Celano E, Salehani A, Malcolm JG, et al. Spinal cord ependymoma: a review of the literature and case series of ten patients. J Neurooncol 2016; 128(3):377–86.
44. Plotkin SR, O'Donnell CC, Curry WT, et al. Spinal ependymomas in neurofibromatosis type 2: a retrospective analysis of 55 patients. J Neurosurg Spine 2011;14(4):543–7.
45. Coy S, Rashid R, Stemmer-Rachamimov A, et al. An update on the CNS manifestations of neurofibromatosis type 2. Acta Neuropathol 2019. https://doi.org/10.1007/s00401-019-02029-5.
46. Kalamarides M, Essayed W, Lejeune JP, et al. Spinal ependymomas in NF2: a surgical disease? J Neurooncol 2018;136(3):605–11.
47. Farschtschi S, Merker VL, Wolf D, et al. Bevacizumab treatment for symptomatic spinal ependymomas in neurofibromatosis type 2. Acta Neurol Scand 2016;133(6):475–80.
48. The response of spinal cord ependymomas to bevacizumab in patients with neurofibromatosis type 2. J Neurosurg Spine 2017;26(4):474–82.
49. Sun B, Wang C, Wang J, et al. MRI features of intramedullary spinal cord ependymomas. J Neuroimaging 2003;13(4):346–51.
50. Fanous AA, Jost GF, Schmidt MH. A nonenhancing world health organization grade ii intramedullary spinal ependymoma in the conus: case illustration and review of imaging characteristics. Global Spine J 2012;2(1):57–64.
51. Kahan H, Sklar EM, Post MJ, et al. MR characteristics of histopathologic subtypes of spinal ependymoma. AJNR Am J Neuroradiol 1996;17(1):143–50.
52. Dauleac C, Messerer R, Obadia-Andre N, et al. Cysts associated with intramedullary ependymomas of the spinal cord: clinical, MRI and oncological features. J Neurooncol 2019;144(2):385–91.
53. Akyurek S, Chang EL, Yu TK, et al. Spinal myxopapillary ependymoma outcomes in patients treated with surgery and radiotherapy at M.D. Anderson cancer center. J Neurooncol 2006;80(2):177–83.
54. Feldman WB, Clark AJ, Safaee M, et al. Tumor control after surgery for spinal myxopapillary ependymomas: distinct outcomes in adults versus children: a systematic review. J Neurosurg Spine 2013;19(4):471–6.
55. Harrop JS, Ganju A, Groff M, et al. Primary intramedullary tumors of the spinal cord. Spine (Phila Pa 1976) 2009;34(22 Suppl):S69–77.
56. Bostrom A, Kanther NC, Grote A, et al. Management and outcome in adult intramedullary spinal cord tumours: a 20-year single institution experience. BMC Res Notes 2014;7:908.
57. Bates JE, Peterson CR 3rd, Yeaney GA, et al. Spinal drop metastasis in myxopapillary ependymoma: a case report and a review of treatment options. Rare Tumors 2014;6(2):5404.
58. Fassett DR, Pingree J, Kestle JR. The high incidence of tumor dissemination in myxopapillary ependymoma in pediatric patients. Report of five cases and review of the literature. J Neurosurg 2005;102(1 Suppl):59–64.
59. Zhao C, Wang C, Zhang M, et al. Primary cerebellopontine angle ependymoma with spinal metastasis in an adult patient: a case report. Oncol Lett 2015;10(3):1755–8.
60. Chandra P, Purandare N, Shah S, et al. "Drop" metastases from an operated case of intracranial anaplastic ependymoma identified on fluoro-2-deoxyglucose positron emission tomography/computed tomography. Indian J Nucl Med 2017; 32(1):68–70.
61. Wostrack M, Ringel F, Eicker SO, et al. Spinal ependymoma in adults: a multicenter investigation of surgical outcome and progression-free survival. J Neurosurg Spine 2018;28(6):654–62.
62. Safaee M, Oh MC, Mummaneni PV, et al. Surgical outcomes in spinal cord ependymomas and the importance of extent of resection in children and young adults. J Neurosurg Pediatr 2014;13(4):393–9.
63. Chamberlain MC. Etoposide for recurrent spinal cord ependymoma. Neurology 2002;58(8):1310–1.

64. Shirato H, Kamada T, Hida K, et al. The role of radiotherapy in the management of spinal cord glioma. Int J Radiat Oncol Biol Phys 1995;33(2): 323–8.
65. Wen BC, Hussey DH, Hitchon PW, et al. The role of radiation therapy in the management of ependymomas of the spinal cord. Int J Radiat Oncol Biol Phys 1991;20(4):781–6.
66. Vera-Bolanos E, Aldape K, Yuan Y, et al. Clinical course and progression-free survival of adult intracranial and spinal ependymoma patients. Neuro Oncol 2015;17(3):440–7.
67. Carter M, Nicholson J, Ross F, et al. Genetic abnormalities detected in ependymomas by comparative genomic hybridisation. Br J Cancer 2002;86(6): 929–39.
68. Fakhrai N, Neophytou P, Dieckmann K, et al. Recurrent spinal ependymoma showing partial remission under Imatimib. Acta Neurochir (Wien) 2004; 146(11):1255–8.
69. Epari S, Bhatkar R, Moyaidi A, et al. Histomorphological spectrum and immunohistochemical characterization of hemangioblastomas: an entity of unclear histogenesis. Indian J Pathol Microbiol 2014;57(4):542–8.
70. Liu A, Jain A, Sankey EW, et al. Sporadic intramedullary hemangioblastoma of the spine: a single institutional review of 21 cases. Neurol Res 2016; 38(3):205–9.
71. Kiyofuji S, Graffeo CS, Yokoyama M, et al. Intramedullary and intratumoral hemorrhage in spinal hemangioblastoma: case report and review of literature. Surg Neurol Int 2018;9:250.
72. Sharma GK, Kucia EJ, Spetzler RF. Spontaneous intramedullary hemorrhage of spinal hemangioblastoma: case report. Neurosurgery 2009;65(3): E627–8 [discussion: E8].
73. Gluf WM, Dailey AT. Hemorrhagic intramedullary hemangioblastoma of the cervical spinal cord presenting with acute-onset quadriparesis: case report and review of the literature. J Spinal Cord Med 2014;37(6):791–4.
74. Filling-Katz MR, Choyke PL, Oldfield E, et al. Central nervous system involvement in Von Hippel-Lindau disease. Neurology 1991;41(1):41–6.
75. Chu BC, Terae S, Hida K, et al. MR findings in spinal hemangioblastoma: correlation with symptoms and with angiographic and surgical findings. AJNR Am J Neuroradiol 2001;22(1):206–17.
76. Miyagami M, Katayama Y. Long-term prognosis of hemangioblastomas of the central nervous system: clinical and immunohistochemical study in relation to recurrence. Brain Tumor Pathol 2004;21(2): 75–82.
77. Park CH, Lee CH, Hyun SJ, et al. Surgical outcome of spinal cord hemangioblastomas. J Korean Neurosurg Soc 2012;52(3):221–7.
78. Mehta GU, Asthagiri AR, Bakhtian KD, et al. Functional outcome after resection of spinal cord hemangioblastomas associated with von Hippel-Lindau disease. J Neurosurg Spine 2010;12(3): 233–42.
79. Mehta GU, Montgomery BK, Maggio DM, et al. Functional outcome after resection of von hippel-lindau disease-associated cauda equina hemangioblastomas: an observational cohort study. Oper Neurosurg (Hagerstown) 2017;13(4):435–40.
80. Sun HI, Ozduman K, Usseli MI, et al. Sporadic spinal hemangioblastomas can be effectively treated by microsurgery alone. World Neurosurg 2014; 82(5):836–47.
81. Biondi A, Ricciardi GK, Faillot T, et al. Hemangioblastomas of the lower spinal region: report of four cases with preoperative embolization and review of the literature. AJNR Am J Neuroradiol 2005;26(4):936–45.
82. Ghobrial GM, Liounakos J, Starke RM, et al. Surgical treatment of vascular intramedullary spinal cord lesions. Cureus 2018;10(8):e3154.
83. Saliou G, Giammattei L, Ozanne A, et al. Role of preoperative embolization of intramedullary hemangioblastoma. Neurochirurgie 2017;63(5): 372–5.
84. Pan J, Ho AL, D'Astous M, et al. Image-guided stereotactic radiosurgery for treatment of spinal hemangioblastoma. Neurosurg Focus 2017;42(1):E12.
85. Daly ME, Choi CY, Gibbs IC, et al. Tolerance of the spinal cord to stereotactic radiosurgery: insights from hemangioblastomas. Int J Radiat Oncol Biol Phys 2011;80(1):213–20.
86. Flanagan EP, O'Neill BP, Porter AB, et al. Primary intramedullary spinal cord lymphoma. Neurology 2011;77(8):784–91.
87. Bini Viotti J, Doblecki S, Luca CC, et al. Primary intramedullary spinal cord lymphoma presenting as a cervical ring-enhancing lesion in an AIDS patient. Open Forum Infect Dis 2018;5(6):ofy128.
88. Okuda T, Hata N, Suzuki SO, et al. Pediatric ganglioglioma with an H3 K27M mutation arising from the cervical spinal cord. Neuropathology 2018. https://doi.org/10.1111/neup.12471.
89. Deora H, Sumitra S, Nandeesh BN, et al. Spinal intramedullary ganglioglioma in children: an unusual location of a common pediatric tumor. Pediatr Neurosurg 2019;54(4):245–52.
90. Gessi M, Dorner E, Dreschmann V, et al. Intramedullary gangliogliomas: histopathologic and molecular features of 25 cases. Hum Pathol 2016;49: 107–13.
91. Lang FF, Epstein FJ, Ransohoff J, et al. Central nervous system gangliogliomas. Part 2: clinical outcome. J Neurosurg 1993;79(6):867–73.
92. Vongveeranonchai N, Zawahreh M, Strbian D, et al. Evaluation of a patient with spinal cord infarction

after a hypotensive episode. Stroke 2014;45(10): e203–5.
93. Lonser RR, Oldfield EH. Spinal cord hemangioblastomas. Neurosurg Clin N Am 2006;17(1):37–44.
94. Lonser RR, Oldfield EH. Microsurgical resection of spinal cord hemangioblastomas. Neurosurgery 2005;57(4 Suppl):372–6 [discussion: 6].
95. McCormick PC. Microsurgical resection of intramedullary spinal cord hemangioblastoma. Neurosurg Focus 2014;37(Suppl 2). https://doi.org/10.3171/2014.V3.FOCUS14306. Video 10.
96. Barzilai O, Lidar Z, Constantini S, et al. Continuous mapping of the corticospinal tracts in intramedullary spinal cord tumor surgery using an electrified ultrasonic aspirator. J Neurosurg Spine 2017; 27(2):161–8.
97. Forster MT, Marquardt G, Seifert V, et al. Spinal cord tumor surgery–importance of continuous intraoperative neurophysiological monitoring after tumor resection. Spine (Phila Pa 1976) 2012;37(16): E1001–8.
98. Cheng JS, Ivan ME, Stapleton CJ, et al. Intraoperative changes in transcranial motor evoked potentials and somatosensory evoked potentials predicting outcome in children with intramedullary spinal cord tumors. J Neurosurg Pediatr 2014; 13(6):591–9.
99. Sala F, Palandri G, Basso E, et al. Motor evoked potential monitoring improves outcome after surgery for intramedullary spinal cord tumors: a historical control study. Neurosurgery 2006;58(6):1129–43 [discussion: 43].
100. Quinones-Hinojosa A, Lyon R, Zada G, et al. Changes in transcranial motor evoked potentials during intramedullary spinal cord tumor resection correlate with postoperative motor function. Neurosurgery 2005;56(5):982–93 [discussion: 93].
101. Mehta AI, Mohrhaus CA, Husain AM, et al. Dorsal column mapping for intramedullary spinal cord tumor resection decreases dorsal column dysfunction. J Spinal Disord Tech 2012;25(4):205–9.
102. Kothbauer KF, Deletis V, Epstein FJ. Motor-evoked potential monitoring for intramedullary spinal cord tumor surgery: correlation of clinical and neurophysiological data in a series of 100 consecutive procedures. Neurosurg Focus 1998;4(5):e1.
103. Verla T, Fridley JS, Khan AB, et al. Neuromonitoring for intramedullary spinal cord tumor surgery. World Neurosurg 2016;95:108–16.
104. Costa P, Peretta P, Faccani G. Relevance of intraoperative D wave in spine and spinal cord surgeries. Eur Spine J 2013;22(4):840–8.
105. Setzer M, Murtagh RD, Murtagh FR, et al. Diffusion tensor imaging tractography in patients with intramedullary tumors: comparison with intraoperative findings and value for prediction of tumor resectability. J Neurosurg Spine 2010;13(3):371–80.
106. Hadjipanayis CG, Stummer W. 5-ALA and FDA approval for glioma surgery. J Neurooncol 2019; 141(3):479–86.
107. Millesi M, Kiesel B, Woehrer A, et al. Analysis of 5-aminolevulinic acid-induced fluorescence in 55 different spinal tumors. Neurosurg Focus 2014; 36(2):E11.
108. Inoue T, Endo T, Nagamatsu K, et al. 5-aminolevulinic acid fluorescence-guided resection of intramedullary ependymoma: report of 9 cases. Neurosurgery 2013;72(2 Suppl Operative): ons159–68 [discussion: ons68].
109. Eicker SO, Floeth FW, Kamp M, et al. The impact of fluorescence guidance on spinal intradural tumour surgery. Eur Spine J 2013;22(6):1394–401.
110. Ewelt C, Stummer W, Klink B, et al. Cordectomy as final treatment option for diffuse intramedullary malignant glioma using 5-ALA fluorescence-guided resection. Clin Neurol Neurosurg 2010;112(4): 357–61.

Surgical Strategies for Chordoma

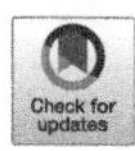

Michiel E.R. Bongers, MD[a,*], Nicolas Dea, MD, MSc, FRCSC[b], Christopher P. Ames, MD[c], Joseph H. Schwab, MD, MS[d]

KEYWORDS

• Chordoma • Resection • Recurrence • Principles • Surgery

KEY POINTS

- Chordomas are rare primary malignant bone neoplasms of the axial skeleton and account for 1% to 4% of all primary malignant bone tumors, with an incidence of 0.08 cases per 100,000 population.
- The best available evidence supports a more aggressive surgical approach to obtain negative margins; this approach is correlated with improved local control and improved survival.
- En bloc resection of chordoma requires multidisciplinary care and surgical planning.

INTRODUCTION

Chordomas are rare tumors of the axial skeleton whose slow growth belies a relentless tumor with a propensity for recurrence and late metastasis. Local control remains an issue with chordoma in spite of aggressive operative management. High local failure rates have led to the exploration of alternative methods of treatment. Radiation continues to gain acceptance as an adjuvant to surgery, and, in some cases, as a standalone treatment. Despite the growing body of radiation literature, operative management remains a commonly used approach in spite of the relatively high morbidity associated with en bloc resection and reconstruction techniques. Systemic therapy remains experimental, but several ongoing clinical trials offer hope for local and distant recurrence.

EPIDEMIOLOGY

Chordomas are rare primary malignant bone neoplasms believed to be derived from the remnants of the embryonic notochord.[1,2] They occur in the axial skeleton, where they are the most common primary bone malignancy. They account for 1% to 4% of all primary malignant bone tumors, with an incidence of 0.08 cases per 100,000 population.[3–6] Chordomas arise most commonly in the sacrum (50%), then the spheno-occipital bone (35%), and lastly the mobile spine (15%).[3,5] Incidence rates were published from a large population-based study; however, these numbers showed a relatively equal distribution (32% spheno-occipital, 33% mobile spine, 29% sacral).[5] Male patients are affected 1.6 times as much as female patients, which is consistent through all age groups.[1] The median age of patients with chordoma found in studies derived from the Surveillance, Epidemiology, and End Results (SEER) Program of the National Cancer Institute was 58.5 years and ranged from 3 to 95 years.[1,5] Genetic studies have shown that the T gene (brachyury) is likely involved in the pathogenesis of chordoma, as nearly every chordoma patient overexpresses this gene.[7,8] In the United

[a] Orthopaedic Oncology Service, Massachusetts General Hospital – Harvard Medical School, Yawkey Building, Room 3.550, 55 Fruit Street, Boston, MA 02114, USA; [b] Division of Spine Surgery, Vancouver General Hospital and the University of British Columbia, Blusson Spinal Cord Center, 6th Floor, 818 West 10th Avenue, Vancouver, British Columbia V5Z 1M9, Canada; [c] Department of Neurological Surgery, University of California, San Francisco, Medical Center, 400 Parnassus Avenue, San Francisco, CA 94143, USA; [d] Orthopaedic Oncology Service, Massachusetts General Hospital – Harvard Medical School, Yawkey Building, Room 3.922, 55 Fruit Street, Boston, MA 02114, USA
* Corresponding author.
E-mail address: michielbongers@gmail.com

Neurosurg Clin N Am 31 (2020) 251–261
https://doi.org/10.1016/j.nec.2019.11.007

States, Caucasians are most commonly affected by chordoma (92%).[5] One reason for the high incidence in Caucasians may be because of the high prevalence (47%) of a specific single-nucleotide polymorphism (SNP) of T Brachyury found in people from northern and western European descent, and thus this SNP might be of prognostic value for chordoma patients.[7] Furthermore, chordoma can have a familial component in some patients, since unique duplications of the T gene have been found in families with 3 or more chordoma cases.[9]

HISTOLOGIC SUBTYPES

Conventional chordoma is the most common subtype and it is characterized by clusters of epithelial cells surrounded by abundant myxoid, extracellular matrix. The cells often have a soap bubble appearance, and the term physaliferous has been applied to their appearance.[10] Lymphocytic infiltrates are found in chordoma, but they are usually constrained to the fibrous septae intervening between tumor lobules. Chondroid chordoma is another subtype that has focal areas of chondroid differentiation. This subtype was thought at one time to have a different phenotype, but the outcomes of chondroid chordomas have not been found to be appreciably different from conventional chordoma.[11] Dedifferentiated chordomas are aggressive tumors with areas of high-grade sarcomatous cells found adjacent to conventional histology. These tumors have a different behavior with high rates of early metastasis and death.[11,12] A third category designated poorly differentiated chordoma is also gaining acceptance. These tumors have not undergone frank dedifferentiation, yet the cells have a more aggressive phenotype than typically seen in conventional chordoma.

There is also a benign class of tumor that has been associated with chordoma, namely the benign notochordal cell tumor (BNCT).[13] These tumors have a sclerotic appearance on radiographs and computed tomography. They are most commonly devoid of soft tissue extension, but this is an area of controversy. One of the key histologic features of these tumors is the lack of myxoid extracellular matrix and epithelioid cells. BNCTs are thought to be benign. They have been found within conventional chordoma, however, and there is some speculation that these are precursors to chordoma.

MANAGEMENT BACKGROUND

Because chordomas most commonly arise in the sacrum, it is useful to focus on the sacrum to gather an understanding of why chordomas are often managed with aggressive surgery. Early reports on the outcomes of chordoma were universally poor. One can imagine the difficulty trying to manage a chordoma in the period before computed tomography or MRI that would make developing an effective operative strategy nearly impossible. It is important to note that surgical intensive care units (ICUs) and blood banking were not common for the better part of the 20th century, which also impeded operative management. For this reason, most chordomas were treated with intralesional subtotal resections often followed with palliative doses of radiation.[14] Recurrence was reported to be over 90%, which is not surprising given that most tumors were not actually removed completely. Unfortunately, recurrent chordoma in the sacrum can be a vexing problem, with progressive growth leading to loss of bowel and bladder function, and neglected tumors would often erode through the skin, leading to pain and foul-smelling wounds. Patients often suffered for long periods of time with these unsolvable problems. Faced with these outcomes, Bertil Stener, from Göteborg, Sweden, began taking a more aggressive approach advocating for en bloc removal of the sacrum.[14] Mid to high sacrectomy would lead to loss of bowel, bladder, and sexual function. However, Stener must have been chastened by what he had witnessed in patients after intralesional resection in order to offer such a radical approach.[15] Although the concept of en bloc resection gained acceptance, it became clear that the morbidity and mortality associated with high sacrectomy was a formidable problem. Still, the data in support of obtaining negative margins were compelling in the short term with improved local control seen in patients treated with en bloc resection and negative margins.[16] More recently, however, data have emerged that suggest that wide resection alone does not guarantee local control. A recent study from 2 large referral centers highlighted the outcomes of 99 cases of primary chordoma in the sacrum. Two issues emerged. First, wide resection was obtained in only roughly 50% of cases and, more importantly, disease-free survival was only 50% at 10 years even after wide resection.[17] Questions naturally arise with these data, and one must wonder why a tumor recurs even after a wide resection. The answer may lie in a report from Japan demonstrating the presence of tumor cells, so-called skip metastases, found outside the main mass of the tumor.[18] These skip metastases were found up to 2 cm outside the main mass, and they were present in 43% of cases. The presence of skip metastases was associated with poor local control in that series.

RADIATION THERAPY

Chordomas have often been regarded to be unresponsive to radiation therapy. However, most historic reports reveal relatively low doses of radiation (< 50 Gy) being used in the salvage setting. It is known that salvaging a recurrent chordoma is difficult in the best circumstances and the use of radiation seemed to have been reserved for these circumstances. It is also accepted that lower doses of radiation are not an effective strategy for chordoma. However, advances in the delivery of radiation have allowed the dose of radiation to be escalated. Doses of over 70 Gy have been advocated by some including Massachusetts General Hospital (MGH). Over time, MGH began to accumulate an experience with using high-dose radiation as an adjuvant to surgery, with outcomes comparing favorably to historical reports.[19] The radiation used at MGH is proton based, which takes advantage of favorable distribution patterns inherent in protons, namely a high dose concentration at the tumor with no exit dose. These factors decrease the off-target impact of radiation, allowing one to increase the dose. More recently, carbon ion radiation has gained acceptance in the management of chordoma. Again, the use of carbon ions takes advantage of the properties inherent in carbon ions to escalate the dose of radiation.[20] Advances in the delivery of photon radiation have also allowed the dosage of radiation to be escalated, and hypofractionated dosing schedules have been advocated to increase the biologic effective dose.[21,22] Local control rates with these various forms of radiation have been more promising within the last 10 years with all 3 methods of radiation both as an adjuvant to surgery and as a standalone treatment. Initially, the morbidity of radiation alone is superior to what one can expect from surgery. It is unclear what the long-term results of radiation will be on nerve function, but it has not been reported be a problem in most patients with the short to mid-term follow up. Similarly, local control rates with radiation alone are promising with short to mid-term follow. Again, it is imperative that patients with chordoma are followed for long periods of time, as chordomas are known to recur much later than most of malignant bone tumors. The uncertainties on the most appropriate treatment of chordoma, with or without radiation, reflects in a management heterogeneity across centers around the world.[23]

PRINCIPLES OF RESECTION

In 1980, the Enneking classification was introduced for patients with primary malignant tumors of the appendicular skeleton.[24] This principle resulted in improvement of local control and increased survival in these patients.[25] Hereafter, this led to the application of the Enneking classification for treatment of primary malignant tumors of the axial skeleton. Because several studies have shown that local recurrence rates decreased and survival rates improved following spinal tumor resection with negative margins, the main goal of surgery became to achieve negative margins confirmed by the musculoskeletal pathology department.[25–32] Based on a combination of tumor grade, tumor extent, and whether or not metastases exist, a surgical margin has been recommended for optimal local control.[33] Because of the malignant nature of chordoma, these tumors should all undergo a wide resection when following the principles of the Enneking classification.[24,25,33] However, the concept of wide margin may be less applicable in the spine, where marginal resection is most common. If marginal or wide margins are obtained, the resection can be called Enneking appropriate (EA); if the surgery resulted in intralesional or contaminated margins, the resection may be termed Enneking inappropriate (EI).[25,28,33] However, as mentioned earlier, recently published literature shows that micro-skip metastases, which are undetectable by current imaging methods, can occur at up to 20 mm from the main tumor.[18] Importantly, skip metastases have only been studied in 1 paper and only in the sacrum. It is unclear if this same concept applies to mobile spine. Nonetheless, despite the concept of skip metastases, the best available evidence supports a more aggressive surgical approach to treat these tumors, and obtaining a negative margin is correlated with improved LC and improved survival.[16,25,32] Evidence-based oncologic principles should therefore be followed until better long-term results from other treatment modalities are available. However, achieving these margins entails a higher morbidity and increased sacrifice of neurologic function. Thus, patient preference should always play a key role in the treatment of these patients.

Operative Considerations

Mobile spine

In the mobile spine, the gold standard for surgical treatment is en bloc spondylectomy including a surrounding layer of healthy soft tissue. Depending on the location of the tumor, several considerations need to be made while planning for surgery.

In the cervical spine, caution must be taken to the many important and adjacent anatomic structures. If functional cervical spinal nerve roots will be removed with the planned operation, the expected loss of motor and sensory function should be discussed including options for correction of the expected deficits, such as tendon transfers. One important vascular structure to consider is the vertebral artery, which travels bilaterally through the foramen transversarium typically beginning at C6 to merge with the contralateral branch to form the basilar artery once it passes through the foramen magnum. Thus, establishing tumor involvement of the vertebral artery in these patients should be included in the preoperative work-up. In addition to preoperative MRI, an angiogram should be performed to determine dominance of the vertebral artery and sufficient collateral blood blow from the uninvolved vertebral artery. High cervical atlantoaxial (C1-2) tumors, which frequently involve at least one of the vertebral arteries, are often more difficult to access than the subaxial spine. Trans- or submandibular approaches are frequently required to expose these tumors. One study shows that these high-cervical surgeries result in more violated margins, higher complication rates, and increased tumor recurrence, as opposed to subaxial resections.[34] The location of the esophagus relative to the tumor is also an important consideration. If one is considering radiation, either as an adjuvant or as a standalone treatment, the esophagus may limit the amount of radiation that can be delivery safely. It is important to discuss the possibility of needing tube feeds and or tracheostomy in the short term after en bloc resection near the trachea and esophagus.

Case example 1 The first case describes the treatment of a cervical chordoma.

A 55-year-old man presented with a large left anterior cervical mass biopsy confirmed to be chordoma. On MRI, the mass involved the anterior segments of C2 to C4, eccentric to the left (**Fig. 1**). The tumor encased the C3 and C4 nerve root and the left vertebral artery. With goals of an en bloc resection, a 2-stage approach was taken. First the patient underwent a posterior approach for an occiput to T2 fusion with posterior column release. Specifically, laminectomy and bilateral fasciectomy were performed to expose the C2 to C5 spinal cord and nerve roots. The left C3 and C4 nerve roots were ligated. The left vertebral artery was tied off superior and inferior to the tumor (**Fig. 2**A). The patient then returned to the operating room for an anterior lateral approach via an oblique incision under the mandible. A combined transcervical and transmandibular approach was taken in order to gain adequate access to the tumor and surrounding structures (**Fig. 2**B). First a discectomy at C4-5 was performed, and osteotomy cuts were made vertically from C4 superiorly into the inferior portion of the C2 body. Then a horizontal osteotomy was made at C2. The tumor was then dissected free and delivered en bloc as a single unit (**Fig. 2**C, D). The anterior column was reconstructed with an expandable cage and anterior plate (**Fig. 3**). At 2-year follow-up, the patient was tumor free and without mechanical complications (**Fig. 4**).

The upper thoracic spine poses a particular problem, because access is complicated by the presence of functional nerve roots, the esophagus, and the great vessels. Collaboration with thoracic surgery is an important component of operative planning in these cases. Sternotomy or sternothoracotomy may be necessary depending on the extent of the tumor. The nerve roots in the mid-thoracic and lower thoracic spine can usually be sacrificed. However, angiography should be considered to help localize the dominant blood supply to the spinal cord. Spinal cord infarction is possible if the dominant artery is disrupted by removing the segmental vessel being used as a conduit. However, an animal model has shown that removal of the dominant spinal artery and the adjacent sets of segmental arteries can be done safely. The animal model did reveal a drop in the blood supply to the spinal cord with

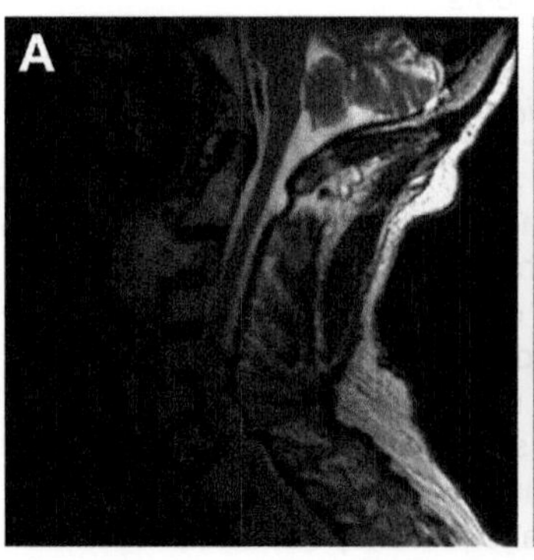

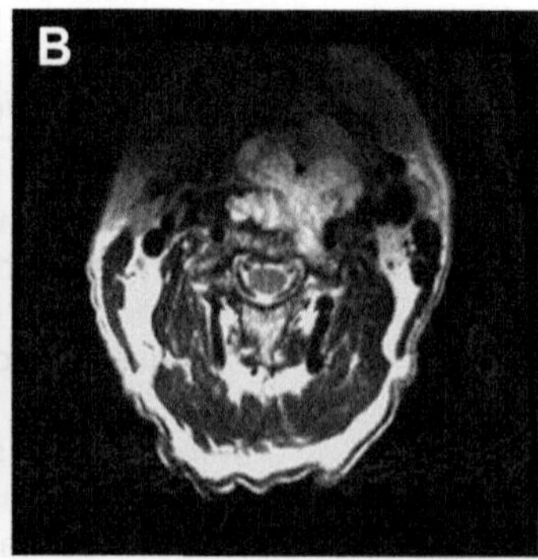

Fig. 1. *(A)* Saggital T2 weighed MRI image of C2-C4 lesion. *(B) Axial* T2 weighed MRI image of C2-C4 lesion.

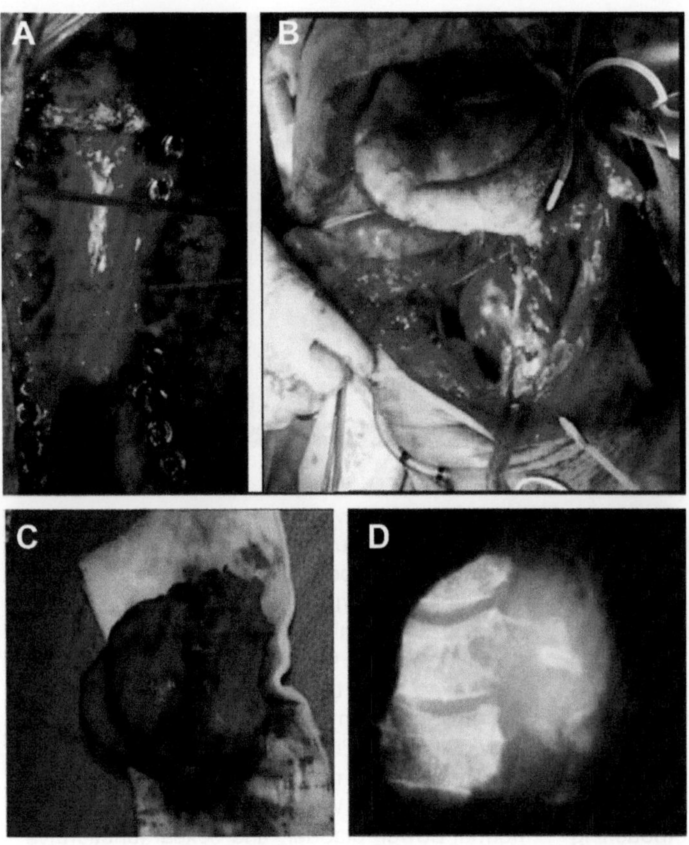

Fig. 2. Intraoperative images of the en bloc resection of the cervical chordoma. (*A*) Vertebral artery is tied off superior and inferior to the tumor. (*B*) Combined transcervical and transmandibular approach using an oblique incision to access the tumor. (*C*) En bloc resected specimen. (*D*) Saggital X-ray of the en bloc resected specimen.

resection of the 3 sets of segmental roots, but it did not correlate with a functional deficit in their dog model.[35,36] The same group followed this with a cases series, where they had knowingly sacrificed the dominant artery and the 2 adjacent roots without having a postoperative deficit.[37] Still,

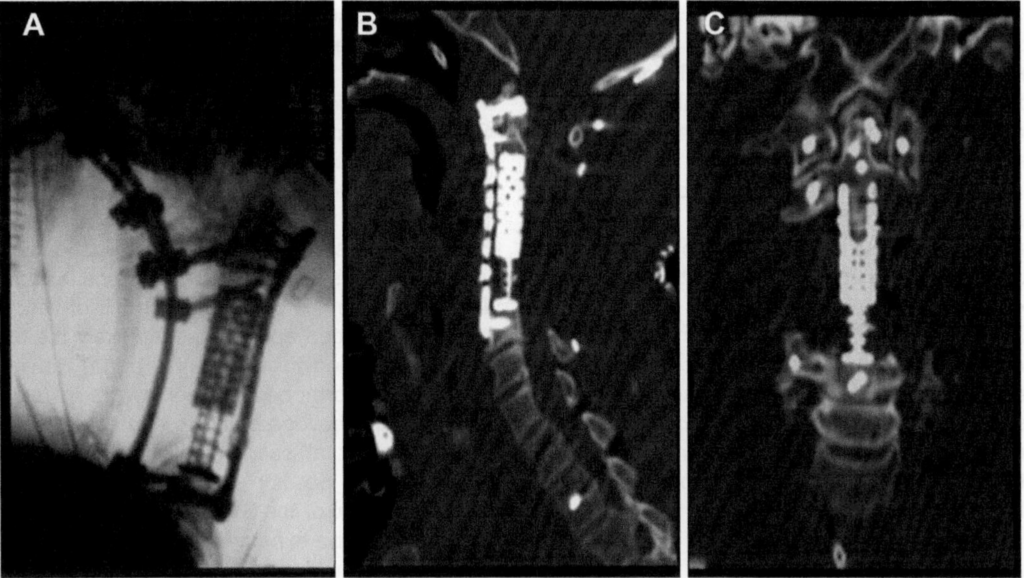

Fig. 3. Anterior column reconstruction using an expandable cage and an anterior plate. (*A*) Saggital fluoroscopic image of instrumentation. (*B*) Saggital CT image of instrumentation. (*C*) Coronal CT image of instrumentation.

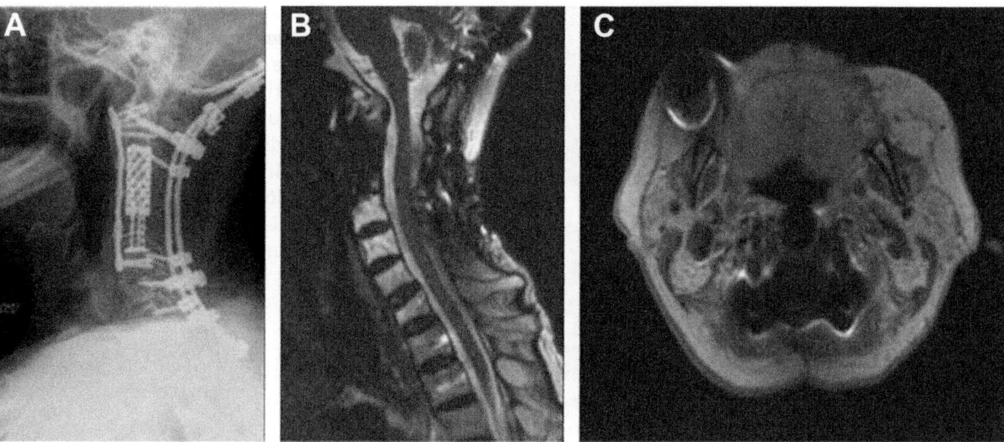

Fig. 4. Radiological imaging at 2 years follow-up.

one must discuss the risks associated with these procedures with the patient. This is particularly true in cases where the spinal cord blood supply may already be compromised, such as in patients with vascular or renal disease or in cases of spinal cord compression.

Thoracic nerve root ligation will have less functional impact compared with the cervical spine, as they innervate muscles of the chest wall and abdomen. Because of abdominal wall denervation, patients often complain of an outpouching of the flank when the lower thoracic roots are excised for tumor removal. The location of the azygous vein and aorta must also be identified, and management of these vessels must be part of the operative plan.

In the lumbar spine, the ligation of nerve roots again becomes more critical, as most exiting nerve roots have their dermatomes in the lower extremities and are also involved in ambulation. Several biomechanical considerations should similarly be taken. First, as the vertebra descend, the weight they need to support increases. Second, the lumbar spine has a much larger range of motion than the thoracic spine. This means that a reconstruction method following resection should be able to withstand more than only the longitudinal forces. The flexion, extension, and torsion to which this part of the body is subject to must also be controlled. The operative plan should include a method for managing vena cava, aorta, and iliac vessels. The ureters are at risk during resection, and placement of stents prior to surgery can help mitigate the risk of inadvertent ligation of the ureter during surgery.

Sacrum

Planning for sacral resection involves deciding where the sacrum must be transected. This is dictated by the tumor, and it has implications on the approach, potential pitfalls, and expected functional outcomes. For instance, a tumor in the coccyx can usually be removed without loss of bowel or bladder function. However, large tumors emanating from the coccyx may compress the rectum, and one must content with this during surgery. Similarly, distal sacral tumors that do not involve S2 or S3 nor the exiting pudendal nerves can be removed with an expectation of relatively normal bowel, bladder, and sexual function.[38–40] These tumors can often be removed from a posterior approach only.[41,42] Because the internal iliac vessels are left intact, one can expect a viable gluteus maximus, and advancing these muscles medially can be an effective means of closure should the situation call for soft tissue reconstruction. These distal tumors are below the large vessels of the pelvis and can usually be removed without risking major vascular injury.

Removing higher sacral tumors that involve the S2 and S3 nerve roots will lead to loss of bowel or bladder function and sexual function.[38] The iliac vessels may be at risk during these approaches, and one must have a plan to content with them. Some favor a staged approach with ligation of the internal iliac vessels followed by a prone resection. Total sacrectomies carry a higher risk of vascular injury, and staged approaches are likely the most common method to manage the aorta. However, Guo and his orthopedic oncology group use an intraoperative balloon pump to decrease bleeding during their total sacrectomies, which they do from a prone position only. Total sacrectomies involve removal of the S1 nerve roots, and plantar flexion should be expected to be weak. One must also suspect that loss of the L5 nerve root, at least functionally, may also occur during resection, leading to dorsiflexion weakness and hip abductor weakness. The soft tissue defect left after total sacrectomy also must be contented with for 2 reasons. First, wound healing is a notorious problem after total sacrectomy, and second, bowel herniation can be a problem if one does not fill the defect.[43,44] One method to do this is to use a tunneled, rectus abdominus, myocutaneous flap.[45]

Case example 2 The second case is that of a recurrent sacral chordoma.

The patient had had an intralesional resection several years earlier and now presents with recurrence along with bowel and bladder dysfunction. The T2 axial and sagittal MRI images shown in **Fig. 5** reveal that the tumor appears to be relatively small with soft tissue extension anteriorly. However, on closer inspection one notes that a lobule of tumor extends nearly to the L5-S1 disc space in the spinal canal. In addition, further assessment of the piriformis muscle in **Fig. 5**A reveals that the tumor extends along the fibers of the muscle as is often the case. One must keep in mind the recent data suggesting that there may be skip metastases and total removal of the piriformis muscle should be planned in this case. The mass abuts the rectum, and one can expect scarring between the tumor and the rectum because of the previous surgery. This should be taken into consideration when one is deciding whether to remove the rectum with the tumor. In this case, the decision was made to remove the rectum with the tumor and to perform a colostomy. As part of their multidisciplinary plan for this patient ,the authors consulted their colleagues in radiation oncology. The authors applied their protocol, which involves 50.4 Gy of proton/photon radiation followed by 30 days rest before stage en bloc resection. This would then be followed up with 19.8 Gy of radiation for a total dose of 70.2 Gy. The protocol utilizes radiation to the gross tumor but also to areas outside the gross tumor including the upper sacrum and lower lumbar spine. The lateral pelvis/supra-acetabulum would also receive radiation. The authors' plan involves removing the entire sacrum with bony cuts lateral to the sacroiliac joints and through the L5-S1 disc space. One must decide whether to reconstruct the bony defect left after the resection. The authors felt that reconstruction made sense in this setting, as they had concern for spinopelvic instability without an osseous connection left between these structures. However, because this patient is being treated with radiation, it was determined that a biologic reconstruction made sense given the known deleterious impact radiation has on bone structure.[46] The authors decided to use a vascularized fibular graft to reconstruct the pelvis. This complicates the surgical plan, since the patient will be prone during the second stage when the tumor will be removed. The authors decided to add a third day of surgery to allow for appropriate positioning of the patient to harvest the vascularized graft.

Stage 1 involved multiple surgeons including colorectal surgery who performed a colostomy. Plastic surgery mobilized the rectus abdominus myocutaneous flap in preparation for pulling it through on stage 2. Colleagues in urology placed stents to aid in identification of the ureters during surgery and thereby helping to protect them from injury. Vascular surgery colleagues mobilized the great vessels and ligated the internal iliac vessels. Also during stage 1, the authors utilized navigation to help guide osteotomies lateral to sacral iliac joint. This involved lateral dissection into the iliacus muscle with identification of the L5 and S1 nerve roots as well as the obturator nerve. The authors made their bony cuts with a 6 mm diamond tip burr. The diamond burr minimized bony bleeding by cauterizing the bone as it works via friction. The authors also removed the L5-S1 disc space.

After making bony cuts, the authors placed a sheet of Gore-Tex dorsal to the great vessels in order to provide an additional measure of safety during stage 2. The patient was then transferred to the ICU for monitoring and stage 2 was planned for 72 hours later.

During stage 2 the patient was positioned prone on a spinal table with the abdomen free. The authors placed the legs in a sling in order to access to the perineum, as the anus was removed with the specimen. A large soft tissue envelop including skin was removed with the tumor (**Fig. 6**). The

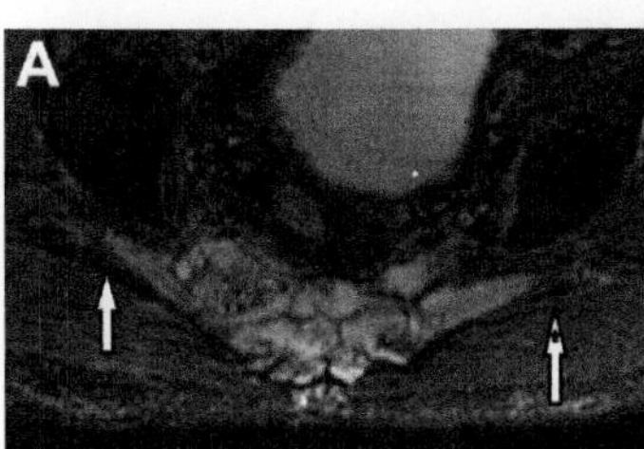

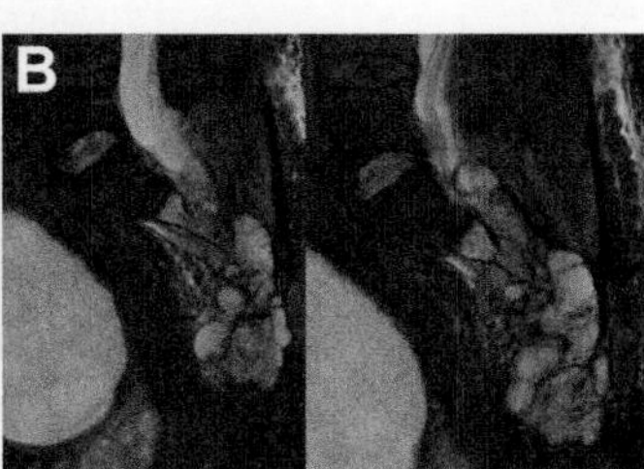

Fig. 5. (*A*) Axial T2 weighed MRI image of recurrent sacral chordoma. The arrows show tumor extension along the fibers of the periformis muscle. (*B*) Sagittal T2 weighed MRI image of recurrent sacral chordoma.

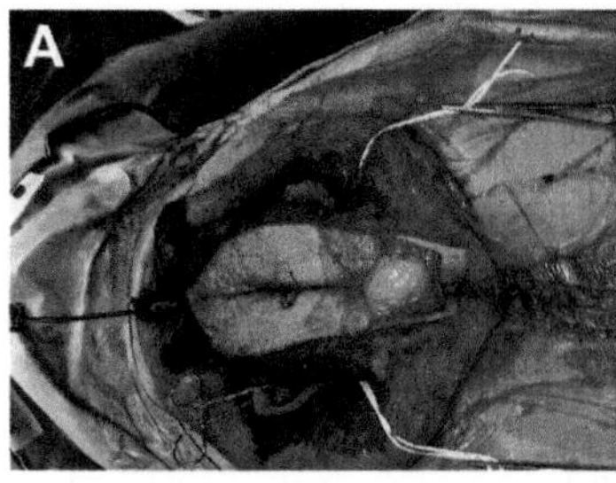
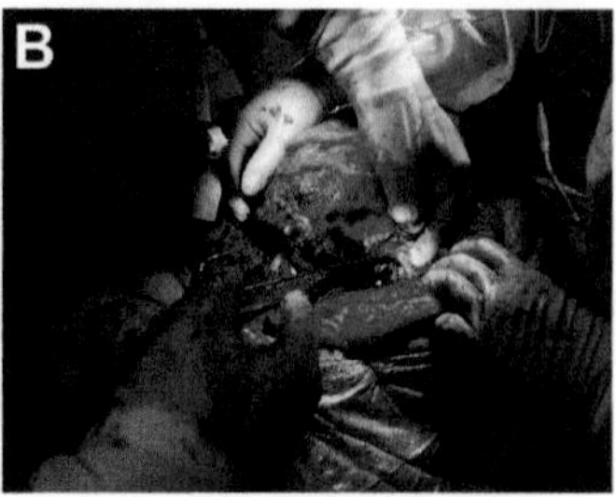

Fig. 6. (*A*) Posterior exposure of sacral chordoma. (*B*) Ligation of the piriformis muscle during sacral chordoma excision.

sciatic nerves were identified, and the piriformis muscle is detached from its insertion into the greater trochanter. Further dissection was carried out whereby the external rotators of the hip were incised allowing visualization of the sacral spine and lateral side wall of the pelvis. The sacral spinous and tuberous ligaments were removed from their bony attachments on the ischium. Dissection was carried ventral to the anus and circumferentially around the anus. Lateral dissection, with protection of the sciatic nerve, allows one to meet up with the plane developed lateral to the rectum in stage 1. Lumbar laminectomy was performed, and the thecal sac was ligated at the level of the L5-S1 disc with the S1 roots removed with the tumor. Navigation was again used during stage 2 to allow an osteotomy to be performed in the ilium aiming for the osteotomy made in stage 1. Once the bone cuts were made, the tumor could gently be tipped dorsally, allowing for better visualization of the anterior structures. The Gore-Tex sheet was encountered at this point. This allowed the authors to ligate further soft tissue pelvis attachments more safely. Once the tumor was resected, the authors assessed the margins grossly with the pathologist, and microscopic margins were also assessed for areas that appeared close. In this case, the authors placed a wound VAC in preparation for stage 3 reconstruction.

Stage 3 started in the supine position for vascularized fibular graft harvest by the authors' colleagues in plastic surgery. The patient was subsequently placed prone, and spinal pelvic fixation was performed. The vascularized graft was cut at an angle (**Fig. 7**) in order to facilitate placement into the caudal endplate of L5 (**Fig. 8**). The other ends of the graft were placed into a small cut into the supra-acetabular region. Once the graft was in place, it was held in place by compressing the spinal pelvic rods. The vascular anastomosis was then carried out by plastic surgery as well as closure by advancing the rectus flap. Final margins were negative. The patient does not have dorsiflexion of his ankles nor plantarflexion of his ankles, and he spent 6 weeks in the hospital before going to a rehabilitation center for another 6 weeks. The morbidity of these procedures cannot be taken lightly, and frank conversation about this can only hope to begin to inform patients about the undertaking with which they are involved.

Quality of life

Quality of life is a personal issue, and what one person will accept another will not. Issues with quality of life are particularly important when one discusses sacral tumors where loss of bowel, bladder, and sexual function can be life-changing events. This loss of function is seen primarily

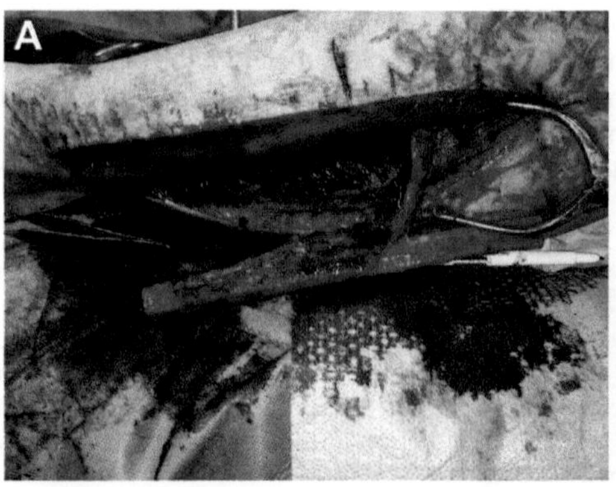
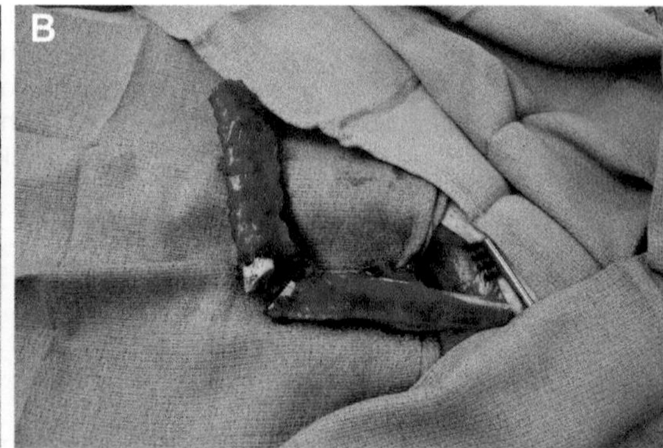

Fig. 7. (*A*) Harvest of the vascularized fibula graft. (*B*) Vascularized fibular graft cut to size and cut in the preferred angle for docking.

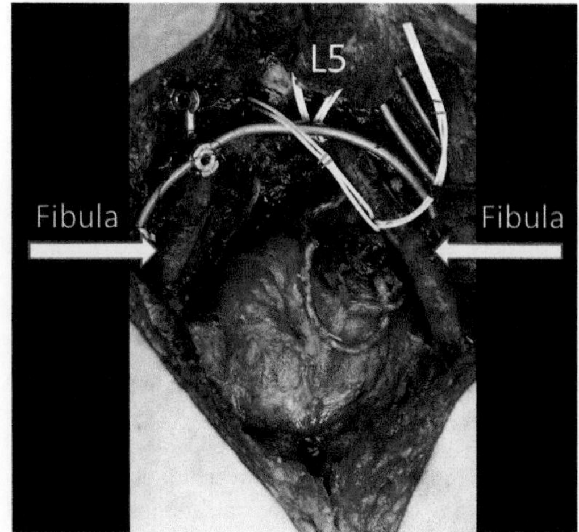

Fig. 8. Inserted and anastomosed vascularized fibula graft docking into the caudal endplate of L5 and earlier performed cuts in the supra-acetabular region bilaterally, with additional instrumentation.

when the S2 and S3 roots or their terminal branches in the pudendal nerve are incised.[47] Several studies have documented the loss of function related to these issues.[39,48,49] It has been shown that the health-related quality of life often recuperates to close to normal values with increasing follow-up, but decreases with disease recurrence.[44] However, the quality-of-life measures do not fully capture the loss of independence some patients express after these operations. The life changes are felt in having to consider how to manage self-catheterization or bowel continence when one is making plans. Quality of life is generally higher in patients who undergo resection of tumors in the mobile spine, but, up to 15% of patients report severe pain and severe impairment of their daily activities. The changes in quality of life are acceptable given the alternative of no treatment, but when compared with radiation alone, some patients opt for the latter.[50]

DISCLOSURE

The authors have nothing to disclose.

REFERENCES

1. Smoll NR, Gautschi OP, Radovanovic I, et al. Incidence and relative survival of chordomas: the standardized mortality ratio and the impact of chordomas on a population. Cancer 2013;119(11): 2029–37.
2. Yakkioui Y, van Overbeeke JJ, Santegoeds R, et al. Chordoma: the entity. Biochim Biophys Acta 2014; 1846(2):655–69.
3. Sundaresan N. Chordomas. Clin Orthop Relat Res 1986;204:135–42.
4. Gokaslan ZL, Zadnik PL, Sciubba DM, et al. Mobile spine chordoma: results of 166 patients from the AOSpine Knowledge Forum Tumor database. J Neurosurg Spine 2016;24(4):644–51.
5. McMaster ML, Goldstein AM, Bromley CM, et al. Chordoma: incidence and survival patterns in the United States, 1973-1995. Cancer Causes Control 2001;12(1):1–11.
6. Fabbri N, Ruggieri P. Chordoma. In: Picci P, Manfrini M, Fabbri N, et al, editors. Atlas of musculoskeletal tumors and tumorlike lesions. Switzerland: Springer International Publishing; 2014. p. 233–8.
7. Bettegowda C, Yip S, Lo S-FL, et al. Spinal column chordoma: prognostic significance of clinical variables and T (brachyury) gene SNP rs2305089 for local recurrence and overall survival. Neuro Oncol 2017;19(3):405–13.
8. Vujovic S, Henderson S, Presneau N, et al. Brachyury, a crucial regulator of notochordal development, is a novel biomarker for chordomas. J Pathol 2006;209:157–65.
9. Yang XR, Ng D, Alcorta DA, et al. T (brachyury) gene duplication confers major susceptibility to familial chordoma. Nat Genet 2009;41(11):1176–8.
10. Nielsen GP, Rosenberg AE. Notochordal tumors; chordoma. In: Nielsen GP, Rosenberg AE, Deshpande V, et al, editors. Diagnostic pathology. Bone. 1st edition. Altona (Canada): Amirsys Publishing; 2013. p. 9–15.
11. Shih AR, Cote GM, Chebib I, et al. Clinicopathologic characteristics of poorly differentiated chordoma. Mod Pathol 2018;31:1237–45.
12. Chugh R, Tawbi H, Lucas DR, et al. Chordoma: the nonsarcoma primary bone tumor. Oncologist 2007; 12(11):1344–50.
13. Nielsen GP, Rosenberg AE. Notochordal tumors: benign notochardal cell tumor. In: Nielsen GP, Rosenberg AE, Deshpande V, et al, editors. Diagnostic pathology. Bone. 1st edition. Altona (Canada): Amirsys Publishing; 2013. p. 4–7.
14. Eriksson B, Gunterberg B, Kindblom L, et al. A clinicopathologic and prognostic study of a Swedish national series. Acta Orthop Scand 1981;52(1):49–58.
15. Stener B, Gunterberg B. High amputation of the sacrum for extirpation of tumors. Principles and technique. Spine (Phila Pa 1976) 1978;3(4): 351–66.
16. Fuchs B, Dickey ID, Yaszemski MJ, et al. Operative management of sacral chordoma. J Bone Joint Surg Am 2005;87(10):2211–6.
17. Radaelli S, Stacchiotti S, Ruggieri P, et al. Sacral chordoma: long-term outcome of a large series of

patients surgically treated at two reference centers. Spine (Phila Pa 1976) 2016;41(12):1049–57.
18. Akiyama T, Ogura K, Gokita T, et al. Analysis of the infiltrative features of chordoma: the relationship between micro-skip metastasis and postoperative outcomes. Ann Surg Oncol 2018;25:912–9.
19. Delaney TF, Liebsch NJ, Pedlow FX, et al. Long-term results of phase II study of high dose photon/proton radiotherapy in the management of spine chordomas, chondrosarcomas, and other sarcomas. J Surg Oncol 2014;110(2):115–22.
20. Imai R, Kamada T, Araki N, Working Group for Bone and Soft Tissue Sarcomas. Carbon ion radiation therapy for unresectable sacral chordoma: an analysis of 188 cases. Int J Radiat Oncol Biol Phys 2016; 95(1):322–7.
21. Pennicooke B, Laufer I, Sahgal A, et al. Safety and local control of radiation therapy for chordoma of the spine and sacrum: a systematic review. Spine (Phila Pa 1976) 2016;41(Suppl 2):S186–92.
22. Jin CJ, Berry-Candelario J, Reiner AS, et al. Long-term outcomes of high-dose single-fraction radiosurgery for chordomas of the spine and sacrum. J Neurosurg Spine 2019;1–10.
23. Dea N, Fisher CG, Reynolds JJ, et al. Current treatment strategy for newly diagnosed chordoma of the mobile spine and sacrum: results of an international survey. J Neurosurg Spine 2018;30(1):119–25.
24. Enneking WF, Spanier SS, Goodman MA. A system for the surgical staging of musculoskeletal sarcoma. Clin Orthop Relat Res 1980;153:106–20.
25. Fisher CG, Saravanja DD, Dvorak MF, et al. Surgical management of primary bone tumors of the spine: validation of an approach to enhance cure and reduce local recurrence. Spine (Phila Pa 1976) 2011;36(10):830–6.
26. Schwab J, Gasbarrini A, Bandiera S, et al. Osteosarcoma of the mobile spine. Spine (Phila Pa 1976) 2012;37(6):E381–6.
27. Boriani S, Gasbarrini A, Bandiera S, et al. En bloc resections in the spine: the experience of 220 patients during 25 years. World Neurosurg 2017;98:217–29.
28. Pombo B, Cristina Ferreira A, Cardoso P, et al. Clinical effectiveness of Enneking appropriate versus Enneking inappropriate procedure in patients with primary osteosarcoma of the spine: a systematic review with meta-analysis. Eur Spine J 2019;1:3.
29. Colangeli S, Muratori F, Bettini L, et al. Surgical treatment of sacral chordoma: en bloc resection with negative margins is a determinant of the long-term outcome. Surg Technol Int 2018;33:343–8.
30. Dekutoski MB, Clarke MJ, Rose P, et al. Osteosarcoma of the spine: prognostic variables for local recurrence and overall survival, a multicenter ambispective study. J Neurosurg Spine 2016;25(1):59–68.
31. Talac R, Yaszemski MJ, Currier BL, et al. Relationship between surgical margins and local recurrence in sarcomas of the spine. Clin Orthop Relat Res 2002;397:127–32.
32. Le Charest-Morin R, Fisher CG, Sahgal A, et al. Primary bone tumor of the spine-an evolving field: what a general spine surgeon should know. Global Spine J 2019;9(1S):108–16.
33. Dea N, Gokaslan Z, Choi D, et al. Spine oncology - primary spine tumors. Neurosurgery 2017;80(3S): S124–30.
34. Molina CA, Ames CP, Chou D, et al. Outcomes following attempted en bloc resection of cervical chordomas in the C-1 and C-2 region versus the subaxial region: a multiinstitutional experience. J Neurosurg Spine 2014;21(3):348–56.
35. Nambu K, Kawahara N, Kobayashi T, et al. Interruption of the bilateral segmental arteries at several levels: influence on vertebral blood flow. Spine (Phila Pa 1976) 2004;29(14):1530–4.
36. Kato S, Kawahara N, Tomita K, et al. Effects on spinal cord blood flow and neurologic function secondary to interruption of bilateral segmental arteries which supply the artery of Adamkiewicz: an experimental study using a dog model. Spine (Phila Pa 1976) 2008;33(14):1533–41.
37. Murakami H, Kawahara N, Demura S, et al. Neurological function after total en bloc spondylectomy for thoracic spinal tumors. J Neurosurg Spine 2010;12(3):253–6.
38. Todd LT, Yaszemski MJ, Currier BL, et al. Bowel and bladder function after major sacral resection. Clin Orthop Relat Res 2002;475(397):36–9.
39. van Wulfften Palthe ODR, Houdek MT, Rose PS, et al. How does the level of nerve root resection in en bloc sacrectomy influence patient-reported outcomes? Clin Orthop Relat Res 2017;475(3): 607–16.
40. Moran D, Zadnik PL, Taylor T, et al. Maintenance of bowel, bladder, and motor functions after sacrectomy. Spine J 2015;15(2):222–9.
41. Fourney DR, Rhines LD, Hentschel SJ, et al. En bloc resection of primary sacral tumors: classification of surgical approaches and outcome. J Neurosurg Spine 2005;3(2):111–22.
42. Ruggieri P, Angelini A, Ussia G, et al. Surgical margins and local control in resection of sacral chordomas. Clin Orthop Relat Res 2010;468(11):2939–47.
43. Charest-Morin R, Flexman AM, Srinivas S, et al. Perioperative adverse events following surgery for primary bone tumors of the spine and en bloc resection for metastases. J Neurosurg Spine 2019;1–8.
44. Dea N, Charest-Morin R, Sciubba DM, et al. Optimizing the adverse event and HRQOL profiles in the management of primary spine tumors. Spine (Phila Pa 1976) 2016;41(Suppl 2):S212–7.
45. Schwab JH, Healey JH, Rose P, et al. The surgical management of sacral chordomas. Spine (Phila Pa 1976) 2009;34(24):2700–4.

46. van Wulfften Palthe O, Jee K-W, Bramer JAM, et al. What is the effect of high-dose radiation on bone in patients with sacral chordoma? A CT study. Clin Orthop Relat Res 2018;476(3):520–8.
47. Phukan R, Herzog T, Boland PJ, et al. How does the level of sacral resection for primary malignant bone tumors affect physical and mental health, pain, mobility, incontinence, and sexual function? Clin Orthop Relat Res 2016;474(3):687–96.
48. van Wulfften Palthe ODR, Janssen SJ, Wunder JS, et al. What questionnaires to use when measuring quality of life in sacral tumor patients: the updated sacral tumor survey. Spine J 2017;17(5):636–44.
49. Schwab JH, Janssen SJ, Paulino Pereira NR, et al. Quality of life after resection of a chordoma of the mobile spine. Bone Joint J 2017;99-B(7):979–86.
50. Chen Y-L, Liebsch N, Kobayashi W, et al. Definitive high-dose photon/proton radiotherapy for unresected mobile spine and sacral chordomas. Spine (Phila Pa 1976) 2013;38(15):E930–6.

Radiation Strategies for Spine Chordoma

Proton Beam, Carbon Ions, and Stereotactic Body Radiation Therapy

David J. Konieczkowski, MD, PhD[a], Thomas F. DeLaney, MD[b], Yoshiya (Josh) Yamada, MD, FRCPC[c,*]

KEYWORDS

• Chordoma • Carbon • Proton • Stereotactic body radiation therapy • Stereotactic radiosurgery • Spine • Sacrum

KEY POINTS

- Surgery alone provides inadequate local control (LC) of spine and sacral chordomas.
- Dose-escalated radiotherapy (RT) with protons, carbon ions, or stereotactic body radiation therapy may improve LC in surgical patients and can be used as definitive-intent therapy in nonsurgical patients.
- The best outcomes are achieved when patients are treated at original presentation and with dose-escalated RT, either as monotherapy or in addition to an en bloc resection.
- When both surgery and RT are used, preoperative RT may be associated with better LC than postoperative RT.
- RT should be considered for all spine and sacral chordoma patients, and decisions regarding RT should be made by a radiation oncologist prior to surgery.

INTRODUCTION

Chordomas are rare, slow-growing malignant mesenchymal tumors that arise along the axial skeleton from the clivus to coccyx from remnants of the embryonic notochord. Chordomas are characterized by, and depend on, expression of the transcription factor brachyury, a master regulator of normal notochord development.[1–4] Chordoma incidence is estimated at less than 1 case per million per year[5–8] and approximately 300 cases per year in the United States. Although chordomas do have metastatic potential, their predominant pattern of growth is local invasion. They thus have appreciable risk of local recurrence (LR),[9,10] which can cause significant morbidity and mortality given their location near spinal cord, cauda equina, and nerve roots. Therefore, in the management of localized disease, achieving local control (LC) is of paramount importance.

Surgical resection traditionally has been the mainstay of therapy for nonmetastatic chordomas. Achieving adequate oncologic margins in these complex locations, however, often is challenging or impossible, and surgery alone has been associated with suboptimal LC. For example, a meta-analysis of published sacral chordoma series from 1980 to 2016, including 1235 patients (80% R0/1 resections and 37% adjuvant RT) found, at 6-year mean follow-up, 43% LR.[10] Similarly, a

[a] Harvard Radiation Oncology Program, Massachusetts General Hospital, 55 Fruit Street, Boston, MA 02114, USA; [b] Department of Radiation Oncology, Massachusetts General Hospital, Harvard Medical School, 55 Fruit Street, Boston, MA 02114, USA; [c] Department of Radiation Oncology, Memorial Sloan Kettering Cancer Center, 1275 York Avenue, New York, NY 10065, USA

* Corresponding author.

E-mail address: yamadaj@mskcc.org

Neurosurg Clin N Am 31 (2020) 263–288
https://doi.org/10.1016/j.nec.2019.12.002

meta-analysis of 167 sacral chordoma cases who underwent surgery at 12 spinal oncology referral centers (81% R0/1 resections and <23% adjuvant RT) found 35% LR at a relatively short 3.2-year median follow-up.[11] Surgery also can be associated with significant toxicity, particularly for high sacral tumors, for which sacrectomy requires sacrifice of S1/2 nerve roots; thus, in a series of 42 sacral chordoma patients from Memorial Sloan Kettering undergoing surgery (89% R0/1 resections and 12% adjuvant RT), in whom LR was 40% at 84-month mean follow-up, complications included 74% self-catheterization, 67% sexual dysfunction, and 29% permanent colostomy.[9]

Given the suboptimal results with surgery alone, the addition of RT often is considered with the goal of improving disease control. There also is a role for RT in definitive-intent treatment of unresected patients. Traditionally, RT doses to spinal tumors have been constrained by the spinal cord radiation tolerance, which is conventionally set at 45 Gy. Photon RT to conventional doses (ie, <70 Gy) in standard fractionation (ie, approximately 1.8 Gy/d), however, is inadequate to achieve LC in these radioresistant tumors. For example, an National Cancer Database (NCDB) analysis of 282 sacral and spinal chordoma patients treated from 2005 to 2010 found that, after R0/1 resection, receipt of adjuvant RT to a median dose of 58 Gy (in 25.9% of patients) was not associated with improved overall survival (OS)[12] (although LC could not be analyzed). Similarly, a meta-analysis of 193 patients undergoing sacrectomy (16% R1) at 4 spinal oncology referral centers found that RT to a median dose of 61.8 Gy was not associated improved LC at 7 years mean follow-up (hazard ratio [HR] 1.13 [0.59–2.17]; P = .71), whereas a trend toward improvement was seen with doses greater than or equal to 70 Gy (HR 0.52 [0.20–1.32]; P = .17), particularly among R1 patients (HR 0.40 [0.16–1.00]; P = .051). Thus, conventional doses of RT remain inadequate to control these challenging and radioresistant tumors.

More recently, advances in RT techniques have allowed safe delivery of significantly higher RT doses. Three major techniques have been used for such dose escalation (**Table 1**): proton therapy, carbon ion therapy, and photon-based stereotactic body radiation therapy (SBRT). Fundamentally, particle therapy (proton and carbon) uses the physical properties of charged particles to increase tumor dose while sparing normal tissue, whereas SBRT uses improvements in localization and conformality of photons to the same end. There are significant differences between these techniques with respect to level of evidence and technical details. Proton therapy, which is supported by 4 prospective and 8 retrospective studies, generally has pursued dose escalation (ie, to >70 gray-equivalent relative biological effectiveness [GyRBE]) using conventionally fractionated RT (eg, 1.8–2.0 GyRBE/d, yielding biologically equivalent doses of 66–76 GyRBE) while treating a significant elective clinical target volume (CTV) expansion to a lower dose to account for microscopic tumor spread (eg, 1 vertebral body or sacral level above/below lesion and 1–2 cm anatomically constrained radial expansions). Carbon ion studies, including 1 prospective and 3 retrospective, generally have used moderate hypofractionation (3–4 GyRBE/d, yielding biologically equivalent doses of 85–105 GyRBE) and more modest CTV expansions (eg, 5 mm anatomically constrained) treated to full dose. The main retrospective SBRT study delivered a single large fraction (24 Gy, yielding a biologically equivalent dose of 156 GyRBE) with no elective CTV expansion (see **Table 1**). Despite such differences, these approaches together offer a significant body of literature supporting the safety and efficacy of dose-escalated RT in the management of spinal and sacral chordomas, which this article discusses.

TECHNICAL ASPECTS OF RADIOTHERAPY FOR CHORDOMAS

Scrupulous attention and significant expertise are required for successful RT for these challenging tumors. Diagnostic imaging should include preoperative (and, where applicable, postoperative) T2 and precontrast and postcontrast T1 magnetic resonance imaging (MRI) sequences to delineate the gross tumor, adjacent areas at risk for microscopic spread, and nearby spinal cord/cauda/sacral nerve roots. T2 and postcontrast T1 MRIs should be 3-D acquisitions or acquired separately in the axial, coronal, and sagittal planes. Diagnostic MRIs should be fused to CT planning images for contouring.

CT simulation with intravenous (IV) contrast is required. For patients with tumor at cord level (L2) or above, contrast myelography at the time of simulation is helpful in delineating (1) the thecal sac (which is generally not at risk of tumor spread and can be excluded from the treatment volume) and (2) the spinal cord (generally the most critical organ at risk). Alternatively, MRI simulation (where available) may achieve the same goals as computed tomography (CT) myelography (and, potentially for the purposes of contouring, as diagnostic MRI).

Principles of immobilization include low intrafraction motion (ie, rigidity), low interfraction

Table 1
Radiation approaches for chordomas of the spine and sacrum

Approach	Typical Fractionation	Typical Total Physical Dose	Typical Total Biologically Equivalent Dose (EQD2)	Typical Elective CTV Expansion	Level of Evidence
Proton	Conventional fractionation (1.8–2.0 GyRBE/day)	70–77.4 GyRBE	EQD2 ~70 GyRBE	Generous Mobile spine: 1 vertebral body above/below, 1–1.5 cm radial (anatomically constrained) to lower dose Sacrum: 1 sacral level above/below; 1.5–2 cm radial (anatomically constrained); consider inclusion of sacrospinous ligaments, piriformis muscles where appropriate; to lower dose	4 prospective, 8 retrospective
Carbon	Moderate hypofractionation (3–4 GyRBE/day)	64–70 GyRBE	EQD2 ~105 GyRBE	Limited 5 mm (anatomically constrained) to full dose	1 prospective, 3 retrospective
SBRT	Single fraction	24 Gy	EQD2 ~150 GyRBE	None	1 retrospective

motion (ie, reproducibility), and patient tolerability. Although institutional practices vary, a reasonable approach is as follows. Cervical (C) and upper thoracic (T) spine patients are simulated supine under a shoulder-length thermoplastic mask with a custom head cup. Lower T and lumbar (L) spinal and sacral patients can be simulated prone; custom vacuum bag immobilization can be considered. During treatment, daily image guidance is mandatory. Although institutional practices vary, because these tumors are located in bony structures, even orthogonal Kilovoltage imaging frequently can provide adequate daily setup imaging. A treatment couch with 6 degrees of freedom is helpful to optimize patient alignment.

For patients treated postoperatively, artifacts due to metallic surgical hardware can obscure both diagnostic and simulation imaging and even may be associated with inferior outcomes.[13] All institutionally available approaches should be used to minimize this issue—for example, comparison to pretreatment studies without hardware, use of both CT and MRI, artifact reduction algorithms, and manual removal of artifact during the treatment planning process. Hardware artifact may be particularly problematic for dose calculations for protons and carbon ions, and delivering some or all postoperative treatment with intensity modulated RT (IMRT)/volumetric modulated arc therapy (VMAT) photons may help mitigate this issue.[14,15] Artifacts also can be minimized at the time of surgery by favoring reconstruction with allografts or cages instead of rods, use of titanium or, where available, carbon fiber when rods are necessary,[16,17] and avoiding rod cross-links at the tumor level.[14,15]

For select operative patients with tumor abutting dura, an intraoperative dural plaque brachytherapy boost (eg, phosphorous-32 or yttrium-90) may allow further dose escalation to the at-risk dural margin[14,15,18,19] Conversely, for patients with bowel directly adjacent to tumor, placement of a presacral spacer prior to RT may allow full coverage of tumor while reducing dose to bowel[20–26]; this approach, however, requires an additional (potentially laparoscopic) surgery.

PROTON

Background

Proton therapy has intrinsic physical properties that allow for high-dose delivery while sparing normal tissue tolerance (**Fig. 1**A). Photons penetrate through the patient, depositing decreasing dose along the entire beam path, according to an exponential decay function. In contrast, protons lose energy continuously in tissue, penetrating to a given depth before stopping altogether. As protons slow to a stop at their end of range, the dose deposited increases dramatically—the Bragg peak phenomenon—and then falls to zero distally. Compared with photon therapy, this property leads to reduced dose to organs at risk distal to the target in the beam path and reduced integral dose to the patient. For this reason, proton therapy has been an attractive technique for dose escalation for radioresistant tumors in close proximity to dose-limiting normal structures, including chordomas of the spine and sacrum. There are 2 main technologies for proton therapy delivery. In passively scattered, for example, double-scatter (DS), proton therapy (**Fig. 1**B), a narrow proton beam is laterally scattered into a homogenous, wide treatment field; a collimation device (aperture or multileaf collimator) achieves lateral conformality to the target volume, whereas a range compensator confers distal conformality. DS is the original proton therapy technology. It can achieve, however, only limited conformality of the high-dose region to the target volume, particularly proximally; this limitation often leads to high skin dose and to difficulty treating target volumes deep and concave to an avoidance structure (eg, a vertebral body relative to the spinal cord). In pencil beam scanning (PBS) proton therapy (**Fig. 1**C), the proton beam is kept in its original narrow size and, instead of being passively scattered, is actively scanned in the lateral dimensions, painting 1 at a time each voxel of tumor at a given

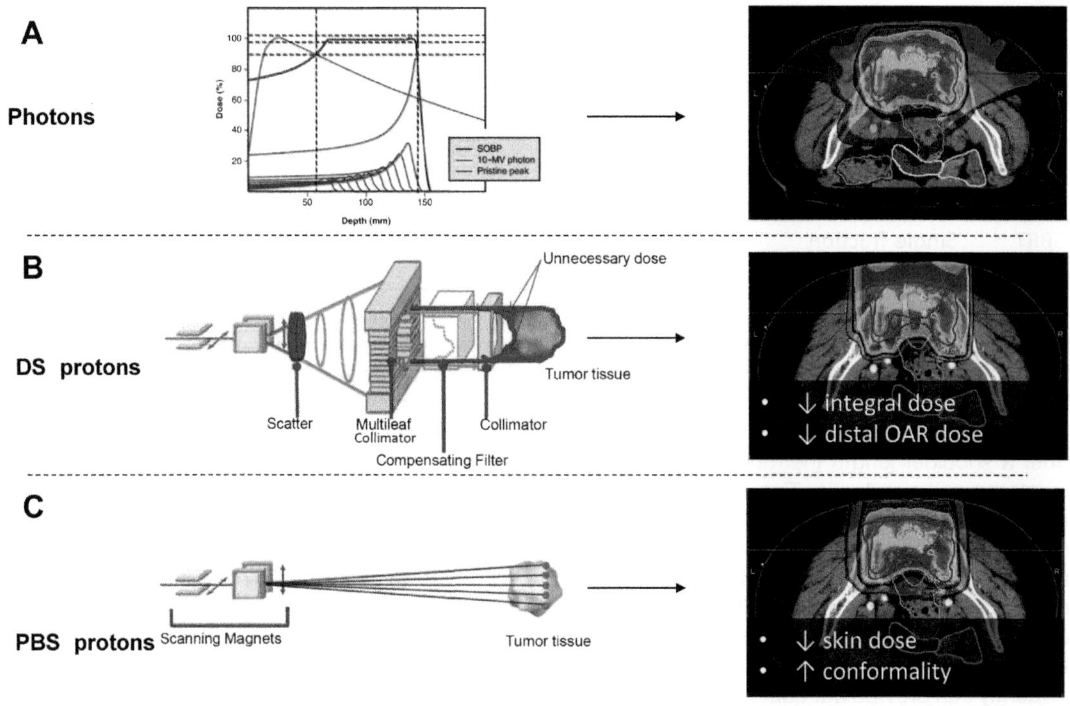

Fig. 1. Raster scanned with magnets and variable energy. (*A*) Photons deposit dose throughout the beam path (*left*), leading to low-dose bath around the target volume (*right*). In contrast, protons deposit dose up until the Bragg peak and then stop (*left*). (*B*) In DS proton therapy, the proton beam is passively scattered in the X and Y directions, given lateral conformality by a collimation device, and given distal conformality by a range compensator. Compared with photon therapy, DS protons permit decreased integral dose to the patient, particularly to organs at risk distal to the target volume in the beam path. (*C*) In PBS proton therapy, the proton beam is actively steered in the X and Y directions. Each voxel of the tumor at a given depth is painted before the beam energy is stepped and the next layer treated. Compared with DS protons, PBS protons permit improved conformality of the high dose to the target volume, particularly proximally, which leads to decreased skin dose. ([*A*] Diagram on the left is from Levin WP, Kooy H, Loeffler JS. Proton beam therapy. Br J Cancer. 2005;93(8):850; with permission; and [*B, C*] Diagram on the left is courtesy of Toshiba Japan). OAR, organs at risk; SOBP, spread-out Bragg peak.

depth. The beam energy then is modulated in order to treat the next layer of tumor. PBS is the current generation of proton therapy technology and, relative to DS, achieves superior high-dose conformality, particularly proximal to the target, leading to decreased skin dose and improved dose distribution around concave targets. In general, the proton literature—including 4 prospective and 8 retrospective studies—has pursued dose escalation (ie, total dose >70 GyRBE) using conventional fractionation (ie, 1.8–2 GyRBE/d) and fairly generous CTV expansions to account for potential microscopic spread.

Prospective Evidence

Postoperative/definitive-intent

Two prospective studies describe outcomes after postoperative or definitive-intent RT (**Table 2**a).

Indelicato and colleagues[27] reported a prospective series[28] from the University of Florida College of Medicine- Jacksonville of 51 patients with sacral (41%) or spinal (39% cervical and 20% thoracolumbar) chordomas (67%) or chondrosarcomas (33%), of which 24% were recurrent after prior surgery. Patients were treated either with definitive-intent RT alone or with surgery followed by postoperative RT, although the percentage of each and the margin status for those undergoing surgery are not reported. Nonetheless, between unresected and R2 resected patients, 53% had gross disease present at the time of RT. Median RT dose was 70.2 GyRBE (range 64.2–75.6), with 67% treated at 1.8 GyRBE daily and 33% at 1.2 GyRBE twice a day. In order to treat potential microscopic tumor spread, an elective CTV expansion of 1 cm to 2 cm (anatomically constrained) around gross tumor volume (GTV) was treated to 45 GyRBE. In order to facilitate comparison across different fractionation regimens used in different studies, delivered doses can be converted into an equivalent dose in 2 GyRBE fractions (EQD2). Assuming an α/β ratio of 2 for chordoma,[29,30] the median EQD2 in this study was 73.5 GyRBE. Patients were treated with either DS or PBS (distribution not reported), with 12% also receiving 3-dimensional (3-D) photons and 33% IMRT photons. Spinal cord planning constraints are not reported. Although no prespecified endpoint is described, with a median follow-up of 3.7 years, 4-year LC was 58%, disease-free survival (DFS) at 4 years (DFS4) 57%, and OS at 4 years (OS4) 72%. On subset analysis, primary lesions had lower local failure (LF) than recurrent lesions (29% vs 81%; P = .01); LF was likewise higher in patients less than or equal to 58 years old (62% vs 26%; P = .04). Toxicities included (2 each) second malignancies and sacral soft tissue necrosis and (1 each) vertebral fracture, necrotic bone cyst, chronic urinary tract infection (UTI), and bilateral radiation nephritis.

Baumann and colleagues[31] reported a prospective phase I/II trial[32] at the University of Pennsylvania in 20 patients with skull base (60%) and spine (40%) chordomas (90%) and chondrosarcomas, of which 5% were recurrent after prior treatment; 85% received surgery followed by postoperative RT, of whom 24% achieved R0/1 and 76% R2 margins; 15% received definitive-intent RT without resection. Median RT dose was 73.8 GyRBE (range 68.4–79.2) in 1.8 GyRBE daily fractions, for a median EQD2 of 70.1 GyRBE. CTV expansions are not reported. Planning constraints were a spinal cord point maximum of 45 GyRBE. The primary outcome was feasibility (no treatment delay >10 d) and safety (<20% acute grade [Gr] 3 toxicity) with secondary outcomes of LC, progression-free survival (PFS), and OS. The primary outcomes were reportedly met (n = 2 acute Gr3 toxicity; feasibility/treatment delays not reported). With a median follow-up of 37 months, LC at 3 years (LC3) was 86%, PFS at 3 years (PFS3) 90%, and OS was not reported. No significant outcome differences by subset were reported.

Preoperative/definitive-intent

Two additional prospective studies from Massachusetts General Hospital have demonstrated promising outcomes after preoperative RT for spinal and sacral chordomas (see **Table 2**b). The theoretic advantage of this approach is that delivering some preoperative RT may sterilize enough tumor clonogens to prevent intraoperative seeding of the operative field; without such seeding, postoperative RT need not cover all surgically manipulated tissues and instead can target a smaller volume around the tumor bed. This principle may be particularly important for spine/sacral chordomas given the extensive surgical approaches frequently required for these tumors, which often include combined anterior/posterior approaches, violation of the pleural and/or peritoneal cavities, and multilevel spinal instrumentation. Covering such an extensive surgical bed to a tumoricidal dose, as postoperative-only RT requires, generally is impossible.

In the first study, DeLaney and colleagues[14,33] reported a phase II trial of DS proton therapy in 50 patients with spine sarcomas, of which 48% were chordomas, 52% sacral, and 28% recurrent after prior surgery. Patients could receive:(1) preoperative RT followed by postoperative RT (recommended, although the number receiving preoperative RT is not reported); (2) postoperative

Table 2
Prospective proton therapy studies

Study	RT Timing	Center and Years Enrolled	Number of Pts	Location	Histology (% Chordoma)	% Recurrent	% Surgery/% Definitive-intent RT (No Surgery) Margin Status Among Surgical Pts	Median RT Dose (Range)	CTV Expansion and Dose	Extracranial CNS Planning Constraints	RT Technology	Median f/u	Prespecified Endpoints	Disease Outcomes	Key Subsets	Other Subsets	Toxicity Outcomes	Notes
Indelicato et al[27]	Post-operative	UF Jacksonville 2007–2013	51	C (39%) T/L (20%) S (41%)	67%	24%	N.R./N.R. N.R.	70.2 GyRBE (64.2–75.6) EQD2 66.7 GyRBE 67% 1.8 GyRBE daily 33% 1.2 GyRBE bid	1–2 cm (anatomically constrained) from pre-operative GTV, to 45 GyRBE	n.r.	DS or PBS (distribution N.R.) 3D (12%) or IMRT (33%) photons permitted	3.7 y	N.R.	LC4 58% PFS4 57% OS4 72%	Primary vs recurrent: LF 29% vs 81% (*P* = .01)	Age ≤ vs >58 y: LF 62% vs 26% (*P* = .04)	N = 2 each second malignancies and sacral soft tissue necrosis N = 1 each vertebral fracture, necrotic bone cyst, chronic UTI, bilateral radiation nephritis	
Baumann et al[31]	Post-operative	Penn 2010–2014	20	60% skull base 15% C 25% S	90%	5%	85%/15% 24% R0/1 76% R2	73.8 GyRBE (68.4–79.2), 1.8 daily EQD2 70.1 GyRBE	n.r.	Spinal cord 45 Gy point maximum	50% DS 50% PBS	37 mo	Primary: Feasibility (no tx delay ≥10d), safety (<20% acute Gr3 toxicity) Secondary: LRFS, PFS, OS	LC3: 86% PFS3: 90% OS: N.R.			N = 2 acute Gr3 N = 1 late Gr3	Met primary feasibility and safety endpoints
DeLaney et al[14,33]	Pre-operative recommended	MGH 1997–2005	50	11% T 26% L 52% S	58%	28%	74%/26% 22% R0 45% R1 32% R2	76.6 GyRBE (59.4–77.4) at 1.8 GyRBE daily EQD2 73.5 GyRBE	CTV1: 1–1.5 cm (anatomically constrained) from pre-operative GTV plus 1 VB above/below (and all surgically manipulated tissues, hardware, drains if postop), to 50.4 GyRBE	Spinal cord point maximum, ≤5 cm length: Center: 54 Gy Surface: 63 Gy Cauda: 70.2; 77.4 if contacting tumor	DS 70% with 3D or IMRT photons (up to 50.4 Gy)	7.3 y	N.R.	LC 5/8: 81%/74% PFS 5/8: 64%/52% OS 5/8: 84%/65%	Primary vs recurrent: LC 5/8 0%/8% vs 50%/n.r., *P* = .005 (chordoma)		Gr3-4 5y/8y 10%/13% 2 sacral neuropathy and 2 erectile dysfunction at >77 Gy to sacral nerve roots	N = 3 received dural plaque brachy-therapy boost (7.5–10 Gy)

									CTV2: pre-operative GTV, to 70.2 GyRBE (77.4 GyRBE if R2)									
Konieczkowski et al[15]	Pre ± post-operative: 79% Post-operative-only: 21%	MGH 2013–2017	60	17% C 8% T 20% L 55% S/C	85%	3%	85%/15% 63% R0 20% R1 10% R0/1 7% R2	Surgical: 64.8 GyRBE (19.8–77.4) EQD2 61.6 GyRBE Definitive-intent RT: 77.4 GyRBE (77.4–79.2) EQD2 73.5 GyRBE All at 1.8 GyRBE daily	Similar to DeLaney et al[14,33]	Surface/central point maximum: C: 67/55 T/L: 63/54 Cauda: 77.4/70.2 S1-S3: 77.4/77.4	PBS up to 19.8 Gy IMRT photons permitted	31 mo	Primary: LC3 Secondary: DFS3, OS3, toxicity	LC 2.5: 93% PFS 2.5: 81% OS 2.5: 92%	Preop vs post-op only RT: RFS 2.5 84% vs 62% (*P* = .003)	Chordoma vs chondrosarcoma: LF 2.5 2.9% vs 26% (*P* = .01) C/T vs L/S: RFS 2.5 64 vs 86% (*P* = .01)	Gr3 26% at 2.5 y (all in surgery + RT group)	N = 6 received dural plaque brachytherapy boost (10 Gy) No LF to date in definitive-intent RT group (p = ns)

Abbreviations: MGH, Massachusetts General Hospital; NS, not significant; Penn, University of Pennsylvania; UF, University of Florida college of Medicine – Jacksonville; VB, vertebral body; 2.5 (as in, LC 2.5), at 2.5 years.

RT (if they had undergone an adequate oncologic resection prior to trial enrollment); or (3) definitive-intent RT if not undergoing resection (24%). Among surgical patients, 22% achieved R0, 45% R1, and 32% R2 margins. Median RT dose was 76.6 GyRBE (median EQD2 73.5 GyRBE), primarily via DS proton therapy, but with up to 50.4 Gy of 3-D or IMRT photons permitted. CTV expansions included low-risk CTV (CTV1), encompassing a 1-cm to 1.5-cm anatomically constrained expansion on the preoperative GTV, 1 vertebral body above and below the preoperative GTV (to account for spread along epidural venous plexus), and, in postoperative cases, all surgically manipulated tissues, hardware, and drain sites, treated to 50.4 GyRBE; high-risk CTV (CTV2), encompassing the preoperative GTV, treated to 70.2 GyRBE; and postoperative gross residual disease treated to 77.4 GyRBE. In patients who received preoperative RT, no attempt was made during postoperative courses to cover all surgically manipulated tissues, drain sites, or hardware because it was felt that the preoperative course adequately controlled the risk of intraoperative tumor seeding in these sites. The spinal cord Dmax over a $\leq$ 5 cm length was limited to 54 GyRBE to cord center and 63 GyRBE to cord surface; cauda was limited to 70.2 GyRBE or 77.4 GyRBE if abutting tumor; 3 patients with tumor directly abutting dura received a 7.5-Gy to 10-Gy boost via high-dose rate (HDR) dural plaque brachytherapy. At a median follow-up of 7.3 years, LC at 5 years and at 8 years (5/8) was 81%/74%, DFS 5/8 was 64%/52%, and OS 5/8 was 85%/65%. On subset analysis, primary versus recurrent chordomas had LF 5/8 of 0%/8% vs 50%/NR (P = .005). There was a trend toward lower LR in R0 versus R1/2 patients (0/8 vs 9/29 patients; P = .11). Analysis by timing of RT (preoperative vs postoperative) was not described. Cumulative Gr3-4 toxicity at 5/8 years was 10%/13%; 2 sacral neuropathies and 2 erectile dysfunctions occurred at doses of greater than 77 GyRBE to sacral nerve roots.

In the second study, which has been presented but not yet published, Konieczkowski and colleagues[15] reported a phase II trial[34] of PBS proton therapy in 60 patients with chordoma (85%) or chondrosarcoma (15%) of the spine (45%) or sacrum (55%); 15% underwent definitive-intent RT and 85% underwent surgery with preoperative RT and/or postoperative RT. Among surgical patients, margins were 63% R0, 20% R1, 10% GTR (R0/1 undefined), and 7% R2. Of surgical patients, 14% received preoperative-only RT, 65% preoperative RT and postoperative RT, and 21% postoperative-only RT. Median doses were 64.8 GyRBE (19.8–77.4) in surgical patients and 77.4 GyRBE (77.4–79.2) for definitive-intent patients. Up to 19.8 Gy of IMRT photons was permitted and 6 patients received 10 Gy HDR dural plaque brachytherapy boost. CTV expansions were similar to prior institutional studies,[14,33] with CTV1 treated to 45 GyRBE to 50.4 GyRBE, CTV2 to 64.8 GyRBE to 70.2 GyRBE, and gross residual disease to 77.4 GyRBE to 79.2 GyRBE. Planning constraints were a surface/central cord point maximum as follows: C spine, 67/55 GyRBE; T/L spine, 63/54 GyRBE; cauda, 77.4/70.2 GyRBE, and S1–S3, 77.4/77.4 GyRBE. The prespecified primary endpoint was LC at 3 years and secondary endpoints DFS and OS at 3 years and toxicity. In the interim abstract report at 2.5 years' median follow-up, LC was 93%, PFS 81%, and OS 92%. Subset analysis was significant for lower LF in chordoma versus chondrosarcoma (2.9% vs 26%, respectively; P = .01), improved recurrence-free survival (RFS) in L/S versus C/T spine (86% vs 64%, respectively; P = .01), and improved RFS among surgical patients who received at least some preoperative RT (85% vs 62%, respectively; P = .003). No LFs were observed in the definitive-intent RT group (P = Non-significant vs surgery group). There were no Gr4–5 toxicities; Gr3 toxicity incidence was 26% at 2.5 years, all in the surgery plus RT group.

Retrospective Evidence

Eight major retrospective series describe outcomes after proton therapy for spinal and sacral chordomas: 2 postoperative (**Table 3**a), 2 preoperative (see **Table 3**b), 2 definitive-intent (see **Table 3**c), and 2 salvage (see **Table 3**d).

Postoperative

The 2 retrospective postoperative studies are discussed here and summarized in **Table 3**a.

Snider and colleagues[13] reported on 100 chordoma patients treated postoperatively with PBS proton therapy at Paul Scherrer Institute in Switzerland from 1997 to 2015. Lesions were 46% C spine, 5% T spine, 12% L spine, and 37% sacrum; 30% of lesions were recurrent. All underwent surgery, with 40% R0/1 and 60% R2 margins. Postoperative proton therapy was delivered to median 74 GyRBE (range 59.4–77 GyRBE), generally delivered in 1.8 GyRBE to 2 GyRBE fractions daily (median EQD2 74 GyRBE). Patients prior to 2008 were treated with a limited, focal CTV expansion (not further specified); due to concern for marginal failures; later patients were treated with a larger, comprehensive CTV expansion (including the surgical bed and 1 vertebral body above/below the GTV, treated to 54 GyRBE).

Table 3
Retrospective proton therapy studies

Study	RT Timing	Center and Years Treated	Number of Pts	Location	Histology (% Chordoma)	% Recurrent	% Surgery/ % Definitive-Intent RT (No Surgery) Margin Status Among Surgical Pts	Median RT Dose (Range) Median EQD2	CTV Expansion and Dose	Extracranial CNS Constraints	RT Technology	Median f/u	Disease Outcomes	Primary vs Recurrent	Key Subsets	Other Subsets	Toxicity Outcomes	Notes
3a: post-operative																		
Snider et al[13]	Post-operative	PSI 1997–2015	100	46% C 5% T 12% L 37% S	100%	30%	100%/0% R0/1 40% R2 60%	74 GyRBE (59.4–77) at 1.8–2 GyRBE daily EQD2 74 GyRBE	focal: "individualized" Comprehensive: surgical bed, 1 VB above/ below GTV To 54 GyRBE	Cord D2% <64GyRBE Central cord (2–3 mm): 54 GyRBE	PBS (12% photons)	65 mo	LC5 63% DFS5 57% OS5 81%		Gross residual disease present vs absent: OS5 76% vs 88%, $P = .05$	Univariate Stabilization hardware present/ absent: LC5/DFS5 /OS5 46%/34% /73% vs 76%/72%/ 87%, $P = .01$/ 0.003/0.01 "focal" CTV vs comprehensive CTV: OS5 71% vs 95%, $P = .01$ Age <55.5 vs ≥55.5: OS5 86% vs 77%, $P = .02$ Multivariate: Incr LC with: decr PTV volume ($P = .005$), no surgical stabilization ($P = .002$) Incr DFS with decr CTV1 C/C length ($P = .008$), no surgical stabilization ($P = .003$) Incr OS with:	8% with acute Gr3 toxicity 5% with late Gr3 toxicity N = 1 s malignancy	Smaller CTVs before 2008 subsequently expanded due to marginal failures lower OS in older patients, without change in other disease endpoints, may reflect competing risks Median follow up in "focal" CTV era (before 2008) 89 mo vs 51.5 mo in "comprehensive" CTV era (after 2008)

(continued on next page)

Table 3 (*continued*)

Study	RT Timing	Center and Years Treated	Number of Pts	Location	Histology (% Chordoma)	% Recurrent	% Surgery/ % Definitive-Intent RT (No Surgery) Margin Status Among Surgical Pts	Median RT Dose (Range) Median EQD2	CTV Expansion and Dose	Extracranial CNS Constraints	RT Technology	Median f/u	Disease Outcomes	Primary vs Recurrent	Key Subsets	Other Subsets	Toxicity Outcomes	Notes
																comprehensive CTV (*P* = .007), no gross residual disease (*P* = .007)		
Youn et al[35]	Post-operative vs definitive	Korea 2007–2015	58	59% skull base 12% C 29% S	100%	N.R.	N.R./N.R. 14% R0/1 86% R2 or biopsy only	69.6 GyRBE (64.8–79.2) at 2.4 GyRBE daily EQD2 76.6 GyRBE	"tumor bed"	Cord median 45 GyRBE; D1% 54 GyRBE	N.R.	42.8 mo	LC5 88% DFS n.r. OS5 88%			LC: C vs non-C (57 vs 93% *P* = .02), dose < vs ≥69.6 (64% vs 93%, *P* = .05) DMFS: S vs non-S (54% vs 100%, *P* = .001), dose < vs ≥69.6 (58% vs 95%, *P* = .016), tumor size < vs ≥5 cm (100% vs 60%, *P* = .001)	No acute Gr3 toxicity reported N = 3 with late Gr3 (skin/sub-cutaneous, rectal, sacral neuropathy, brainstem injury)	Excellent LC may reflect majority skull base (97% LC in this series)
3b: pre-operative																		
Rotondo et al[18]	Pre-operative (19.8–50.4) + post-operative	MGH 1982–2011	126	T 12.6% L 31.5% S 55.9%	100%	25%	93%/7% R0 27% R1 45% R2 24%	72.4 GyRBE (46.3–83.6), typically at 1.8–2 GyRBE daily	Similar to DeLaney et al[14,33]	n.r. but generally per 19095372, 24752878	DS + photons	47 mo	LC5 62% OS5 81%	LC5 68% vs 49% (*P* = .058)	R0/1 vs R2 margin OS5 88% vs 66% (*P* = .017) Preop RT vs not:	More prior surgeries: LC HR 1.44 (1.03 = 2.02, *P* = .034)	N = 50≥ Gr3 compli-cations (n = 17 wound infection,	Intra-operative boost: 7 HDR dural plaque (median 10 Gy),

								EQD2 68.4 GyRBE							LC5 85% vs 56% (P = .019) (primary only)	En bloc vs intralesional resection: LC5 72% vs 55% (P = .016)	6 insufficiency fractures, 4 neuropathy); no myelopathy	4 IORT e- (median 10 Gy), 4 LDR brachytherapy (median 42 Gy) 0/28 recurrences among primary tumors treated with preop RT and en bloc resection
Wagner et al[19]	Low-dose preoperative + postoperative	MGH 1982–2006	48	71% S 21% spine 8% appendicular	52%	29%	100%/0% R0 44% R1 12% R2 44%	Preop: 20 GyRBE (9–29.4) Postop: 50.4 GyRBE (18–61.2) Total: 70.4 GyRBE, typically at 1.8–2 GyRBE daily EQD2 66.7 GyRBE	Similar to DeLaney et al[14,33]	n.r. but generally per 19095372, 24752878	DS and/or photons	31.8 mo	LC5 72% DFS5 54% OS5 65%	LC5 89% vs 18%, P = .001 DFS5 72% vs 30% (P = .001)	R0/1 vs R2: DFS5 (P = .07)		21% delayed wound healing and delayed PORT "notable" late toxicity in 4/37 pts (2 sacral fractures, 1 lymphedema, 1 RT proctitis)	7 pts with dural plaque boost
3c: definitive-intent																		
Kabolizadeh et al[36]	Definitive-intent	MGH 1975–2012	40	C 22% T 3% L 8% S 27% Para-axial: 30%	100%	0%	0%/100% n/a	77.4 GyRBE (64.7–79.2) at 1.8–2 GyRBE daily EQD2 75.2 GyRBE	Similar to DeLaney et al[14,33]	Cord surface/ center: C: 67/55 GyRBE T/L: 63/54 GyRBE	DS + photons	50.3 mo	LC5 85% DFS n.r. OS5 82%			Tumor volume OS (P = .008), DSS (P = .023), DF (P = .044) Dose: OS (P = .032)	N = 10 sacral fractures, 6 sacral neuropathy, 1 bowel fistula	
Aibe et al[22]	Definitive-intent	Hyogo 2009–2015	33	100% S	100%	0%	0%/100% n/a	70.4 GyRBE at 2.2 GyRBE daily EQD2 73.9 GyRBE	5mm from GTV (anatomically constrained), full dose	Cord Dmax 48 GyRBE	DS	37 mo	LC3 89% DFS3 82% OS3 93%			S2 or above vs below S2: LC3 76% vs 100%, P = .05	Gr3: N = 1 acute (dermatitis) and n = 5 late (pain, sacral fracture, ileus)	33% with presacral spacer placement

(continued on next page)

Table 3
(continued)

Study	RT Timing	Center and Years Treated	Number of Pts	Location	Histology (% Chordoma)	% Recurrent	% Surgery/% Definitive-Intent RT (No Surgery) Margin Status Among Surgical Pts	Median RT Dose (Range) Median EQD2	CTV Expansion and Dose	Extracranial CNS Constraints	RT Technology	Median f/u	Disease Outcomes	Primary vs Recurrent	Key Subsets	Other Subsets	Toxicity Outcomes	Notes
3d: salvage																		
MacDonald et al[37]	Post-operative vs definitive-intent	Indiana 2005–2012	16	50% clivus 12% C 19% T/L 19% S	100%	100% (88% prior surgery + RT, 12% prior RT only)	50%/50% N.R.	75.6 GyRBE (71.2–79.2) 88% at 1.8–2.0 GyRBE daily 12% at 1–1.2 GyRBE bid EQD2 75.6 GyRBE	n.r.	n.r.	DS	24 mo	LC2 85% DFS2 n.r. OS2 80%			None	n = 1 acute Gr3 laryngeal edema n = 1 acute Gr4 obstructive hydrocephalus n = 1 late Gr3 brainstem radionecrosis n = 2 late Gr4 brainstem stroke, CSF leak with meningitis	
Holliday et al[38]	58% salvage 42% post-operative	MDACC 2006–2012	19	68% S	68%	58%	42%/48% Adjuvant: R0: 0% R1: 62% R2: 38%	Adjuvant: 70 GyRBE (56–70.2) Salvage: 70 GyRBE (60–78) At 2 GyRBE daily EQD2 70 GyRBE	n.r.	n.r.	DS	34.5 mo	LC2 58% PFS2 52% OS2 93%	LC2 88% vs 45% ($P = .061$) PFS2 75% vs 45% ($P = .198$) OS2 88% vs 100% ($P = .228$)	Gross disease vs no (20% vs 79% recurrence, $P = .025$	Adjuvant vs salvage: S vs non-S (84% vs 16%, $P = .004$) Surgery-RT interval (25 vs 2.5 mo, $P = .025$)	No differences between approaches	Adjuvant group had: Less sacral location (25% vs 100%, $P = .0005$) Less gross disease (38% vs 100%, $P = .0003$) Longer surgery-RT interval (2.5 vs 32.6 mo, $P = .00007$) Less hardware (63% vs 100%, $P = .05$)

Abbreviations: Decr, decreased; DF, distant failure; Gr >= 3. Gr2-3; Incr, increased; IORT, intra-operative radiotherapy; MSKCC: Memorial Sloan Kettering Cancer Center; MV: Megavoltage; NA,

Dose constraints were maximum dose to 2% (D2%) less than 64 GyRBE to the T2 MRI-delineated spinal cord and 54 GyRBE to the central 2 mm to 3 mm of cord. At a median follow-up of 65 months, LC at 5 years (LC5) was 63%, DFS at 5 years (DFS5) 57%, and OS at 5 years (OS5) 81%. On subgroup analysis, presence vs absence of stabilization hardware was associated with inferior outcomes respectively (LC5 46% vs 76%; *P* = .001; DFS5 34% vs 72%; *P* = .003; and OS5 73% vs 87%; *P* = .01) as was presence vs absence of gross residual disease respectively (OS5 76% vs 88%; *P* = .05). Focal versus comprehensive treatment era (OS5 71% vs 95%; *P* = .01) and age less than 55.5 (OS5 86% vs 77%; *P* = .02) also were associated with worse outcomes, although both relationships to OS may be confounded by competing mortality risks. On multivariate analysis, surgical hardware was associated with worse LC and DFS (*P* = .002 and *P* = .003), smaller planning target volume (PTV) with improved LC (*P* = .005), smaller craniocaudal length with improved DFS (*P* = .008), and comprehensive CTV treatment and absence of gross residual disease with improved OS (*P* = .007 for both); 8% acute and 5% late Gr3 toxicity were reported with 1 second malignancy.

Youn and colleagues[35] reported on 58 chordoma patients (59% skull base, 12% C spine, and 29% sacrum) treated in Korea from 2007 to 2015 in the postoperative or definitive-intent setting. The percentage of patients undergoing surgery is not reported, but 14% achieved an R0/1 resection whereas 86% had gross residual disease (due to either R2 resection or biopsy only). Patients received proton therapy (technology not reported) to a median dose of 76.6 GyRBE (range 64.8–79.2 GyRBE) in 2.4-GyRBE daily fractions (EQD2 76.6 GyRBE). CTV expansion included the tumor bed but is not described further. Dose constraints were a median cord dose of 45 GyRBE and cord Maximum dose to 1% (D1%) 54 GyRBE. At median 42.8-month follow-up, LC5 was 88%, DFS5 was not reported, and OS5 was 88%. Subset analysis was significant for worse LC5 in C spine versus non–C spine (57% vs 93%, respectively; *P* = .02). Dose less than 69.6 GyRBE versus greater than or equal to 69.6 GyRBE was associated with worse LC (64% vs 93%, respectively; *P* = .05) and DMFS (58% vs 95%, respectively; *P* = .016). Better DMFS also was seen in nonsacral versus sacral patients (100% vs 54%, respectively; *P* = .001) and in tumors less than 5 em versus greater than or equal to 5 cm (100% vs 60%%, respectively; *P* = .001). No acute and 3 late Gr3 toxicities were reported (including skin/subcutaneous, rectal, sacral neuropathy, and brainstem injury). Favorable outcomes in this series may reflect the high percentage of skull base lesions, which had 97% LC in this study.

Preoperative

Both retrospective preoperative series are from Massachusetts General Hospital (see **Table 3**b).

In the first series, Rotondo and colleagues[18] describe 126 patients with chordoma (56% sacral, 44% spine, and 25% recurrent) treated from 1982 to 2011 predominantly with preoperative RT (19.8–50.4 GyRBE), surgery, and postoperative RT. Treatment was by mixed DS protons and photons; 15 patients received a boost with HDR dural plaque, intraoperative electrons, or low-dose rate (LDR) brachytherapy; 47% of patients underwent preoperative RT (19.8–50.4 GyRBE), surgery (27% R0, 45% R1, and 24% R2 margins), and postoperative RT, with a median total dose of 72.4 GyRBE (46.3–83.6) (median EQD2 68.4 GyRBE). CTV expansions and planning constraints were similar to those used in prior institutional studies.[14,33] In patients who received preoperative RT, no attempt was made during postoperative courses to cover all surgically manipulated tissues, drain sites, or hardware because it was felt that the preoperative course adequately controlled the risk of intraoperative tumor seeding in these sites. At a median follow-up of 47 months, LC5 was 62% and OS5 81%. There was a trend toward better LC5 in primary versus recurrent disease (68% vs 49%, respectively; *P* = .058) and significantly better LC in patients with fewer prior surgeries (HR 1.44 [1.03–2.02]; *P* = .034). En bloc versus intralesional resection was associated with improved LC5 (72% vs 55%, respectively; *P* = .016) and R0/1 versus R2 margin with improved OS5 (88% vs 66%, respectively; *P* = .017). Among patients with primary (nonrecurrent) disease, LC5 was higher among patients receiving at least some preoperative RT (85% vs 56%, respectively; *P* = .019). There were no recurrences among 28 primary tumors diagnosed by core biopsy and treated with at least some preoperative RT followed by en bloc resection. There were 50 greater than or equal to Gr3 complications, including 17 wound infections, 6 fractures, and 4 neuropathies; no myelopathy was observed.

In the other series, Wagner and colleagues[19] describe a subset of 48 patients treated with low-dose (median 20 Gy, range 9–29.4 Gy) preoperative RT, resection (44% R0, 12% R1, and 44% R2), and postoperative RT (median 50.4 Gy additional, range 18–61.2) (median EQD2 66.7 GyRBE). CTV expansions and planning constraints were similar to those used in other institutional studies[14,33];

again, the postoperative course did not cover all surgically manipulated tissues, drain sites, or hardware. The rationale for this low-dose preoperative approach is that, although these preoperative doses are lower than used in the prospective trials discussed previously, they still may be sufficient to prevent intraoperative tumor seeding, yet are low enough minimize postoperative wound healing complications. The postoperative boost is then intended to sterilize areas of likely positive margin around the tumor bed but (unlike with postoperative-only RT) need not cover all surgically manipulated tissues because the risk of iatrogenic intraoperative seeding has been minimized by the preoperative RT course. Seven patients also received an HDR dural plaque brachytherapy boost. At 32-month median follow-up, LC5 was 72%, DFS5 54%, and OS5 65%. LC5 and DFS5 were significantly higher for primary versus recurrent disease (89% vs 18% and 72% vs 30%, respectively; $P = .001$ for both comparisons); there also was a trend toward improved DFS5 in R0/1 versus R2 resections ($P = 0.07$). 21% experienced wound healing issues that delayed initiation of PORT; notable late toxicities arose in 4 of 37 evaluable patients, including 2 sacral fractures, 1 lymphedema, and 1 RT proctitis.

Definitive-intent

The 2, retrospective definitive-intent studies are discussed here and summarized in **Table 3**c.

Kabolizadeh and colleagues[36] describe 40 patients with sacral chordoma treated receiving definitive-intent RT without surgery between 1975 and 2012 at Massachusetts General Hospital. Lesions were 22.5% C spine, 2.5% T spine, 7.5% L spine, and 67.5% sacral. Patients received a mix of DS protons and photons to a median dose of 77.4 GyRBE (64.7–79.2) (EQD2 75.2 GyRBE). CTV expansions were similar to those used in other institutional studies.[14,33] Cord planning constraints to surface/center were 67/55 GyRBE for C spine and 63/54 GyRBE for T/L spine. At a median follow-up of 50.3 months, LC5 was 85%, DFS5 was not reported, and OS5 was 82%. On subset analysis, tumor volume was associated with OS ($P = .008$), DSS ($P = .023$), and distant failure ($P = .044$), and dose with OS ($P = .032$). Toxicity included 10 sacral fractures, 6 sacral neuropathies, and 1 enteric fistula.

Aibe and colleagues[22] reported the Hyogo, Japan, experience with 33 patients with sacral chordoma treated with definitive-intent DS proton therapy between 2009 and 2015. None underwent resection, although 33% underwent presacral spacer placement. RT dose was 70.4 GyRBE in 32 fractions of 2.2 GyRBE (EQD2 73.9 GyRBE). CTV was a 5-mm anatomically constrained from GTV, treated to full dose. Cord planning constraint was Point maximum dose (Dmax) 48 GyRBE. At a median follow-up of 37 months, LC3 was 89%, DFS at 3 years (DFS3) 82%, and OS at 3 years (OS3) 93%. On subset analysis, tumors involving S2 or above were associated with worse LC (76% vs 100%; $P = .05$). One acute Gr3 (dermatitis) and 5 late Gr3 toxicities (pain, sacral fracture, and ileus) were reported.

Salvage

The 2 retrospective salvage studies are discussed here and summarized in **Table 3**d.

McDonald and colleagues[37] reported the Indiana University experience with salvage RT for 16 patients after prior surgery plus RT (88%) or prior RT alone (12%) for chordomas of the skull base (50%) and spine (12% C, 19% T/L, and 19% S). 50% received definitive-intent reirradiation and 50% received surgery followed by reirradiation; margin status for surgical patients is not reported. Patients received a median of 75.6 GyRBE (range 71.2–79.2 GyRBE) using DS proton therapy (EQD2 75.6 GyRBE). CTV expansions and cord planning constraints were not reported. At a median follow-up of 24 months, LC at 2 years (LC2) was 85%, DFS was not reported, and OS at 2 years (OS2) was 80%. No subset outcome differences were reported. Toxicities included 1 acute Gr3 laryngeal edema, 1 acute Gr4 obstructive hydrocephalus, 1 late Gr3 brainstem radionecrosis, 1 late Gr4 brainstem stroke, and 1 late Gr4 CSF leak with meningitis.

Holliday and colleagues[38] reported a series of 9 adjuvant and 10 salvage patients (68% chordoma) treated with DS proton therapy at MD Anderson Cancer Center from 2006 to 2015. In the adjuvant patients, surgical margins were 62% R1 and 38% R2. Median RT dose was 70 GyRBE in 2 GyRBE fractions in both groups (EDQ2 70 GyRBE); CTV expansions and cord constraints were not reported. At a median follow-up of 34.5 months, LC2 was 58%, PFS at 2 years (PFS2) 52%, and OS2 93%. Remarkably given the small number of patients, patients treated in the adjuvant vs salvage setting had a borderline significant trend toward improved LC (88% vs 45%; $P = .061$). Adjuvant patients had less sacral disease, less gross disease, and a shorter surgery-RT interval than salvage patients; in the setting of confounding between these variables and treatment group, these variables were also associated with improved outcomes. No toxicity differences were reported between groups.

Toxicity

In addition to the toxicity outcomes reported for individual studies discussed previously, several additional studies have analyzed toxicity outcomes.

Stieb and colleagues[39] reviewed plans for 76 patients treated at Paul Scherrer Institute for spinal (68% C, 22% T, and 9% L) chordoma (72%) or chondrosarcoma using PBS proton therapy (median dose 73.9 GyRBE, range 59.4–75.2) from 2000 to 2014. No patient had prior RT or concurrent systemic therapy. Planning constraints for the cord surface were D2% 64 GyRBE, or 60 GyRBE for target volumes longer than 3 vertebrae, and, for the central cord (defined as the geometrically central 2–3 mm), D2% 60 GyRBE. D2% was preferred for constraints as it was judged more reliable than point Dmax. The delivered median Dmax and median D2% to the cord surface were 58.7 GyRBE (48.3–75.9) and 52.7 GyRBE (43.1–73.8) respectively and to the central cord 52.7 GyRBE (32.3–73.3) and 52.0 GyRBE (25.3–73.1) respectively. At a median follow-up of 66 months, there was 5% acute radiation neurotoxicity (n = 1 Gr1 and n = 3 Gr2) and 16% late neurotoxicity (n = 7 Gr1, n = 4 Gr2, and n = 1 Gr4). The single late Gr4 toxicity was a patient with pretreatment spinal cord compression causing tetraplegia who improved after decompressive surgery and then redeveloped tetraplegia 17 months after RT; this patient received Dmax/D2% 57.8/54.9 to the surface and 54.1/52.7 to the central cord. Among all patients, there was no significant correlation between surface or central DMax or D2% or length of CTV and toxicity, although trends toward association with Gr greater than or equal to 2 late neurotoxicity were observed for Dmax and D2% to the surface and central cord. The investigators, therefore, propose adoption of surface D2% = 64 GyRBE and central D2% = 54 GyRBE for continued clinical use.

Two articles also report the Massachusetts General Hospital toxicity experience. In the first, Marucci and colleagues[40] reviewed plans for 85 patients with cervical spine or cervical-occipital junction chordomas or chondrosarcomas treated with combined proton (DS)/photon RT (mean 76.3 GyRBE, range 68.9–83) between 1982 and 2000. Planning constraints for most patients were a Dmax to cord surface/center of 67 GyRBE/55 GyRBE, respectively; 13 patients were treated on a dose escalation study, which permitted Dmax to cord surface/center of 70/58 GyRBE. At a median follow-up of 41 months, there were 15.2% Gr1–2 and 4.7% Gr3 spinal cord toxicities. Although summary statistics for the entire cohort are not reported, there were no significant differences in any dosimetric parameter between patients with and without toxicity (eg, Dmax center 55.0 ± 2.5 vs 54.4 ± 3.2 GyRBE respectively; P = .41; Dmax surface 66.4 ± 2.8 vs 66.2 ± 3.4 GyRBE respectively; P = .65). In contrast, on both univariate and multivariate analysis, number of prior surgeries was significantly associated with cord toxicity (P = .026).

Chowdhry and colleagues[41] reviewed plans for 68 patients with tumors of the cervical and 20% thoracolumbar) spine (43% chordoma) treated between 2002 and 2013 with mixed photon/proton plans to a median dose of 72 GyRBE (range 59.4–78.2). 24% were treated both preoperatively (median 36 GyRBE) and postoperatively, with the remainder treated postoperatively only; 15% of patients received an HDR dural plaque brachytherapy boost, and 16% received chemotherapy. Of 68 total patients, 23 had complete dosimetric information available. Although summary statistics for cord dosimetry are not reported, 8 patients experienced greater than or equal to Gr3 cord toxicity. Of these, 4 were due to surgery, 3 due to tumor progression, and only 1 potentially due to RT. This patient presented with cord compression and underwent surgery, chemotherapy, and RT without initial toxicity. Three years after completing RT, he was diagnosed with myelodysplastic syndrome and received azacytidine and a bone marrow transplant. Thereafter, he developed transient paralysis, which subsequently improved partially with physical therapy. Cord doses in this patient were D5 cc 45 Gy, D2 cc 50 Gy, and D1 cc 52 Gy.

Insufficiency fractures are an additional risk after high-dose RT with or without surgery. Osler and colleagues[42] reported on 62 patients with sacral chordoma who received RT with (44) or without (18) surgery between 1992 and 2013. Fracture rates were 47% overall, including 76% in high sacrectomy plus RT patients, 0% in low sacrectomy plus RT patients, and 22% in RT-alone patients.

Together, these analyses suggest that—in the context of scrupulous care and significant experience in simulation, contouring, planning, and delivery—doses substantially in excess of conventional cord constraints can be used safely.

Future Directions

Other than those discussed later, no prospective studies for proton therapy in spine/sacral chordomas currently are listed on clinicaltrials.gov. Avenues for future investigation may include using PBS to deliver simultaneous integrated boost via moderate hypofractionation; evaluation of preoperative-only RT (instead of split-course preoperative and postoperative), particularly in comparison to postoperative-only RT; and the integration of novel systemic therapies with concurrent RT.[4,43]

CARBON

Background

RT with carbon ions, which are heavy charged particles, shares proton therapy's physical advantage of the Bragg peak. Compared with proton therapy, carbon ion therapy also achieves a sharper lateral penumbra (due to reduced multiple Coulomb scattering), at the cost of increased dose beyond the Bragg peak (due to downstream fragmentation of the carbon nucleus). In addition to its physical properties, however, carbon ion therapy has a theoretic biological advantage over both proton and photon therapy: it is more densely ionizing (ie, higher linear energy transfer), leading to more clustered DNA breaks, more efficient cell kill for a given physical radiation dose (ie, higher relative biological effectiveness), and effective killing despite tumor hypoxia (ie, lower oxygen enhancement ratio). Thus, carbon ion therapy may represent a promising treatment modality, particularly for hypoxic and radioresistant tumors such as chordoma. Carbon ion therapy currently is available only in a few centers worldwide and none in the United States. The major primary evidence for the use of carbon ion therapy in spine/sacrum chordoma includes 1 prospective and 3 retrospective single-institutional series, described later and summarized in **Table 4**. All have used significantly hypofractionated regimens of 3 GyRBE to 4 GyRBE per fraction to a limited CTV expansion (eg, 5 mm). This is markedly higher than the fraction sizes used in proton therapy and, for a given physical dose in GyRBE, results in a significantly higher biologically equivalent dose; accordingly, there have been some reports of toxicity with these regimens.[23,25] Also, in contrast to the majority of the proton literature, CTV expansions in carbon ion studies (to account for microscopic tumor spread) typically have been very modest.

Primary Evidence

Definitive-intent

The largest and only prospective series (see **Table 4**a), from the National Institute of Radiological Sciences/Heavy Ion Medical Accelerator in Chiba, Japan, reported the results of definitive-intent carbon ion therapy for 188 patients with sacral chordoma treated from 1996 to 2013.[23] This retrospective pooled analysis encompasses 2 prospective trials, the first a phase I–II dose escalation protocol (1996–2000) and the second a phase II fixed-dose study (2000–present). Patients received a median 67.2 GyRBE in 16 fractions 4 days per week (the dose of the ongoing phase II study; EQD2 104.1 GyRBE); dose range during the dose escalation study was 64 GyRBE to 73.6 GyRBE, with higher doses subsequently discontinued due to skin and neurologic toxicity. CTV was a 5-mm anatomically constrained expansion from GTV, treated to full dose. Cauda/sacral nerve root planning constraints were not reported. Beam technology was DS. No prior RT was permitted, but it is not reported whether any lesions were recurrent after prior surgery. At a median follow-up of 62 months, LC5 was 77.2%, DFS5 50.3%, and OS5 81%. No significant differences in outcome were seen on subset analysis; 6 patients sustained Gr3 peripheral nerve toxicity, 4 of these at the 73.6 GyRBE dose level, and 2 patients experienced Gr4 skin toxicity (dose level not reported). Of note, 20 patients underwent pretreatment diverting colostomy, and 10 patients had presacral spacers placed.[20,21]

The remaining retrospective carbon ion series are summarized in **Table 4**b.

Wu and colleagues[44] reported retrospective results from the Shanghai Proton and Heavy Ion Center. Here, 21 patients with sarcomas of the axial skeleton (76% chordoma and 90% sacral) were treated from 2015 to 2018 to a median total dose of 69 GyRBE (range 57–80) in 18 fractions to 25 fraction using PBS technology (EQD2 86.3 GyRBE). CTV was a 5-mm expansion from GTV, treated to full dose. Spinal cord planning constraint was Dmax less than 40 GyRBE; 62% of patients had recurrent disease after prior surgery and/or RT and none had prior treatment of the current presentation. At a median follow-up of 21.8 months, LC2 was 85.2%, DFS at 2 years (DFS2) 80.4%, and OS2 100%. No significant differences in outcomes were seen on subset analysis. No Gr3–4 toxicities were reported.

Demizu and colleagues[25] reported retrospective results from the Hyogo Ion Beam Medical Center for 96 patients with unresectable or incompletely resected pelvic sarcomas (58% chordoma and 90% primary) treated from 2005 to 2014; 10% underwent R2 resection prior to RT. Patients received carbon RT (39 patients) or proton RT (52 patients), with modality selected based on target coverage. An initial 40% were treated with 70.4 GyRBE/16 fraction (EQD2 112.6 GyRBE); due to skin and neurologic toxicity with this regimen, the remaining 60% received 70.4 GyRBE in 32 fraction (EQD2 73.9 GyRBE). CTV was a 5-

Table 4
Prospective and retrospective carbon ion studies

Study	RT Timing	Center and Years Enrolled	Number of Pts	Location	Histology % Chordoma	% Recurrent	% Surgery/% Definitive-Intent RT (No Surgery) Margin Status Among Surgical Pts	Median RT Dose (Range)	CTV Expansion and Dose	Extracranial CNS Planning Constraints	Treatment Technology	Median f/u	Disease Outcomes	Key Subsets	Other Subsets	Toxicity Outcomes	Notes
4a: Prospective																	
Imai et al[23]	Definitive -intent	Chiba 1996–2013	188	100% S	100%	NR	0%/100% n/a	67.2 GyRBE (64–73.6) in 4–4.6 GyRBE fx, 4 d per week EQD2 104.1 GyRBE	5mm from GTV (anatomically constrained), full dose	n.r.	DS	62 mo	LC5 77.2 DFS5 50.3 OS5 81.1		none	N = 2 Gr4 skin N = 6 Gr3 neuropathy	11% with pre-RT diverting colostomy 5% with spacer placement
4b: retrospective																	
Wu 3et al[44]	Definitive-intent	Shanghai 2015–2018	21	90% S 5% T 5% pelvis	76% (n = 16)	62%	0%/100% n/a	69 GyRBE (57–80) in 3.2 GyRBE fx (schedule not described) EQD2 86.3 GyRBE	5mm from GTV, full dose	Dmax 40 GyRBE	PBS	21.8 mo	LC2 85.2 DFS2 80.4% OS2 100%		none	No Gr3-4 reported	
Demizu et al[25]	90% definitive-intent 10% post-operative (R2)	Hyogo 2005–2014	96	100% S	58% (n = 56)	10%	10%/90% 100% R2	40%: 70.4 GyRBE in 4.4 GyRBE fx (EQD2 112.6 GyRBE) 60%: 70.4 GyRBE in 2.2 GyRBE fx (EQD2 73.92 GyRBE) (schedule not described)	5mm from GTV, full dose	Dmax 42 GyRBE (16 fx) Dmax 48 GyRBE (32 fx)	DS 57% proton, 43% carbon	32 mo	LC3 92% DFS3 72% OS3 83%	Primary vs recurrent: PFS, HR 1.34–9.54 for recurrent, $P = .011$ Cox MV	Chordoma vs other OS (0.098–0.895, $P = .031$ Cox MV) PTV ≤500 cm3 PFS (HR 0.110–0.513, $P<.001$ Cox MV) Prior sacral chordoma series: Male vs female (PFS, $P = .029$ log-rank univariate)	24% Gr ≥3 acute 25% Gr ≥3 late (50% in 16 fx, 9% in 32 fx)	42% spacer placement
Uhl et al[45]	43% definitive 57% post-operative	Heidelberg 2009–2012	56	100% S	100%	27%	57%/43% 41% R0/1 59% R2	66 GyRBE (60–74) (EQD2 82.5 GyRBE) Carbon only (n = 33): 60–66 GyRBE at 3 Gy/fx Carbon + photon (n = 23): 50–52 Gy at 2 Gy/fx photon + 15–24 GyRBE at 3 GyRBE/fx carbon	n.r.	n.r.	Carbon: PBS Photon: IMRT or tomo-therapy	25 mo	LC2 75 DFS2 NR OS2 100	Primary vs recurrent: LC2 85% vs 47%, $P = .001$ log-rank univariate	Male vs female (LC2 85% vs 60%, $P = .03$ log-rank univariate)	No Gr3-4 reported (relative to pre-RT baseline)	52% sacral fractures (ungraded) at 35.5 mo f/u (Bostel et al[46])

mm expansion from GTV, treated to full dose. Cord constraints were Dmax 42 GyRBE for the 16-fraction regimen and Dmax 48 GyRBE for the 32-fraction regimen; 42% had a presacral spacer placed prior to RT. At a median follow-up of 32 months, LC3 was 92%, DFS3 72%, and OS3 83%. In a Cox multivariable analysis, chordoma histology was associated with improved OS (HR 0.098–0.895; P = .031); primary (vs recurrent) tumor (HR 0.105–0.747; P = .011) and PTV less than or equal to 500 cm3 (HR 0.110–0.513; P<.001) were associated with improved PFS; 24% of patients experienced grade greater than or equal to 3 acute dermatitis and 25% experienced late grade greater than or equal to 3 effects, including 50% in the 16-fraction group and 9% in the 32-fraction group. These results are similar to those previously published from the same institution using a smaller subset of primary sacral chordomas,[24] although in that analysis, male sex was associated with significantly better PFS (point estimates not reported; P = .029).

Postoperative

Only 1 series reports on a significant number of patients treated in the postoperative setting. Uhl and colleagues[45] reported on 56 sacral chordoma patients (27% recurrent after prior surgery) treated at the Heidelberg Ion Beam Therapy Center between 2009 and 2012; 57% had surgery followed by postoperative RT, of whom 41% had R0/1 and 59% R2 margins. Patients received either (1) carbon ion therapy alone to 60 GyRBE to 66 GyRBE in 3-Gy fractions, or (2) photon RT to 50 Gy to 52 Gy in 2-Gy fractions followed by a carbon ion boost of 15 GyRBE to 24 GyRBE in 3 GyRBE fractions. median total dose was 66 Gy (EQD2 82.5 GyRBE); no planning constraints are reported. CTV expansions were not specified. Carbon ion technology was PBS, and photon technology was IMRT or tomotherapy. At a median follow-up of 25 months, LC was 75% and OS 100%; DFS was not reported. LC2 was better in primary versus recurrent tumors (85% vs 47%; P = .001) and in men versus women (85% vs 60%; P = .03). At the time of initial publication, no new Gr3–4 toxicities were reported relative to the pre-RT baseline. Subsequently, at a median follow-up of 35.5 months, sacral insufficiency fractures were reported in 52%; grade was not reported, but 34% of patients with fractures were symptomatic.[46]

Preoperative

Published experience with preoperative carbon ion therapy is limited to an Italian case series of 2 patients without follow-up data.[47]

Future Directions

Given this evidence, carbon ion therapy seems a promising modality for the treatment of spine and sacral chordomas, although direct comparison to the results of proton studies is difficult given the markedly different fractionation regimens and CTV expansions.

The ongoing single-institution phase II ISAC trial[48] at Heidelberg randomizes patients with sacral chordoma (either unresected or after R2 resection) to PBS proton versus carbon ion therapy, treating to 64 GyRBE in 16 fractions (EQD2 96 GyRBE).[30] CTV expansion will be an anatomically constrained 2-cm expansion on GTV plus, in postoperative cases, surgically manipulated tissues; cauda dose constraint is 60 GyRBE (EQD2). The primary endpoint of this study is grade greater than or equal to 3 toxicity prior to 12 months or treatment discontinuation for any reason. The study was opened in 2013 with an originally projected accrual time of 2 years; no results have yet been reported. This study thus adopts both the markedly hypofractionated approach of some carbon ion centers and the more generous CTV expansions typical of the conventionally fractionated proton literature. Given that experience with proton hypofractionation is very limited, and—even with smaller CTV expansions—some carbon ion centers have moved toward more conventional fractionation due to toxicity concerns,[24,25] tolerability of this treatment protocol needs to be carefully assessed. Ultimately, the optimum fractionation regimen and CTV expansion for both carbon ion and protons likely will remain ongoing questions.

The European Espace de Traitement Oncologique par Ions Légers dans le cadre Européen (ETOILE) study[49] randomizes patients with unresectable non–skull base chordoma, adenoid cystic carcinoma of the head and neck, or other sarcomas (except skull base chondrosarcoma) between (a) photon therapy with or without proton therapy versus (b) carbon ion therapy, with a primary outcome of 5-year PFS. Finally, the ongoing European Sacral Chordoma: Surgery Versus Definitive Radiation Therapy in Primary Localized Disease (SACRO) study[50] randomizes patients with localized sacral chordoma to surgery with or without RT versus RT alone, with RT delivered by carbon ion, proton, or mixed proton/photon therapy, with a primary endpoint of 5-year PFS. Details of these study designs and RT regimens have not been published in a peer-reviewed journal.

STEREOTACTIC BODY RADIATION THERAPY

Background

Stereotactic body radiation therapy (SBRT) is a treatment paradigm, typically photon-based, that delivers radiation to extracranial targets in 1 to 5 fractions (according to US billing definitions) at high dose per fraction. (Stereotactic radiosurgery and stereotactic RT refer, respectively, to single-fraction and multifraction treatments delivered in a similar paradigm to intracranial targets, although these terms sometimes also are used to refer to treatment of targets in the spine.) In contrast to fractionated photon or particle RT, elective target volume expansions for SBRT (ie, CTV, to account for microscopic spread) typically are small or nonexistent. By using highly rigid and reproducible immobilization, precise setup imaging (eg, cone beam CT[51]), and careful calibration of the treating linear accelerator, stereotactic accuracy can be achieved and expansion margins for setup uncertainty (ie, PTV) also can be minimized (typically to 2 mm or less). In addition, modern treatment planning allows generation of highly conformal plans with steep dose gradients. Together, these advances have minimized the spatial uncertainty of RT, allowing delivery of higher doses of radiation to the tumor while limiting radiation dose, and, thus, the risk of radiation complications, to the surrounding normal tissues. Thus, for example, for appropriately selected spinal chordomas, it generally is possible to treat gross tumor to 24 Gy in a single fraction while maintaining the spinal cord point Dmax to less than 14 Gy.

Several factors make SBRT theoretically appealing for the treatment of histologies resistant to conventionally fractionated radiation. First, although the physical dose delivered with SBRT is often lower than that with conventional fractionation, the biologically equivalent dose is comparable or higher, because larger fraction sizes are more likely to cause lethal damage (eg, double-strand breaks) to tumor cell DNA. Second, unlike conventionally fractionated RT, high dose (>8 Gy) per fraction RT leads to endothelial apoptosis in tumor vasculature,[52,53] provoking an ischemia/reperfusion injury that inhibits tumor double-strand breaks repair.[54] Third, high dose per fraction RT is likely immunostimulatory, whereas conventionally fractionated radiation likely is immunosuppressive.[53,55,56]

In light of its combination of spatial precision and efficacy in radioresistant histologies, SBRT may be a particularly promising approach for treatment of spinal/sacral chordomas. Several single-institutional retrospective studies have reported experience with SBRT for this indication and are described later, with 1 main study—which treated in a single fraction and with no CTV expansion—reporting the largest and most current experience.

Low-Dose Stereotactic Body Radiation Therapy

Initial experiences with low-dose SBRT for spinal/sacral chordomas were disappointing.

Henderson and colleagues[57] reported a retrospective single-institution cohort of 18 chordoma patients treated at Georgetown with low-dose SBRT using the CyberKnife platform. Tumors were 44% spinal, 39% clival, and 17% sacral. Median SBRT dose was 35 Gy in 5 fractions (range 24–40 Gy) (EQD2 78.8 Gy). CTV expansion was 1 cm from GTV. With a median follow-up of 5.8 years, LC5 was 59%.[57]

Jiang and colleagues[58] reported a retrospective single-institution cohort of 20 patients treated at Stanford Cancer Institute between 1994 and 2010 with low-dose SBRT using CyberKnife; 45% were recurrent at time of treatment; 65% of lesions were clival, 20% spinal (10% C, 5% T, and 5% L), and 15% sacral. Median SBRT dose was 32.5 Gy in 5 fractions (range 20 Gy in 1 fraction to 50 Gy in 5 fractions) (EQD2 69.0 Gy). CTV expansion was not reported. With a median follow-up of 34 months, LC was 55%.

Moving from 5 fraction to single-fraction treatment, Jung and colleagues[59] reported a single-institution retrospective cohort of 8 patients and 12 lesions treated at Cleveland Clinic with SBRT for chordomas. Lesions were 83% spinal (33% C and 50% L) and 17% sacral. 58% of lesions underwent surgery. SBRT delivered median 16 Gy (range 11–16 Gy) in 1 fraction (EQD2 72 Gy). CTV expansions included the entire involved vertebral body but no other expansions. At a short median follow-up of 9.7 months, LC had already fallen to 75%.

The markedly inferior results with low-dose SBRT compared with fractionated proton therapy, despite apparently equivalent EQD2s, may reflect inaccuracy of the linear-quadratic model used to calculated EQD2 at large fraction sizes and/or other differences in treatment approach (eg, more generous CTV expansions in the fractionated proton literature).

High-Dose Stereotactic Body Radiation Therapy

Given these disappointing results with low-dose SBRT, other groups have investigated dose escalation. Two single-institution retrospective series form the bulk of the current experience with high-dose SBRT for chordoma; the larger such study is summarized in **Table 5**.

Table 5
Retrospective SBRT study

Study	RT Timing	Center and Years Treated	Number of Pts	Location	Histology % Chordoma	% Recurrent	% Surgery/% Definitive-Intent RT (No Surgery) Margin Status Among Surgical Pts	Median RT Dose (Range)	CTV Expansion and Dose	Extracranial CNS Planning Constraints	Treatment Technology	Median f/u	Disease Outcomes	Significant Subsets	Toxicity Outcomes
Jin et al[61]	34% pre-operative 31% post-operative 34% definitive-intent	MSKCC 2006–2017	36	20% C 9% T 20% L 51% S	100%	0%	65%/35% 30% R2 decompression 22% intralesional R0/1 47% en bloc R0/1	24 Gy/1 fx EQD2 156 Gy	Per Cox et al[62]; next normal marrow space adjacent to tumor within involved vertebral level	Dmax 14 Gy	Photon SBRT	38.8 mo	LC3 86% OS3 90%	Decompression surgery vs other: LC HR 4.05 (0.64–25.8, $P = .14$)	26% late Gr ≥3 RT toxicity 13% Gr ≥3 surgical toxicity Gr2/3 toxicity for en bloc vs other surgery: 73%/18% vs 29%/20%, $P = .03$

In the first, updating and expanding on an initial report of promising 2-year LC after SBRT for chordomas,[60] Jin and colleagues[61] reported a single-institution retrospective cohort of 35 previously untreated chordoma patients treated with SBRT at Memorial Sloan Kettering from 2006 to 2017. Tumors were 49% spinal (20% C, 9% T, and 20% L) and 51% sacral. 34% received preoperative SBRT, 31% postoperative SBRT, and 34% definitive-intent SBRT without surgery.

Of surgical patients, 30% underwent decompressive/separation surgery only (ie, intralesional R2 resections), 22% underwent GTR via intralesional curettage, and 47% en bloc resections (resulting in 72% R0, 20% R1, and 9% R2 margins). Select surgical patients (number not reported) with significant epidural disease received 10 Gy HDR dural plaque brachytherapy at the time of surgery. Mobile spine tumors were treated with SBRT to 24 Gy in 1 fraction (EQD2 156 Gy); 3 patients with sacral tumors were treated with 18 Gy to 21 Gy in 1 fraction to limit dose to adjacent bowel. CTV expansions followed published spine SBRT guidelines[62] and generally included the next adjacent normal marrow space within the involved vertebral level. Spinal cord point Dmax was constrained to 14 Gy. **Fig. 2** provides an example of a postoperative SBRT case.

At a median follow-up of 38.8 months, LC3 was 86% and OS3 90%; among patients treated with 24 Gy, LC3 was 96% (**Fig. 3**). Disease outcomes did not differ significantly by extent of surgery, although on univariate analysis, there was a trend toward worse LC among those undergoing only decompressive surgery (HR 4.05, 0.64–25.8; $P = .14$). There was no difference in LC between sacral patients undergoing preoperative SBRT followed by en bloc resection (which achieved 100% LC) versus those undergoing SBRT alone ($P = .30$). Overall, the 25 patients who had gross residual disease after surgery or received definitive-intent RT without surgery achieved 88% LC.

Among all patients, there were no acute Gr greater than or equal to 3 RT toxicities; 26% experienced late Gr greater than or equal to 3 RT toxicity, including soft tissue or bone necrosis; fracture; recurrent laryngeal nerve palsy; sacral neuropathy; and second malignancy. Among surgical

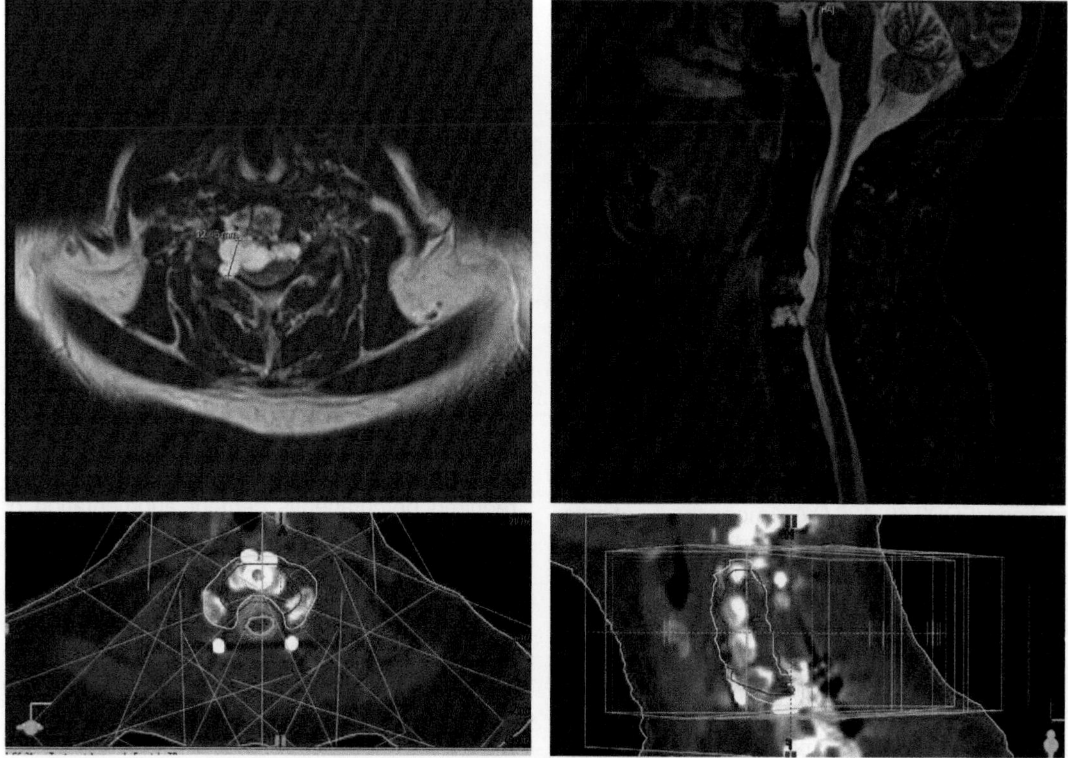

Fig. 2. A 57-year-old woman who presented with chordoma causing spinal cord compression at C4-C6, as seen on pre-operative axial (top left) and sagittal (top right) T2 weighted MRI. En bloc resection was not possible and she underwent surgical decompression and fixation. Post-operatively, she received 24 Gy in a single fraction from C4-C6 (bottom row: target and spinal cord volume and SBRT beam arrangement in axial (bottom left) and sagittal (bottom right) views). At 9 years' follow-up, the patient remains well without evidence of recurrence.

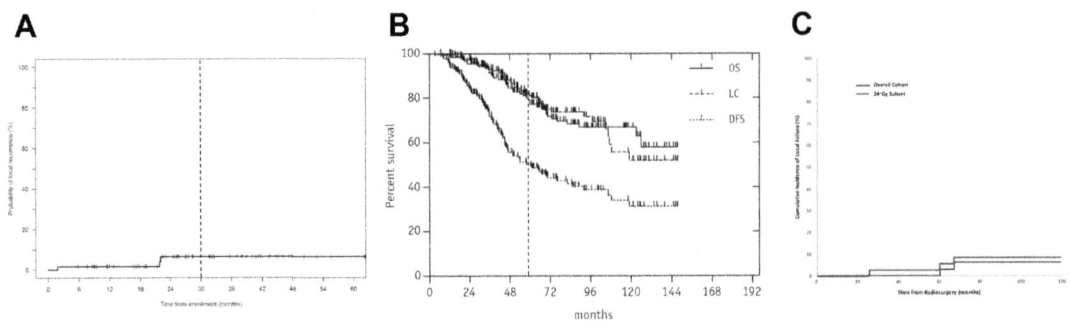

Fig. 3. LC/LF after proton therapy, carbon ion therapy, or SBRT for chordoma. (*A*) LF at 2.5 years of spine/sacral chordomas treated with proton therapy was 6.5% (median follow-up 30 months).[15] (*B*) LC at 5 years of sacral chordomas treated with carbon ion therapy was 77.2% (median follow-up 62 months). (*C*) LC at 3 years of spine/sacral chordomas treated with SBRT was 86% (median follow-up 38.8 months). (*From* [*B*] Imai R, Kamada T, Arak N, et al. Carbon ion radiation therapy for unresectable sacral chordoma: an analysis of 188 cases. Int J Radiat Oncol Biol Phys. 2016;95(1):325; with permission; and [*C*] Jin CJ, Berry-Candelario J, Reiner A, et al. Long-term outcomes of high-dose single-fraction radiosurgery for chordomas of the spine and sacrum. J Neurosurg Spine. 2019;Oct 18:1–10; with permission). cum.inc, cumulative incidence.

patients, 13% had Gr greater than or equal to 3 surgical toxicity (all sepsis). Overall toxicity was higher among patients who underwent en bloc resection (73% Gr2 and 18% Gr3) versus separation or intralesional surgery (29% Gr2 and 20% Gr3) ($P = .03$).

Overall, these data suggest that high-dose SBRT, with or without surgery, can lead to promising LC for spinal and sacral chordomas with a favorable toxicity profile.

In the postoperative and salvage settings, Lockney and colleagues[63] reported a retrospective cohort of 12 patients with spine chordomas treated with single-fraction or multifraction SBRT from 2004 to 2016 at Memorial Sloan Kettering. Lesions were 50% C, 33% T, and 17% L spine; 58% had recurrent disease. These patients were unsuitable for en bloc resection and were treated instead with intralesional resection with gross residual disease, followed by SBRT; 43% also underwent HDR dural plaque brachytherapy for significant epidural disease. SBRT doses were 24 Gy/1 fraction in 50% (EQD2 156 Gy); the remainder were treated with 24 Gy to 36 Gy in 3 fractions (EQD2 60–126 Gy). Among the 5 patients with primary (nonrecurrent) disease, median follow-up was 66 months, actuarial OS2 80%, and crude LC at last follow-up 80%. Among the 7 patients with recurrent disease, median follow-up was 11 months, actuarial OS2 86%, and crude LC at last follow-up 57%. There were 33% Gr3 and 8% Gr4 toxicities in total; major surgery-related and radiation-related complications occurred in 18% and 27% of patients. Although patient numbers are small, these results suggest that, among patients unsuitable for en bloc resection, intralesional separation surgery (with gross residual disease) followed by SBRT can achieve meaningful LC, particularly in primary disease.[63]

Toxicity

In addition to the toxicity results described previously, other studies have reported long term toxicity following spine SBRT for other indications.

Moussazadeh and colleagues[64] reported a retrospective experience from Memorial Sloan Kettering of 31 patients with spinal tumors who were treated with SBRT (24 Gy $\times$ 1) to 36 total lesions and survived at least 5 years. Spinal cord point Dmax was constrained to 14 Gy. There were no grade greater than or equal to 2 acute toxicities. At a median follow-up of 6.1 years, late Gr2 toxicity ($\geq$3 months after treatment) included 8 cases (22.2%) of mild neuropathy (presenting at median 14.2 mo) and 2 (5.6%) of myalgias/myositis (presenting at median 7.5 mo). no Gr3–4 toxicities were observed; 36% of treated spinal levels developed vertebral compression fractures at a median of 25.7 months, of which 38% required percutaneous cement augmentation or surgery.[64]

Cox and colleagues[65] also reported the retrospective Memorial Sloan Kettering experience with SBRT esophageal toxicity. Among 182 patients with tumors abutting the esophagus who received SBRT (median 24 Gy $\times$ 1) between 2003 and 2010, at a median follow-up of 12 months, acute grade greater than or equal to 3 esophageal toxicity was 1.1% and late grade greater than or equal to 3 esophageal toxicity was 6.0%. Based on this experience, the investigators propose constraints, including a D2.5 cc of 14 Gy,[65] Although this series did not include chordoma patients, thoracic chordoma patients are at risk for similar complications when treated with SBRT, and care should be exercised in this setting.

Finally, Yamada and colleagues[66] reported a retrospective cohort of 811 lesions in 657 patients treated with spine SBRT at Memorial Sloan Kettering between 2003 and 2015. At a median RT dose of 24 Gy in 1 fraction and a mean follow-up of 27 months, the rate of myelopathy was 0.42%. Thus, even with long-term follow-up, rates of spinal cord injury with high-dose spine SBRT are very low in experienced hands.[66]

Future Directions

There is thus a growing body of literature that supports the use of SBRT for the treatment of spinal and sacral chordomas in the preoperative, postoperative, definitive-intent, and salvage settings.

Like with conventionally fractionated RT, SBRT dose escalation appears to lead to improved LC. This gain in local tumor control, however, needs to be weighed against a likely higher—but by no means prohibitive—rate of complications.

Unlike for conventionally fractionated RT, there are insufficient data to evaluate outcomes by timing of SBRT relative to surgery. Emerging long-term follow-up does suggest, however, that high-dose SBRT provides durable LC of tumors not suitable for en bloc resection. Thus, like for conventionally fractionated RT, there may be an important role for SBRT in the management of patients for whom an en bloc resection would be infeasible or highly morbid.

Two studies involving SBRT in chordoma currently are ongoing. The first, enrolling patients with recurrent or metastatic chordoma, is a nonrandomized phase I/II trial of nivolumab with or without concurrent SBRT.[67] The second is a randomized phase II trial of a yeast-brachyury vaccine with or without concurrent RT (SBRT or conventionally fractionated).[68] These studies may provide further insight into the interaction between high-dose SBRT, the immune system, and the key molecular drivers of chordoma.

SUMMARY

Taken together, these studies suggest several principles for the integration of surgical and RT management of spinal and sacral chordomas.

First, given the inadequate LC achieved with surgery alone,[9–11] RT should be considered part of the treatment paradigm for all chordomas of the spine and sacrum, regardless of resection or margin status. Decisions regarding RT should be made by a radiation oncologist experienced in treating chordomas, and, given the potential importance of preoperative RT (discussed later), this evaluation should take place before surgery.

Second, outcomes for primary tumors are significantly better than for recurrent tumors, regardless of specific RT approach.[14,18,19,25,27,38,45] Thus, every effort should be made to achieve LC at the initial presentation.

Third, presence of gross residual disease after an intralesional excision often is associated with inferior outcomes despite proton beam RT although this has not been found with SBRT.[13,15,18,19,38,61] Unresected patients, however, treated with definitive-intent RT alone—either high-dose conventionally fractionated proton therapy or SBRT—can have relatively favorable outcomes.[22–25,36,44,45] Thus, if surgery is undertaken, en bloc oncologic resection with negative margins (at least R1 but preferably R0) should be the goal. For patients in whom the only surgical option is an intralesional excision or a highly morbid oncologic resection, definitive-intent RT—via proton therapy, carbon ion therapy, or SBRT—may represent a reasonable alternative. In cases in which urgent surgery is required (eg, symptomatic spinal cord compression or mechanical instability), 2 different strategies have been used. First, if an en bloc resection is not feasible, low-dose preoperative RT (eg, 19.8 Gy) can be considered with the goal of decreasing the risk of intraoperative seeding[19]; whether or not such treatment is delivered, postoperative RT is certainly necessary (although smaller postoperative fields can be used if low-dose preoperative treatment has been given). Second, separation surgery or intralesional gross total resection followed by high-dose SBRT is a viable option.[61]

Fourth, both studies that have compared preoperative to postoperative proton therapy have shown improved outcomes with a component of preoperative RT[15,18]; an additional study has shown excellent outcomes in preoperative RT without direct comparison to postoperative RT,[14] and a meta-analysis has suggested a trend toward improved LC with both preoperative RT and postoperative RT that was not seen with postoperative RT only.[69] Although no prospective study has been designed specifically to compare preoperative versus postoperative RT, the theoretic and practical advantages, favorable outcomes, and acceptable toxicity of preoperative RT suggest that this paradigm should be both strongly considered in clinical use and formally evaluated in trials moving forward.

Fifth, for both conventionally fractionated proton therapy and SBRT, dose escalation is an important determinant of durable LC.

Finally, given the significant multidisciplinary expertise required for successful management of these challenging tumors, and the importance of adequate oncologic treatment in the primary setting, referral to a specialized center with significant chordoma experience is critical at the time of initial diagnosis.

ACKNOWLEDGMENTS

The authors are grateful to Dr Nicolas Depauw and Dr Kathryn Held for their input on the particle therapy physics and radiation biology content, respectively.

DISCLOSURE

D.J. Konieczkowski and T.F. DeLaney: no disclosures. Y. Yamada: Chordoma Foundation, Medical Advisory Board; BrainLab, Consultant; and University of Wollongong, Consulting Professor.

REFERENCES

1. Vujovic S, Henderson S, Presneau N, et al. Brachyury, a crucial regulator of notochordal development, is a novel biomarker for chordomas. J Pathol 2006;209(2):157–65.
2. Pillay N, Plagnol V, Tarpey PS, et al. A common single-nucleotide variant in T is strongly associated with chordoma. Nat Genet 2012;44(11):1185–7.
3. Tarpey PS, Behjati S, Young MD, et al. The driver landscape of sporadic chordoma. Nat Commun 2017;8(1):890.
4. Sharifnia T, Wawer MJ, Chen T, et al. Small-molecule targeting of brachyury transcription factor addiction in chordoma. Nat Med 2019;25(2):292–300.
5. Bakker SH, Jacobs WCH, Pondaag W, et al. Chordoma: a systematic review of the epidemiology and clinical prognostic factors predicting progression-free and overall survival. Eur Spine J 2018;27(12):3043–58.
6. Huang JF, Chen D, Zheng XQ, et al. Conditional survival and changing risk profile in patients with chordoma: a population-based longitudinal cohort study. J Orthop Surg Res 2019;14(1):181.
7. Yu E, Koffer PP, DiPetrillo TA, et al. Incidence, treatment, and survival patterns for sacral chordoma in the United States, 1974-2011. Front Oncol 2016;6:203.
8. Kerr DL, Dial BL, Lazarides AL, et al. Epidemiologic and survival trends in adult primary bone tumors of the spine. Spine J 2019;19(12):1941–9.
9. Schwab JH, Healey JH, Rose P, et al. The surgical management of sacral chordomas. Spine (Phila Pa 1976) 2009;34(24):2700–4.
10. Kerekes D, Goodwin CR, Ahmed AK, et al. Local and distant recurrence in resected sacral chordomas: a systematic review and pooled cohort analysis. Global Spine J 2019;9(2):191–201.
11. Varga PP, Szövérfi Z, Fisher CG, et al. Surgical treatment of sacral chordoma: prognostic variables for local recurrence and overall survival. Eur Spine J 2015;24(5):1092–101.
12. Yolcu Y, Wahood W, Alvi MA, et al. Evaluating the role of adjuvant radiotherapy in the management of sacral and vertebral chordoma: results from a national database. World Neurosurg 2019;127:e1137–44.
13. Snider JW, Schneider RA, Poelma-Tap D, et al. Long-term outcomes and prognostic factors after pencil-beam scanning proton radiation therapy for spinal chordomas: a large, single-institution cohort. Int J Radiat Oncol Biol Phys 2018;101(1):226–33.
14. DeLaney TF, Liebsch NJ, Pedlow FX, et al. Long-term results of Phase II study of high dose photon/proton radiotherapy in the management of spine chordomas, chondrosarcomas, and other sarcomas. J Surg Oncol 2014;110(2):115–22.
15. Konieczkowski DJ, Chen YLE, Bernstein KD, et al. Prospective phase II study of scanned beam proton therapy for spine sarcomas. Int J Radiat Oncol Biol Phys 2018;102(3, Supplement):e325–6.
16. Mastella E, Molinelli S, Magro G, et al. Dosimetric characterization of carbon fiber stabilization devices for post-operative particle therapy. Phys Med 2017;44:18–25.
17. Ringel F, Ryang Y-M, Kirschke JS, et al. Radiolucent carbon fiber-reinforced pedicle screws for treatment of spinal tumors: advantages for radiation planning and follow-up imaging. World Neurosurg 2017;105:294–301.
18. Rotondo RL, Folkert W, Liebsch NJ, et al. High-dose proton-based radiation therapy in the management of spine chordomas: outcomes and clinicopathological prognostic factors. J Neurosurg Spine 2015;23(6):788–97.
19. Wagner TD, Kobayashi W, Dean S, et al. Combination short-course preoperative irradiation, surgical resection, and reduced-field high-dose postoperative irradiation in the treatment of tumors involving the bone. Int J Radiat Oncol Biol Phys 2009;73(1):259–66.
20. Takahashi M, Fukumoto T, Kusunoki N, et al. Particle beam radiotherapy with a surgical spacer placement for unresectable sacral chordoma. Gan To Kagaku Ryoho 2010;37(12):2804–6 [in Japanese].
21. Lorenzo C, Andrea P, Barbara V, et al. Surgical spacer placement prior carbon ion radiotherapy

(CIRT): an effective feasible strategy to improve the treatment for sacral chordoma. World J Surg Oncol 2016;14(1):211.
22. Aibe N, Demizu Y, Sulaiman NS, et al. Outcomes of patients with primary sacral chordoma treated with definitive proton beam therapy. Int J Radiat Oncol Biol Phys 2018;100(4):972–9.
23. Imai R, Kamada T, Araki N, et al. Carbon ion radiation therapy for unresectable sacral chordoma: an analysis of 188 cases. Int J Radiat Oncol Biol Phys 2016;95(1):322–7.
24. Mima M, Demizu Y, Jin D, et al. Particle therapy using carbon ions or protons as a definitive therapy for patients with primary sacral chordoma. Br J Radiol 2014;87(1033):20130512.
25. Demizu Y, Jin D, Sulaiman NS, et al. Particle therapy using protons or carbon ions for unresectable or incompletely resected bone and soft tissue sarcomas of the pelvis. Int J Radiat Oncol Biol Phys 2017;98(2):367–74.
26. Yoon SS, Chen Y-L, Kambadakone A, et al. Surgical placement of biologic mesh spacers prior to external beam radiation for retroperitoneal and pelvic tumors. Pract Radiat Oncol 2013;3(3): 199–208.
27. Indelicato DJ, Rotondo RL, Begosh-Mayne D, et al. A prospective outcomes study of proton therapy for chordomas and chondrosarcomas of the spine. Int J Radiat Oncol Biol Phys 2016;95(1):297–303.
28. Proton Therapy for Chordomas and/or Chondrosarcomas. Available at: https://ClinicalTrials.gov/show/NCT00797602. Accessed February 22, 2020.
29. Elsasser T, Kramer M, Scholz M. Accuracy of the local effect model for the prediction of biologic effects of carbon ion beams in vitro and in vivo. Int J Radiat Oncol Biol Phys 2008;71(3):866–72.
30. Uhl M, Edler L, Jensen AD, et al. Randomized phase II trial of hypofractionated proton versus carbon ion radiation therapy in patients with sacrococcygeal chordoma-the ISAC trial protocol. Radiat Oncol 2014;9:100.
31. Baumann BC, Lustig RA, Mazzoni S, et al. A prospective clinical trial of proton therapy for chordoma and chondrosarcoma: Feasibility assessment. J Surg Oncol 2019;120(2):200–5.
32. Proton Radiation for Chordomas and Chondrosarcomas. Available at: https://ClinicalTrials.gov/show/NCT01449149. Accessed February 22, 2020.
33. DeLaney TF, Liebsch NJ, Pedlow FX, et al. Phase II study of high-dose photon/proton radiotherapy in the management of spine sarcomas. Int J Radiat Oncol Biol Phys 2009;74(3):732–9.
34. High Dose Intensity Modulated Proton Radiation Treatment +/- Surgical Resection of Sarcomas of the Spine, Sacrum and Base of Skull. Available at: https://ClinicalTrials.gov/show/NCT01346124. Accessed February 22, 2020.
35. Youn SH, Cho KH, Kim J-Y, et al. Clinical outcome of proton therapy for patients with chordomas. Radiat Oncol J 2018;36(3):182–91.
36. Kabolizadeh P, Chen Y-L, Liebsch N, et al. Updated outcome and analysis of tumor response in mobile spine and sacral chordoma treated with definitive high-dose photon/proton radiation therapy. Int J Radiat Oncol Biol Phys 2017;97(2):254–62.
37. McDonald MW, Linton OR, Shah MV. Proton therapy for reirradiation of progressive or recurrent chordoma. Int J Radiat Oncol Biol Phys 2013;87(5): 1107–14.
38. Holliday EB, Mitra HS, Somerson JS, et al. Postoperative proton therapy for chordomas and chondrosarcomas of the spine: adjuvant versus salvage radiation therapy. Spine (Phila Pa 1976) 2015; 40(8):544–9.
39. Stieb S, Snider JW, Placidi L, et al. Long-term clinical safety of high-dose proton radiation therapy delivered with pencil beam scanning technique for extracranial chordomas and chondrosarcomas in adult patients: clinical evidence of spinal cord tolerance. Int J Radiat Oncol Biol Phys 2018;100(1): 218–25.
40. Marucci L, Niemierko A, Liebsch NJ, et al. Spinal cord tolerance to high-dose fractionated 3D conformal proton-photon irradiation as evaluated by equivalent uniform dose and dose volume histogram analysis. Int J Radiat Oncol Biol Phys 2004; 59(2):551–5.
41. Chowdhry VK, Liu L, Goldberg S, et al. Thoracolumbar spinal cord tolerance to high dose conformal proton-photon radiation therapy. Radiother Oncol 2016;119(1):35–9.
42. Osler P, Bredella MA, Hess KA, et al. Sacral insufficiency fractures are common after high-dose radiation for sacral chordomas treated with or without surgery. Clin Orthop Relat Res 2016;474(3): 766–72.
43. Cote GM, Barysauskas CM, DeLaney TF, et al. A phase 1 study of nilotinib plus radiation in high-risk chordoma. Int J Radiat Oncol Biol Phys 2018; 102(5):1496–504.
44. Wu S, Li P, Cai X, et al. Carbon ion radiotherapy for patients with extracranial chordoma or chondrosarcoma - initial experience from shanghai proton and heavy ion center. J Cancer 2019;10(15):3315–22.
45. Uhl M, Welzel T, Jensen A, et al. Carbon ion beam treatment in patients with primary and recurrent sacrococcygeal chordoma. Strahlenther Onkol 2015; 191(7):597–603.
46. Bostel T, Nicolay NH, Welzel T, et al. Sacral insufficiency fractures after high-dose carbon-ion based radiotherapy of sacral chordomas. Radiat Oncol 2018;13(1):154.
47. Matsumoto T, Imagama S, Ito Z, et al. Total spondylectomy following carbon ion radiotherapy to treat

chordoma of the mobile spine. Bone Joint J 2013;95-b(10):1392–5.
48. Ion irradiation of sacrococcygeal chordoma. Available at: https://ClinicalTrials.gov/show/NCT01811394. Accessed February 22, 2020.
49. Randomized carbon ions vs standard radiotherapy for radioresistant tumors. Available at: https://ClinicalTrials.gov/show/NCT02838602. Accessed February 22, 2020.
50. Sacral chordoma: surgery versus definitive radiation therapy in primary localized disease. Available at: https://ClinicalTrials.gov/show/NCT02986516. Accessed February 22, 2020.
51. Katsoulakis E, Kumar K, Laufer I, et al. Stereotactic body radiotherapy in the treatment of spinal metastases. Semin Radiat Oncol 2017;27(3):209–17.
52. Park HJ, Griffin RJ, Hui S, et al. Radiation-induced vascular damage in tumors: implications of vascular damage in ablative hypofractionated radiotherapy (SBRT and SRS). Radiat Res 2012;177(3):311–27.
53. Song CW, Kim M-S, Cho LC, et al. Radiobiological basis of SBRT and SRS. Int J Clin Oncol 2014; 19(4):570–8.
54. Bodo S, Campagne C, Thin TH, et al. Single-dose radiotherapy disables tumor cell homologous recombination via ischemia/reperfusion injury. J Clin Invest 2019;129(2):786–801.
55. Lee Y, Auh SL, Wang Y, et al. Therapeutic effects of ablative radiation on local tumor require CD8+ T cells: changing strategies for cancer treatment. Blood 2009;114(3):589–95.
56. Filatenkov A, Baker J, Mueller AMS, et al. Ablative tumor radiation can change the tumor immune cell microenvironment to induce durable complete remissions. Clin Cancer Res 2015;21(16):3727–39.
57. Henderson FC, McCool K, Seigle J, et al. Treatment of chordomas with CyberKnife: georgetown university experience and treatment recommendations. Neurosurgery 2009;64(2 Suppl):A44–53.
58. Jiang B, Veeravagu A, Lee M, et al. Management of intracranial and extracranial chordomas with CyberKnife stereotactic radiosurgery. J Clin Neurosci 2012;19(8):1101–6.
59. Jung EW, Jung DL, Balagamwala EH, et al. Single-fraction spine stereotactic body radiation therapy for the treatment of chordoma. Technol Cancer Res Treat 2017;16(3):302–9.
60. Yamada Y, Laufer I, Cox BW, et al. Preliminary results of high-dose single-fraction radiotherapy for the management of chordomas of the spine and sacrum. Neurosurgery 2013;73(4):673–80 [discussion: 680].
61. Jin CJ, Berry-Candelario J, Reiner AS, et al. Long-term outcomes of high-dose single-fraction radiosurgery for chordomas of the spine and sacrum. J Neurosurg Spine 2019;18:1–10.
62. Cox BW, Spratt DE, Lovelock M, et al. International Spine Radiosurgery Consortium consensus guidelines for target volume definition in spinal stereotactic radiosurgery. Int J Radiat Oncol Biol Phys 2012; 83(5):e597–605.
63. Lockney DT, Shub T, Hopkins B, et al. Spinal stereotactic body radiotherapy following intralesional curettage with separation surgery for initial or salvage chordoma treatment. Neurosurg Focus 2017;42(1):E4.
64. Moussazadeh N, Lis E, Katsoulakis E, et al. Five-year outcomes of high-dose single-fraction spinal stereotactic radiosurgery. Int J Radiat Oncol Biol Phys 2015;93(2):361–7.
65. Cox BW, Jackson A, Hunt M, et al. Esophageal toxicity from high-dose, single-fraction paraspinal stereotactic radiosurgery. Int J Radiat Oncol Biol Phys 2012;83(5):e661–7.
66. Yamada Y, Katsoulakis E, Laufer I, et al. The impact of histology and delivered dose on local control of spinal metastases treated with stereotactic radiosurgery. Neurosurg Focus 2017;42(1):E6.
67. Nivolumab with or without stereotactic radiosurgery in treating patients with recurrent, advanced, or metastatic chordoma. Available at: https://ClinicalTrials.gov/show/NCT02989636. Accessed February 22, 2020.
68. QUILT-3.011 Phase 2 Yeast-Brachyury Vaccine Chordoma. Available at: https://ClinicalTrials.gov/show/NCT02383498. Accessed February 22, 2020.
69. Houdek MT, Rose PS, Hevesi M, et al. Low dose radiotherapy is associated with local complications but not disease control in sacral chordoma. J Surg Oncol 2019;119(7):856–63.

New Prospects for Molecular Targets for Chordomas

Mohammad Zeeshan Ozair, PhD, MD[a], Pavan Pinkesh Shah, BS[b], Dimitrios Mathios, MD[b], Michael Lim, MD[b], Nelson Moss, MD[c,*]

KEYWORDS

• Chordoma • Brachyury • Molecular targeted therapy • Notochord
• Receptor tyrosine kinase (RTKs) • Immunotherapy

KEY POINTS

- Chordomas are benign, highly recurrent tumors of the midline skeleton.
- The molecular changes involved in chordomas include genomic rearrangements and alterations in receptor tyrosine kinase signaling, cell cycle regulation, epigenetic modulators, and the transcription factor Brachyury.
- Chordoma cells are exquisitely dependent on the transcription factor Brachyury for maintenance.
- Although surgical resection and radiation remain first-line treatments for primary chordomas, molecular targeted therapy with signaling inhibitors have shown some benefit in recurrent chordomas.
- Immunotherapies, including Brachyury vaccination and checkpoint inhibition, have shown promising results in early studies.

INTRODUCTION

Chordomas are rare, low-grade tumors of the bone that originate in the midline axial skeleton. They comprise about 3% of primary bone tumors, 20% of primary spinal tumors, and have a predilection to occur in men more than women (2:1 ratio).[1–3] They are typically seen in adults 50 to 60 years of age, but they can occur earlier. Even though they are histologically benign and indolent tumors, chordomas are locally aggressive and have a strong propensity to recur.[2] As slow growing tumors, they are resistant to low-dose conventionally fractionated external beam radiation and highly resistant to conventional chemotherapies. Together with their anatomic location adjacent to the brain stem, cranial nerves, and spinal cord, this property results in their associated morbidity and mortality.

Most chordomas occur in 3 regions of the neuraxis: the sacrum, the skull base clivus, and the mobile spine, with an almost even distribution.[2] Clival chordomas may be more likely to occur in younger patients (<50 years), whereas spinal chordomas typically present in older patients.[2] In advanced cases, chordomas can also metastasize to body sites, including lung, bone marrow, skin, and brain.

Several lines of evidence suggest that chordomas arise from the vestiges of the notochord. This evidence includes their distribution in regions that have been shown to contain remnants of notochord in the midline, such as the vertebral bodies of the spine and the clivus[1,2,4]; their dependence on the transcription factor TBXT (T-Box Transcription Factor T, also known as Brachyury; described later), which is known to be required for notochord differentiation in the embryo[5]; the

[a] Laboratory of Stem Cell Biology and Molecular Embryology, The Rockefeller University, 1230 York Avenue, New York, NY 10065, USA; [b] Department of Neurosurgery, Johns Hopkins University School of Medicine, 733 North Broadway, Baltimore, MD 21287, USA; [c] Department of Neurosurgery, Memorial Sloan Kettering Cancer Center, 1275 York Avenue, New York, NY 10065, USA
* Corresponding author.
E-mail address: mossn@mskcc.org

Neurosurg Clin N Am 31 (2020) 289–300
https://doi.org/10.1016/j.nec.2019.11.004

histologic similarities of benign notochordal cell tumors (which can transform into chordomas) to the embryonic notochordal cells[1,6]; and the development of chordomas in a zebrafish model by overexpression of human RAS^{V12} oncogene in the notochord.[7,8]

Traditionally, the mainstay of treatment of chordoma is en bloc resection, although this is often associated with morbidity and is not always possible because of neurovascular involvement. Stereotactic radiosurgery, carbon ion, and proton beam radiation in the stand-alone or neoadjuvant/adjuvant settings are also in common use with good local control rates.[2,9,10] At present, the median survival of patients with chordoma is 7.7 years across all races and genders.[3] Several ongoing trials are attempting to use pathway inhibitors in conjunction with the aforementioned modalities for recurrent or advanced chordomas. In addition, immunotherapies, including TBXT-directed vaccination and checkpoint inhibition, have been attempted. This article discusses the major pathways that have been implicated in the pathogenesis of chordoma, with an emphasis on molecular vulnerabilities that therapies on the horizon are attempting to exploit.

HISTOPATHOLOGY AND GENETICS OF CHORDOMAS

Histopathologically, chordomas manifest as epithelioid physaliferous cells with rounded nuclei and enlarged intracellular vacuoles.[2] Chordomas can manifest different degrees of atypia on histopathology, but 3 categories are recognized: (1) classic, which appear as described earlier; (2) dedifferentiated, which lack identifying cellular characteristics; and (3) chondroid, which have features of both chondromas and chondrosarcomas. Classic chordomas show immunoreactivity for Brachyury, S100, cytokeratins, as well as the epithelial membrane antigen MUC1.[2] The combination of Brachyury and cytokeratin immunostaining is considered to be diagnostic and pathognomonic for chondromas (sensitivity, 98%; specificity, 100%).[11]

Like other tumors, chordomas are cytogenetically heterogeneous and karyotypically diverse. They feature complex rearrangements of the genome, including chromosomal gains and deletions, genome-wide copy number changes, and chromothripsis.[1,12–14] The most common deletions are observed on chromosome 3p, whereas gains are most often seen in 7q.[1] However, chordomas harbor a low overall mutational rate and a general paucity of driver genes, with about 15 somatic point mutation events/exome. This mutational rate coincides with the slow-growing nature of these tumors and suggests that chordoma cells are initially transformed by dosage changes in a limited number of genes and pathways. Among the mutations that are found in chordomas, the tumor suppressor phosphatase and tensin homolog (PTEN) is inactivated in about three-quarters of all tumors, whereas loss of the cell cycle regulators CDKN2A and CDKN2B is seen in up to 70% of chordomas.[1] Inactivating mutations of p53 and RB are also frequently observed, as are mutations in the epidermal growth factor receptor (EGFR), vascular endothelial growth factor (VEGF), and platelet-derived growth factor (PDGF) pathways. Because of the recent availability of biologic inhibitors of these pathways, several trials are attempting to test the role of molecular targeted therapies (MTTs) in advanced or recurrent chordomas. These trials are discussed in detail later.

Several studies have also documented frequent gene duplications and other mutations in the TBXT gene in both sporadic and familial chondromas, implicating the Brachyury protein.[15–18] Thus, Brachyury is the major transcription factor that regulates chordoma formation, and is detailed later in this article. Apart from TBXT, other mutations have been detected in epigenetic regulators that modulate genome-wide chromatin accessibility, including Brachyury, by 1 of 3 mechanisms: remodeling nucleosome topology, modulating histone modifications, or via DNA methylation. These commonly mutated or deleted genes include SMARCB1, SETD2, PBRM1, EP300, KDM6A, and ARID1B.[12,19] Thus, modulators of chromatin structure are also targets of therapies for chordomas, and the mechanisms of these agents are discussed later.

BRACHYURY IS A DRIVER OF CHORDOMA PATHOGENESIS

TBXT (Brachyury) is an evolutionarily conserved T-box transcription factor that regulates gene regulation through its N terminus, which contains the T-box binding domain. It is expressed in the posterior part of the developing embryo, where it is essential for many aspects of development, such as specification of the mesoderm and its derivatives, migration of mesoderm into the primitive streak, proliferation, epithelial to mesenchymal transition (EMT), as well as induction of primordial germ cell fates in mice.[20–22] Mouse Brachyury knockout embryos fail to develop mesodermal derivatives and are embryonic lethal by E13.5.[23,24] In adults, brachyury expression is normally restricted to the testis and some parts of the thyroid.[25,26]

In the embryo, the notochord is derived from the mesoderm between the third and fourth week of development in humans (postconception days 15–30; E7.0–E8.5 in mice).[27] The notochord lies ventral to the spinal cord and is essential for establishment of the anterior-posterior and dorsoventral axis of the embryo. It does this by releasing and creating a gradient of sonic hedgehog signaling.[28] In adults, the notochord has largely disappeared, except for remnants in the intervertebral disc, the vertebral bodies, and the clivus.[29] The formation of the notochord during development also requires Brachyury expression, where it seems to specifically promote EMT but not proliferation of these cells.[30]

Multiple lines of evidence have shown that TBXT is a critical gene in chordoma pathogenesis. Brachyury is expressed in all chordomas, as detected by RNA sequencing and immunostaining.[31] In addition, some 97% of patients with chordoma harbor a germline single nucleotide polymorphism (SNP) rs2305089 (p. Gly177Asp) in the T-box domain, which leads to enhanced DNA binding and higher expression of its target genes and autotranscription.[32] Furthermore, duplications of the TBXT allele are also present in familial chordomas and some sporadic chordomas.[15–18] In addition, genetic loss-of-function screens for toxicity have shown that Brachyury is the most highly enriched target in multiple chordoma lines, suggesting that chordoma cells are addicted to Brachyury expression for their survival.[5] Lastly, knockdown of Brachyury with shRNA reverses the chordoma phenotype by preventing EMT and inducing growth arrest and senescence of cell lines.[17,33,34] Note that even though the Gly177Asp SNP is found in a large subset of the population, almost all of these people do not develop chordomas, suggesting that the TBXT SNP yields a cellular advantage but is itself insufficient, requiring interaction with other molecular factors to drive chordomagenesis. This suggestion is supported by experiments in zebrafish, in which activation of receptor tyrosine kinases (RTKs) in notochordal cells could lead to chordomagenesis in vivo, but Brachyury overexpression alone does not.[8]

Although it is currently unclear how Brachyury contributes to transformation of notochord remnants, clinicians are beginning to understand how Brachyury enables local aggressiveness of chordomas. Sharifnia and colleagues[5] showed that, in chordoma cell lines and primary tumors, Brachyury binds to large clusters of enhancers that regulate developmental and cancer-related genes. These clusters are called superenhancers and characteristically contain islands of H3K4 acetylation, which mark active enhancers of genes. These superenhancers were typically associated with genes that are highly expressed in chordomas, such as extracellular matrix (ECM)–related genes, Brachyury, HoxA, and EGFR. Brachyury expression was specifically targeted with inhibitors of CDK9 and CDK7/12/13, which are known to be involved in actively transcribed genes and which associate with superenhancers. These inhibitors included THZ1, NVP-2, dinaciclib, and alvocidib, which are all preclinical agents. Loss of Brachyury either by cyclin-dependent kinase (CDK) inhibition or genetic knockout led to a strong decrease in notochord markers, including SOX9 and COL2A1; loss of cell cycle progression genes; growth arrest; and cell death. Thus, targeting Brachyury with a new generation of specific CDK inhibitors seems to be an attractive avenue for future treatment of chordoma.

Brachyury has been previously shown to act as an oncogene in numerous malignancies, including lung and squamous cell carcinomas, sarcomas, germ cell tumors, hematologic cancers, and brain tumors.[26,33,35–38] It confers its oncogenic properties in cells by regulating a diverse array of target genes that hijack its developmental role in promoting stemness, migration, and EMT. In chordomas and other cancers, Brachyury has been shown to upregulate expression and protein stabilization of the oncoprotein Yes-associated protein (YAP), decrease the tumor suppressor PTEN, increase EMT genes such as SNAIL, and attenuate cell cycle progression in tumor initiating cells by suppressing p21, cyclin D1, and pRb.[5,17,33,38–40] Together this network of changes promotes invasiveness of tumor cells and confers radioresistance and chemoresistance. For these reasons, Brachyury has become an attractive target for pharmacotherapeutics as well as immunotherapies.[2,19,41]

EPIGENETIC REGULATORS IN CHORDOMAS

There are many chromatin modifications that affect gene expression in cells. Of these, H3K27 trimethylation (H3K27me3) and H3K9 dimethylation (H3K9me2) are considered to be repressive chromatin because they reduce transcription. In addition, a variant of histone H3, H3.3, which differs by only 4 amino acids, has been shown to be selectively recruited to nucleosomes of actively transcribed genes.[42,43] In contrast, H3K4me3, H3K36me3, and H3K4 acetylation (H3K4ac) are considered to be active chromatin marks because they positively regulate transcription (**Fig. 1**A). Imbalances in histone marks, particularly H3K27 methylation, have been well established to contribute to oncogenesis. This imbalance can

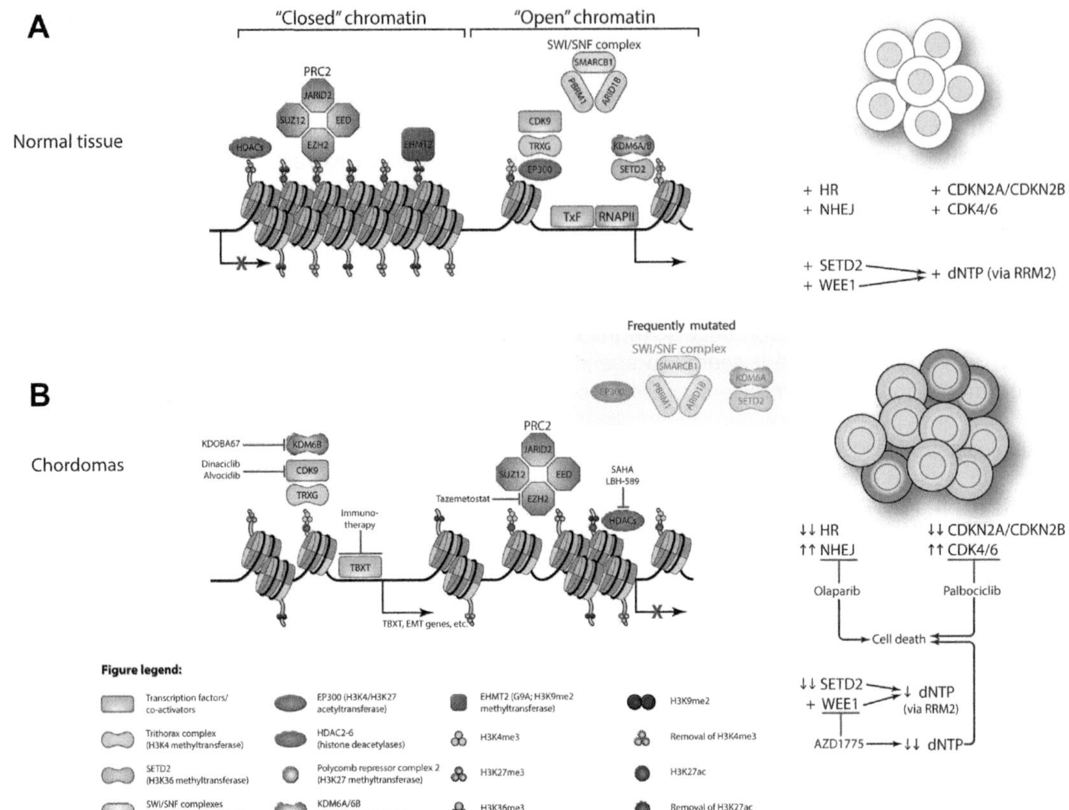

Fig. 1. Cellular and epigenetic changes in chordoma and therapeutic opportunities. (*A*) Open and closed chromatin and associated epigenetic modulators and transcription factors in normal cells. (*Right*) The presence of normal homologous recombination (HR), nonhomologous end-joining (NHEJ), cell cycle regulators (CDKN2A, CDKN2B, and CDK4/6), and the H3K36 methyltransferase SETD2 in these cells. (*B*) In chordoma cells, mutations in epigenetic regulators and transcription factors alter the distribution of open and closed chromatin and lead to genome-wide alterations in the epigenetic signature. Together with mutations in the HR, CDKN2A/2B, and SETD2 pathways, this results in uncontrolled proliferation of cells. The drugs shown in (*B*) are being used in trials to target the compensatory changes in these pathways in tumor cells to revert the chordoma cells to induce cell senescence or death. CDK, cyclin dependent kinase; dNTP, deoxynucleotide triphosphate; HDAC, histone deacetylase, H3K4/27; histone 3 lysine 4/27; PRC2, polycomb repressor complex 2, SWI/SNF, Switch/sucrose nonfermentable.

occur by loss of the EZH2/PRC2 complex, which acts as an H3K27 histone methylation writer, or by overexpression and gain-of-function mutations in this complex, or by loss of antagonists such as H3K27 histone demethylases.[44]

Brachyury as a transcription regulator is known to interact extensively and directly with histone modulators. During development, Brachyury promotes permissive chromatin for transcription by recruitment of methyltransferases at H3K4 sites and demethylases to H3K27 sites and histone deacetylases[45] (see **Fig. 1**A). A conserved tyrosine residue in the N terminus of the protein has been shown to be essential for its ability to recruit these histone modifiers.

Expression of Brachyury within chordomas has been shown to depend on recruitment of two H3K27 histone demethylases, KDM6A (UTX) and KDM6B (JMJD3), to the TBXT locus.[46] Pharmacologic inactivation with KDOBA67 or genetic deletion of these demethylases results in downregulation of Brachyury and its target genes in both chordoma cell lines as well as primary chordomas[46] (**Fig. 1**B). The target genes include cell cycle genes resulting in a strong reduction in growth and cell viability. Moreover, this effect is caused by a genome-wide loss of repressive chromatin marks such as H3K27me3 and H3K9me2 and gain of active chromatin marks such as H3K4me3 and H3.3 in the absence of any change in promoter methylation of TBXT.[46] This finding suggests that, at least in chordomas, loss of promoter methylation of Brachyury does not play a large role in disease pathogenesis.

Previous studies have also shown that primary and recurrent chordomas express multiple histone deacetylases (HDACs), particularly high levels of HDAC6.[47,48] Treatment of a chordoma cell line with panhistone deacetylase inhibitors such as SAHA and LBH-589 resulted in increased cell death.[48] Thus, modulation of histone modifiers with drugs that inhibit H3K4 acetylation or H3K27 trimethylation might represent an intriguing new approach to targeting chordomas (see **Fig. 1**B). Our work, including unpublished data (Nelson et al., 2015), shows intact repressive H3K27 trimethylation, hypotrimethylated (derepressed) H3K36, and H3K4 hypermethylation by histone mass spectrometry in chordoma compared with a basket of cancer cell lines and a primary tumor sample.[49]

In addition to the histone modifiers discussed earlier, SETD2, a H3K36 methyltransferase, is found on chromosome 3p, which, as mentioned earlier, is frequently deleted in chordomas.[12] The H3K36me3 mark activates transcription and mediates DNA repair by homologous recombination; therefore, SETD2 acts as a tumor suppressor gene. Loss of SETD2 function has been observed in many cancers, including renal, breast, and lung, and in gliomas.[50–53] The absence of SETD2 leads to a detectable loss of H3K36 trimethylation in chordomas lacking this gene.[12] This finding presents another therapeutic opportunity because previous studies have shown that H3K36me3-deficient cancers can be targeted and killed by WEE1 inhibitors such as AZD1775 by deoxynucleotide triphosphate (dNTP) starvation[54] (see **Fig. 1**B).

Other epigenetic regulators that are frequently deleted in pediatric chordomas include SMARCB1,[12,55] which is a unit of a large SWI/SNF complex that alters nucleosome topology by physically unwrapping DNA from histones (see **Fig. 1**A). SMARCB1 is a tumor suppressor and an antagonist of the EZH2, and its loss leads to an imbalance in H3K27 methylation.[56] Because of this interaction, phase II clinical trials are currently being conducted in patients with SMARCB1-deleted chordomas with an inhibitor of EZH2, tazemetostat (NCT02601950) (see **Fig. 1**A, **Table 1**). Notably, tazemetostat treatment resulted in responses in a case series of 2 pediatric patients with chordomas.[19,56]

MOLECULAR TARGETED THERAPIES FOR CHORDOMAS

Although management with conventional chemotherapeutic agents has been reported for chordomas, a systematic review of the literature suggests that chordomas are largely insensitive to traditional agents such as cisplatin, alkylating agents, camptothecin, or anthracyclines.[2] RTKs have been shown to be variably mutated and/or overexpressed in chordomas in both primary tumors and cell lines and are thought to be variably important in the initiation and progression of chordomas. To date, MTTs have been attempted clinically in at least 4 signaling pathways[19]: (1) platelet-derived growth factor receptor (PDGFR) and stem cell factor receptor (KIT), targeted by imatinib and dasatinib; (2) vascular endothelial growth factor receptor (VEGFR), targeted by sorafenib, pazopanib, and sunitinib; (3) EGFR and human epidermal growth factor receptor 2 (HER2/neu), targeted by gefitinib, lapatinib, erlotinib, and cetuximab; (4) phosphatidylinositol 3-kinase (PI3K)/AKT/PTEN/mammalian target of rapamycin (mTOR) pathway, targeted by sirolimus and temsirolimus (**Fig. 2**).

In most instances, these drugs have been used in clinical trials on patients with advanced disease, who have either local relapse or metastasis. Because of the limited number of patients involved in these trials and a lack of long-term follow-up in many cases, the interpretation of efficacy of MTTs needs to be restrained. Furthermore, response to treatments has been measured because radiological criteria are often variable between studies. Notwithstanding these caveats, PDGFR inhibitors such as imatinib have been described as first-line MTT agents, although the effects on progression-free survival and overall survival have been modest, with a median progression-free survival of about 9.9 months.[19] In cases in which imatinib therapy failed, EGFR inhibitors such as erlotinib seem to achieve a good response. A systematic review of published studies suggested that the use of monotherapy with 1 tyrosine kinase inhibitor (such as PDGFR inhibitors) were an acceptable first-line treatment of advanced disease with limited adverse effects.[19] In the same review, combination treatments were the recommendation for drug-resistant advanced chordomas, either with 2 tyrosine kinase inhibitors or 1 tyrosine kinase inhibitor and an mTOR inhibitor, with the exact choice of agents depending on the pathways expressed by individual patients' tumors. Among MTTs on the horizon, 1 particular small-molecule inhibitor of the EGFR pathway, afatinib, shows promise because of its ability not just to inhibit EGFR but also to promote Brachyury degradation in multiple chordoma cell lines and inhibit growth of xenotransplant tumors in vivo[57] (see **Fig. 2**). This observation has led to a clinical trial (NCT03083678). Whether MTTs can be beneficial in primary chordomas, either as

Table 1
Active immunotherapy trials including patients with chordoma

Trial Registration Number	Study Title	Type/Phase	Agent/Intervention
NCT02383498	A Randomized, Double-blind, Phase 2 Trial of GI-6301 (Yeast-Brachyury Vaccine) Versus Placebo in Combination with Standard of Care Definitive Radiotherapy in Locally Advanced, Unresectable, Chordoma	Phase II	Biologic: GI-6301 vaccine (yeast-Brachyury) Other: GI-6301 placebo Radiation: radiotherapy
NCT03595228	A Phase 2 Trial of BN-Brachyury and Radiation Therapy in Patients with Advanced Chordoma	Phase II	Biologic: BN-Brachyury (Brachyury vaccine) plus radiation
NCT03623854	A Signal Finding Phase 2 Study of Nivolumab (Anti-PD-1; BMS-936558; ONO-4538) and Relatlimab (Anti-LAG-3 Monoclonal Antibody; BMS-986016) in Patients with Advanced Chordoma	Phase II	Biologic: nivolumab (anti–PD-1) Biologic: relatlimab (anti–LAG-3)
NCT02989636	Phase I Safety Study of Stereotactic Radiosurgery with Concurrent and Adjuvant PD-1 Antibody Nivolumab in Subjects with Recurrent or Advanced Chordoma	Phase I	Biologic: nivolumab (anti–PD-1) Radiation: stereotactic radiosurgery
NCT02601950	A Phase II, Multicenter Study of the EZH2 Inhibitor Tazemetostat in Adult Subjects with INI1-negative Tumors or Relapsed/Refractory Synovial Sarcoma	Phase II	Drug: tazemetostat (for chordomas with SMARCB1/INI1 loss)
NCT02601937	A Phase 1 Study of the EZH2 Inhibitor Tazemetostat in Pediatric Subjects with Relapsed or Refractory INI1-negative Tumors or Synovial Sarcoma	Phase I	Drug: tazemetostat (for chordomas with INI1 loss)
NCT02193503	An Open Phase I Clinical Study Assessing Safety and Tolerability of MVX-ONCO-1 in Patients with Solid Tumor Who Are Not/Not Any Longer Amenable to Standard Therapy	Phase I	Other: MVX-ONCO-1 (autologous tumor cell vaccine + GM-CSF)
NCT03349983	An Open-label Phase 1 Trial to Evaluate the Safety and Tolerability of a Modified Vaccinia Ankara (MVA) Priming Followed by Fowlpox Booster Vaccines Modified to Express Brachyury and T-cell Costimulatory Molecules (MVA-BN-Brachyury/FPV-Brachyury)	Phase I	Biologic: MVA-BN-Brachyury/FPV-Brachyury (Brachyury vaccine)

(*continued on next page*)

Table 1
(*continued*)

Trial Registration Number	Study Title	Type/Phase	Agent/Intervention
NCT03886311	The TNT Protocol: A Phase 2 Study Using Talimogene Laherparepvec, Nivolumab and Trabectedin as First, Second/Third Line Therapy for Advanced Sarcoma, Including Desmoid Tumor and Chordoma	Phase II	Biologic: talimogene laherparepvec (IMLYGIC) (oncolytic virus) Biologic: nivolumab (anti–PD-1) Drug: trabectedin (chemotherapy inhibiting DNA binding of a family of transcription factors)
NCT03874455	Tazemetostat Expanded Access Program for Adults with Solid Tumors	—	Drug: tazemetostat (for chordomas with SMARCA4/INI1 loss)
NCT03173950	Phase II Trial of the Immune Checkpoint Inhibitor Nivolumab in Patients with Select Rare CNS Cancers	Phase II	Biologic: nivolumab (anti–PD-1)
NCT02815995	A Phase II Multi-arm Study to Test the Efficacy of Immunotherapeutic Agents in Multiple Sarcoma Subtypes	Phase II	Biologic: durvalumab (anti–PD-1) Biologic: tremelimumab (anti-CTLA4)

Abbreviations: BN, Bavarian Nordic; CTLA4, cytotoxic T-lymphocyte-associated protein 4; GM-CSF, granulocyte-macrophage colony-stimulating factor; PD-1, programmed cell death protein 1.

stand-alone treatment or in combination with surgery and/or irradiation, needs to be addressed in future trials.

Activation of the signal transducer and activator of transcription 3 (STAT3) pathway and its downstream targets has also been observed in chordoma samples by multiple groups using microarray and immunohistochemistry for phospho-STAT3[58–60] (see **Fig. 2**). Several studies have shown that inhibition of phosphorylated STAT3 using small-molecule inhibitors affects the viability of chordoma cell lines in vitro.[60–63] Although inhibitors of STAT3 still await preclinical studies in animal models, they represent another molecularly exploitable target for future treatments.

In addition to the genes and pathways mentioned earlier, deletions in CDKN2A and CDKN2B are also frequently observed in chordomas.[12,55] The products of these genes (INK4A, ARF, CDKN2B) are tumor suppressors that regulate the cell cycle by regulating the activity of CDK4/6 and protect P53. The loss of these genes results in activation of CDK4/6 and the RB oncogene and uncontrolled cell division, which explains why inhibitors of CDK4/6 such as palbociclib can inhibit proliferation of chordoma cell lines and xenografts efficiently[64,65] (see **Fig. 1**). An ongoing phase II clinical trial is testing the efficacy of palbociclib in chordoma (NCT03110744).

In a recent study of chordomas from patients who were refractory to MTTs, whole-genome and whole-exome sequencing identified large structural rearrangements in the genome. These rearrangements were present with biallelic inactivation of DNA repair genes such as BRCA2, NBN, and CHEK2, and genome-wide mutational signatures and genomic instability that together pointed toward defective homologous recombination (HR) in these chordomas.[14] In 1 case of recurrent disease, treatment with the poly ADP ribose polymerase (PARP) inhibitor olaparib was attempted. PARP1 is required for repair of single-stranded nicks in the genome, and HR-deficient cells are particularly dependent on this pathway for maintaining genome integrity, making them vulnerable to PARP inhibition (see **Fig. 1**). In this case, olaparib led to disease stability and clinical improvement in the patient's spinal cord symptoms for 5 months. However, after 10 months on the drug, a PARP1 resistance mutation developed that restored its enzymatic activity even in the presence of olaparib. Although it is unclear whether the defects in HR repair are a feature of chordomas generally or a consequence of repeated radiotherapy regimens that are used in advanced chordomas such as those being studied here, this case report presents a new clinically actionable vulnerability for future MTT study.

Overall, the body of recent work identifying molecular vulnerabilities has yielded encouraging

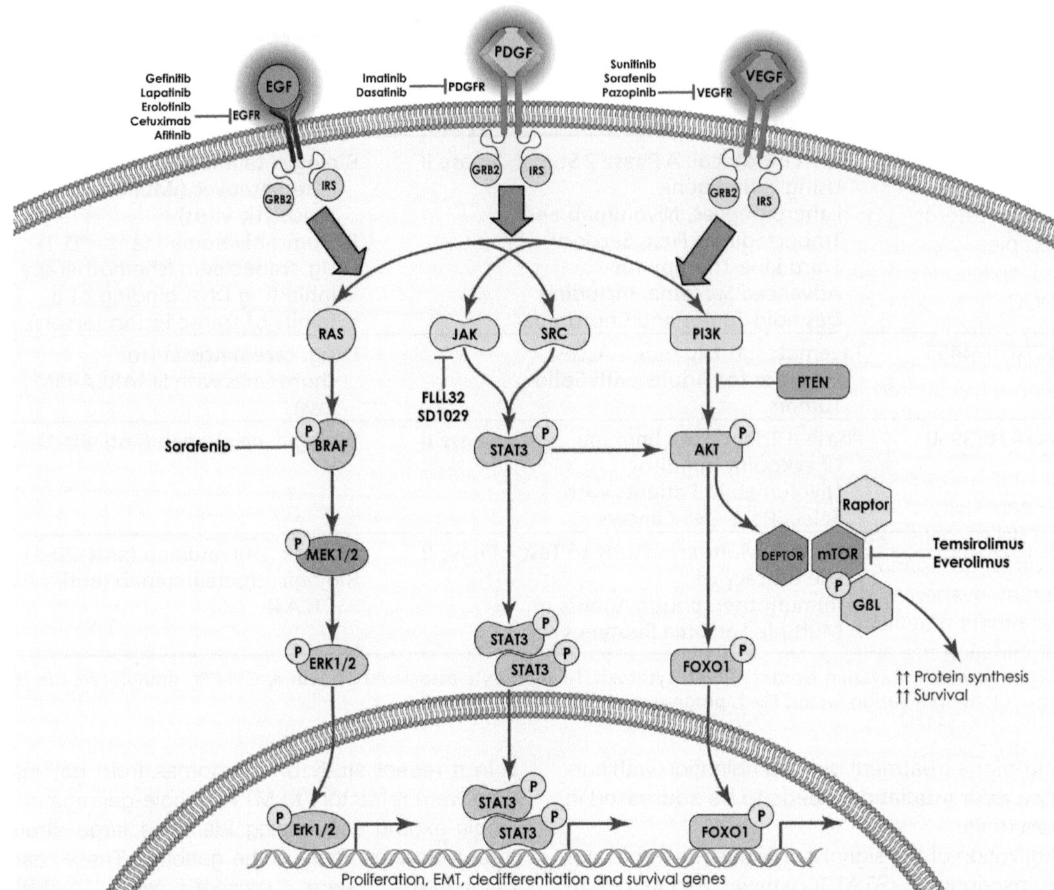

Fig. 2. Molecular pathways targeted in chordomas. The 3 major signaling pathways that have been targeted in chordomas. Components of these pathways are frequently mutated in chordomas, resulting in overactivation that results in increased proliferation upstream of the changes described in **Fig. 1**. Of these pathways, inhibitors to all three RTKs have been used in clinical trials of advanced or recurrent chordomas, as have RAS/MEK/ERK and PI3K/AKT/PTEN/mTOR inhibitors. JAK/STAT3 inhibitors have shown cell death and reduced proliferation in chordoma cell lines in vitro. EGF, epidermal growth factor; ERK, extracellular signal regulated kinase; GRB2, Growth Factor Receptor Bound Protein 2; IRS, Insulin Receptor Substrate; JAK, janus kinase; MEK, MAP kinase/ERK kinase, SRC, Sarcoma oncogene.

early results; however, this remains a work in progress and requires additional validation, drug delivery paradigms, and potentially additional discovery.

THE CHORDOMA IMMUNE MICROENVIRONMENT

Despite chordoma's resistance to traditional chemotherapy and radiation, immunotherapy is a promising avenue in its treatment. The rationale for this includes immune microenvironment characterization studies showing the presence of lymphocytes and macrophages, and the expression of programmed cell death protein 1 (PD-1)/programmed death-ligand 1 (PD-L1) pathway proteins in both primary and recurrent chordomas.[66–68] PD-L1 is constitutively expressed at low levels in chordoma cell lines and immunohistochemically evident, to a variable degree, in 95% of 78 tissue samples (and in some 43% to a high degree).[66,68] In addition, in 1 study, PD-L1 expression was shown to be higher on macrophages than on tumor cells, suggesting that modification of the tumor microenvironment may make therapeutic sense.[68]

PRECLINICAL STUDIES IN IMMUNOTHERAPY FOR CHORDOMAS

Emerging preclinical data have shown some promising results. Several studies have begun exploring the use of antibody-dependent cellular cytotoxicity (ADCC) in chordoma immunotherapy using monoclonal antibodies (mAbs). Fujii and colleagues[67,69] showed significantly increased ADCC lysis in chordoma cell lines cocultured with natural killer cells in the setting of avelumab (anti–PD-L1 mAb) and cetuximab (anti-EGFR mAb). In addition, PD-L1 upregulation further increased ADCC lysis of tumor cells. These results suggest that avelumab may be useful as monotherapy and/or in conjunction with other immune therapies capable of PD-L1 upregulation.[67] Fujii and colleagues[69] also showed enhancement of ADCC lysis with irradiated high-affinity natural killer (haNK) effector cells, which express a high-affinity variant of CD16. haNK cells are currently being investigated in multiple clinical trials for various cancer types (NCT03387085, NCT03853317, NCT03387111, NCT03586869). In addition, olaparib (described earlier) increased the sensitivity of chordoma cells to ADCC by natural killer cells with cetuximab and avelumab in vitro.[70] Olaparib has been approved for *BRCA* mutant ovarian and breast cancer. This agents and others may have roles in future ADCC-based combination therapies.

CLINICAL STUDIES IN IMMUNOTHERAPY FOR CHORDOMAS

Early anecdotal clinical experience with immunotherapy for chordomas has shown some promising results. Migliorini and colleagues[71] reported the results of a series of 3 patients with previously treated and relapsing chordoma who received immunotherapeutic agents. They reported 6 months of response with pembrolizumab in the first patient, 9 months of response with nivolumab (both are anti–PD-1 mAbs) in the second patient, and 19 months of response with the MVX-ONCO-1 vaccine (irradiated autologous tumor cells and allogeneic granulocyte-macrophage colony-stimulating factor–producing cells) in the third patient, with radiographic improvement of the tumor burden and symptomatic relief of the patients' symptoms in all 3 cases.[71]

Initial results from completed clinical trials also show encouraging results. Brachyury, the key regulator described earlier, has emerged as a promising target for immune therapies given its tumor cell specificity with limited normal-tissue expression, and immunogenicity.[38,39,72–75] A phase 1 trial evaluating a yeast-Brachyury vaccine, GI-6301, in multiple tumor types showed enhanced Brachyury-specific CD4 and/or CD8 T-cell responses in 2 of 3 patients with chordoma in the highest dose cohort, and 4 of 7 patients in the second highest dose cohort.[76] Importantly, some disease control was shown in 2 patients with chordoma (1 partial response and 1 mixed response). Both clinical responders had received prevaccination radiation (each approximately 3 months before enrollment). In conjunction with preclinical evidence that radiation modulates the tumor microenvironment,[77] this finding served as the rationale for a phase 2 study assessing clinical response in patients randomized to receive radiation alone or radiation with the yeast-Brachyury vaccine (NCT02383498).

Another phase 1 trial assessed a different Brachyury vaccine built on the modified vaccinia Ankara (MVA) vector, and coding for the expression of Brachyury plus 3 costimulatory molecules (B7.1, ICAM-1, and LFA-3).[78] The assessed outcomes were safety and the generation of Brachyury-specific $CD8^+$ and $CD4^+$ T-cell responses. Six of 11 patients with chordoma showed some Brachyury-specific T-cell response before treatment. Five of these 6 patients saw a heightened Brachyury-specific T-cell response postvaccination, and all 5 patients without baseline response developed a response postvaccination. Disappointingly, most patients did not maintain a Brachyury-specific immune response. Thus, 2 more clinical trials (NCT03595228 and NCT03349983) have been planned to assess Brachyury-specific T-cell response when the vaccine is followed by a fowlpox vector booster. Importantly, both the yeast-Brachyury and MVA-Brachyury vaccines seem to be well tolerated, with no dose-limiting toxicities seen in either trial.[76,78]

There are additionally several ongoing trials evaluating the effect of immune checkpoint blockade as monotherapies and as strategic combination therapies (see **Table 1**). NCT02989636 is a phase I trial designed to assess the use of nivolumab in conjunction with stereotactic radiosurgery for treatment of recurrent or advanced chordomas. NCT03623854 is a phase II trial assessing the effect of a combination of anti–LAG-3 and anti–PD-1 mAbs for patients with advanced chordoma.

Additional targeted therapies that act through immunomodulatory mechanisms have been explored. For example, the EZH2 inhibitor tazemetostat (described earlier) suppresses many immune cell functions, downregulates chemokines, and prevents natural killer cell maturation. A patient with SMARCB1/INI1-negative, poorly differentiated chordoma treated with tazemetostat had a durable response lasting more than 2 years and had a significant increase of CD4 and CD8 T-cell populations.[56] There are ongoing adult and pediatric basket trials including patients with chordoma for tazemetostat (see **Table 1**).

In summary, there are encouraging early data supporting a role for immunotherapy in the treatment of chordoma, but these are not yet validated in efficacy trials against standard therapies. Lessons learned from other tumor types (eg, melanoma and lung cancers) will likely inform both discovery efforts and the design of rational clinical trials. For example, defining the unique tumor-immune interactions in chordoma, both in the primary setting and at recurrence, will likely play a key role, and biomarkers (eg, checkpoint expression) can be anticipated to identify patients most likely to benefit from particular immunotherapies. In addition, as with other cancer types, any immunomodulatory or tumor-specific immunotherapy will likely play a part in a multimodality treatment paradigm including surgical sampling/resection and external beam radiation, at least initially.

ACKNOWLEDGMENTS

M.Z. Ozair was supported by NIH grant 1RF1MH120026-01 and the Robertson Therapeutic Development Fund. N. Moss was supported by the Chordoma Foundation.

DISCLOSURE

The authors have nothing to disclose.

REFERENCES

1. Sun X, Hornicek F, Schwab JH. Chordoma: an update on the pathophysiology and molecular mechanisms. Curr Rev Musculoskelet Med 2015;8(4):344–52.
2. Walcott BP, Nahed BV, Mohyeldin A, et al. Chordoma: current concepts, management, and future directions. Lancet Oncol 2012;13(2):e69–76.
3. Smoll NR, Gautschi OP, Radovanovic I, et al. Incidence and relative survival of chordomas: the standardized mortality ratio and the impact of chordomas on a population. Cancer 2013;119(11):2029–37.
4. Salisbury JR, Deverell MH, Cookson MJ, et al. Three-dimensional reconstruction of human embryonic notochords: clue to the pathogenesis of chordoma. J Pathol 1993;171(1):59–62.
5. Sharifnia T, Wawer MJ, Chen T, et al. Small-molecule targeting of brachyury transcription factor addiction in chordoma. Nat Med 2019;25(2):292–300.
6. Kreshak J, Larousserie F, Picci P, et al. Difficulty distinguishing benign notochordal cell tumor from chordoma further suggests a link between them. Cancer Imaging 2014;14:4.
7. Burger A, Vasilyev A, Tomar R, et al. A zebrafish model of chordoma initiated by notochord-driven expression of HRASV12. Dis Model Mech 2014;7(7):907–13.
8. D'Agati G, Cabello EM, Frontzek K, et al. Active receptor tyrosine kinases, but not Brachyury, are sufficient to trigger chordoma in zebrafish. Dis Model Mech 2019;12(7) [pii:dmm039545].
9. Lockney DT, Shub T, Hopkins B, et al. Spinal stereotactic body radiotherapy following intralesional curettage with separation surgery for initial or salvage chordoma treatment. Neurosurg Focus 2017;42(1):E4.
10. Yamada Y, Laufer I, Cox BW, et al. Preliminary results of high-dose single-fraction radiotherapy for the management of chordomas of the spine and sacrum. Neurosurgery 2013;73(4):673–80 [discussion: 680].
11. Oakley GJ, Fuhrer K, Seethala RR. Brachyury, SOX-9, and podoplanin, new markers in the skull base chordoma vs chondrosarcoma differential: a tissue microarray-based comparative analysis. Mod Pathol 2008;21(12):1461–9.
12. Wang L, Zehir A, Nafa K, et al. Genomic aberrations frequently alter chromatin regulatory genes in chordoma. Genes Chromosomes Cancer 2016;55(7):591–600.
13. Stephens PJ, Greenman CD, Fu B, et al. Massive genomic rearrangement acquired in a single catastrophic event during cancer development. Cell 2011;144(1):27–40.
14. Groschel S, Hubschmann D, Raimondi F, et al. Defective homologous recombination DNA repair as therapeutic target in advanced chordoma. Nat Commun 2019;10(1):1635.
15. Yang XR, Ng D, Alcorta DA, et al. T (brachyury) gene duplication confers major susceptibility to familial chordoma. Nat Genet 2009;41(11):1176–8.
16. Tarpey PS, Behjati S, Young MD, et al. The driver landscape of sporadic chordoma. Nat Commun 2017;8(1):890.
17. Presneau N, Shalaby A, Ye H, et al. Role of the transcription factor T (brachyury) in the pathogenesis of sporadic chordoma: a genetic and functional-based study. J Pathol 2011;223(3):327–35.
18. Kelley MJ, Shi J, Ballew B, et al. Characterization of T gene sequence variants and germline duplications in familial and sporadic chordoma. Hum Genet 2014;133(10):1289–97.
19. Meng T, Jin J, Jiang C, et al. Molecular targeted therapy in the treatment of chordoma: a systematic review. Front Oncol 2019;9:30.
20. Aramaki S, Hayashi K, Kurimoto K, et al. A mesodermal factor, T, specifies mouse germ cell fate by directly activating germline determinants. Dev Cell 2013;27(5):516–29.
21. Lolas M, Valenzuela PD, Tjian R, et al. Charting Brachyury-mediated developmental pathways during early mouse embryogenesis. Proc Natl Acad Sci U S A 2014;111(12):4478–83.

22. Irie N, Weinberger L, Tang WW, et al. SOX17 is a critical specifier of human primordial germ cell fate. Cell 2015;160(1–2):253–68.
23. Chesley P. Development of the short-tailed mutant in the house mouse. J Exp Zool 1935;70(3):429–59.
24. Showell C, Binder O, Conlon FL. T-box genes in early embryogenesis. Dev Dyn 2004;229(1):201–18.
25. Edwards YH, Putt W, Lekoape KM, et al. The human homolog T of the mouse T(Brachyury) gene; gene structure, cDNA sequence, and assignment to chromosome 6q27. Genome Res 1996;6(3):226–33.
26. Hamilton DH, Fernando RI, Schlom J, et al. Aberrant expression of the embryonic transcription factor brachyury in human tumors detected with a novel rabbit monoclonal antibody. Oncotarget 2015;6(7): 4853–62.
27. de Bree K, de Bakker BS, Oostra RJ. The development of the human notochord. PLoS One 2018; 13(10):e0205752.
28. Balmer S, Nowotschin S, Hadjantonakis AK. Notochord morphogenesis in mice: current understanding & open questions. Dev Dyn 2016;245(5): 547–57.
29. McCann MR, Tamplin OJ, Rossant J, et al. Tracing notochord-derived cells using a Noto-cre mouse: implications for intervertebral disc development. Dis Model Mech 2012;5(1):73–82.
30. Zhu J, Kwan KM, Mackem S. Putative oncogene Brachyury (T) is essential to specify cell fate but dispensable for notochord progenitor proliferation and EMT. Proc Natl Acad Sci U S A 2016;113(14): 3820–5.
31. Vujovic S, Henderson S, Presneau N, et al. Brachyury, a crucial regulator of notochordal development, is a novel biomarker for chordomas. J Pathol 2006;209(2):157–65.
32. Pillay N, Plagnol V, Tarpey PS, et al. A common single-nucleotide variant in T is strongly associated with chordoma. Nat Genet 2012;44(11):1185–7.
33. Shah SR, David JM, Tippens ND, et al. Brachyury-YAP regulatory axis drives stemness and growth in cancer. Cell Rep 2017;21(2):495–507.
34. Hsu W, Mohyeldin A, Shah SR, et al. Generation of chordoma cell line JHC7 and the identification of Brachyury as a novel molecular target. J Neurosurg 2011;115(4):760–9.
35. Kilic N, Feldhaus S, Kilic E, et al. Brachyury expression predicts poor prognosis at early stages of colorectal cancer. Eur J Cancer 2011;47(7):1080–5.
36. Imajyo I, Sugiura T, Kobayashi Y, et al. T-box transcription factor Brachyury expression is correlated with epithelial-mesenchymal transition and lymph node metastasis in oral squamous cell carcinoma. Int J Oncol 2012;41(6):1985–95.
37. Roselli M, Fernando RI, Guadagni F, et al. Brachyury, a driver of the epithelial-mesenchymal transition, is overexpressed in human lung tumors: an opportunity for novel interventions against lung cancer. Clin Cancer Res 2012;18(14):3868–79.
38. Huang B, Cohen JR, Fernando RI, et al. The embryonic transcription factor Brachyury blocks cell cycle progression and mediates tumor resistance to conventional antitumor therapies. Cell Death Dis 2013; 4:e682.
39. Fernando RI, Litzinger M, Trono P, et al. The T-box transcription factor Brachyury promotes epithelial-mesenchymal transition in human tumor cells. J Clin Invest 2010;120(2):533–44.
40. Nelson AC, Pillay N, Henderson S, et al. An integrated functional genomics approach identifies the regulatory network directed by brachyury (T) in chordoma. J Pathol 2012;228(3):274–85.
41. Palena C, Polev DE, Tsang KY, et al. The human T-box mesodermal transcription factor Brachyury is a candidate target for T-cell-mediated cancer immunotherapy. Clin Cancer Res 2007;13(8):2471–8.
42. Szenker E, Ray-Gallet D, Almouzni G. The double face of the histone variant H3.3. Cell Res 2011; 21(3):421–34.
43. Ahmad K, Henikoff S. The histone variant H3.3 marks active chromatin by replication-independent nucleosome assembly. Mol Cell 2002;9(6): 1191–200.
44. Martinez-Garcia E, Licht JD. Deregulation of H3K27 methylation in cancer. Nat Genet 2010;42(2):100–1.
45. Beisaw A, Tsaytler P, Koch F, et al. BRACHYURY directs histone acetylation to target loci during mesoderm development. EMBO Rep 2018;19(1): 118–34.
46. Cottone L, Hookway ES, Cribbs A, et al. Epigenetic inactivation of oncogenic brachyury (TBXT) by H3K27 histone demethylase controls chordoma cell survival. bioRxiv 2018;432005.
47. Lee DH, Zhang Y, Kassam AB, et al. Combined PDGFR and HDAC inhibition overcomes PTEN disruption in chordoma. PLoS One 2015;10(8): e0134426.
48. Scheipl S, Lohberger B, Rinner B, et al. Histone deacetylase inhibitors as potential therapeutic approaches for chordoma: an immunohistochemical and functional analysis. J Orthop Res 2013;31(12): 1999–2005.
49. Moussazadeh N, Berman SH, Laufer I, et al. Epigenetic profiling reveals a unique histone code in chordoma. Neurosurgery 2016;63(Clinical Neurosurgery Supplement 1):208.
50. Viaene AN, Santi M, Rosenbaum J, et al. SETD2 mutations in primary central nervous system tumors. Acta Neuropathol Commun 2018;6(1):123.
51. Walter DM, Venancio OS, Buza EL, et al. Systematic in vivo inactivation of chromatin-regulating enzymes identifies Setd2 as a potent tumor suppressor in lung adenocarcinoma. Cancer Res 2017;77(7): 1719–29.

52. Fontebasso AM, Schwartzentruber J, Khuong-Quang DA, et al. Mutations in SETD2 and genes affecting histone H3K36 methylation target hemispheric high-grade gliomas. Acta Neuropathol 2013;125(5):659–69.
53. Wagner EJ, Carpenter PB. Understanding the language of Lys36 methylation at histone H3. Nat Rev Mol Cell Biol 2012;13(2):115–26.
54. Pfister SX, Markkanen E, Jiang Y, et al. Inhibiting WEE1 selectively kills histone H3K36me3-deficient cancers by dNTP starvation. Cancer Cell 2015; 28(5):557–68.
55. Choy E, MacConaill LE, Cote GM, et al. Genotyping cancer-associated genes in chordoma identifies mutations in oncogenes and areas of chromosomal loss involving CDKN2A, PTEN, and SMARCB1. PLoS One 2014;9(7):e101283.
56. Gounder MM, Zhu G, Roshal L, et al. Immunologic correlates of the abscopal effect in a SMARCB1/INI1-negative poorly differentiated chordoma after EZH2 inhibition and radiotherapy. Clin Cancer Res 2019;25(7):2064–71.
57. Magnaghi P, Salom B, Cozzi L, et al. Afatinib is a new therapeutic approach in chordoma with a unique ability to target EGFR and brachyury. Mol Cancer Ther 2018;17(3):603–13.
58. Bosotti R, Magnaghi P, Di Bella S, et al. Establishment and genomic characterization of the new chordoma cell line Chor-IN-1. Sci Rep 2017;7(1):9226.
59. Tauziede-Espariat A, Bresson D, Polivka M, et al. Prognostic and therapeutic markers in chordomas: a study of 287 tumors. J Neuropathol Exp Neurol 2016;75(2):111–20.
60. Yang C, Schwab JH, Schoenfeld AJ, et al. A novel target for treatment of chordoma: signal transducers and activators of transcription 3. Mol Cancer Ther 2009;8(9):2597–605.
61. Jahanafrooz Z, Stallinger A, Anders I, et al. Influence of silibinin and beta-beta-dimethylacrylshikonin on chordoma cells. Phytomedicine 2018;49:32–40.
62. Wang AC, Owen JH, Abuzeid WM, et al. STAT3 inhibition as a therapeutic strategy for chordoma. J Neurol Surg B Skull Base 2016;77(6):510–20.
63. Yang C, Hornicek FJ, Wood KB, et al. Blockage of Stat3 with CDDO-Me inhibits tumor cell growth in chordoma. Spine (Phila Pa 1976) 2010;35(18): 1668–75.
64. Liu T, Shen JK, Choy E, et al. CDK4 expression in chordoma: a potential therapeutic target. J Orthop Res 2018;36(6):1581–9.
65. Levy J. Chordoma foundation in vivo drug screening program. Chordoma Foundation; 2018. Available at: https://figshare.com/projects/Chordoma_Foundation_In_Vivo_Drug_Screening_Program/25948. Accessed August 13, 2019.
66. Feng Y, Shen J, Gao Y, et al. Expression of programmed cell death ligand 1 (PD-L1) and prevalence of tumor-infiltrating lymphocytes (TILs) in chordoma. Oncotarget 2015;6(13):11139–49.
67. Fujii R, Friedman ER, Richards J, et al. Enhanced killing of chordoma cells by antibody-dependent cell-mediated cytotoxicity employing the novel anti-PD-L1 antibody avelumab. Oncotarget 2016;7(23):33498–511.
68. Mathios D, Ruzevick J, Jackson CM, et al. PD-1, PD-L1, PD-L2 expression in the chordoma microenvironment. J Neurooncol 2015;121(2):251–9.
69. Fujii R, Schlom J, Hodge JW. A potential therapy for chordoma via antibody-dependent cell-mediated cytotoxicity employing NK or high-affinity NK cells in combination with cetuximab. J Neurosurg 2018; 128(5):1419–27.
70. Fenerty KE, Padget M, Wolfson B, et al. Immunotherapy utilizing the combination of natural killer- and antibody dependent cellular cytotoxicity (ADCC)-mediating agents with poly (ADP-ribose) polymerase (PARP) inhibition. J Immunother Cancer 2018;6(1):133–47.
71. Migliorini D, Mach N, Aguiar D, et al. First report of clinical responses to immunotherapy in 3 relapsing cases of chordoma after failure of standard therapies. Oncoimmunology 2017;6(8):e1338235.
72. David JM, Hamilton DH, Palena C. MUC1 upregulation promotes immune resistance in tumor cells undergoing brachyury-mediated epithelial-mesenchymal transition. Oncoimmunology 2016;5(4):e1117738.
73. Hamilton DH, Litzinger MT, Fernando RI, et al. Cancer vaccines targeting the epithelial-mesenchymal transition: tissue distribution of brachyury and other drivers of the mesenchymal-like phenotype of carcinomas. Semin Oncol 2012;39(3):358–66.
74. Larocca C, Cohen JR, Fernando RI, et al. An autocrine loop between TGF-beta 1 and the transcription factor brachyury controls the transition of human carcinoma cells into a mesenchymal phenotype. Mol Cancer Ther 2013;12(9):1805–15.
75. Miettinen M, Wang Z, Lasota J, et al. Nuclear brachyury expression is consistent in chordoma, common in germ cell tumors and small cell carcinomas, and rare in other carcinomas and sarcomas: an immunohistochemical study of 5229 cases. Am J Surg Pathol 2015;39(10):1305–12.
76. Heery CR, Singh BH, Rauckhorst M, et al. Phase I trial of a yeast-based therapeutic cancer vaccine (GI-6301) targeting the transcription factor brachyury. Cancer Immunol Res 2015;3(11):1248–56.
77. Gameiro SR, Ardiani A, Kwilas A, et al. Radiation-induced survival responses promote immunogenic modulation to enhance immunotherapy in combinatorial regimens. Oncoimmunology 2014;3(5): e28643.
78. Heery CR, Palena C, McMahon S, et al. Phase I study of a poxviral TRICOM-based vaccine directed against the transcription factor brachyury. Clin Cancer Res 2017;23(22):6833–45.

Printed and bound by CPI Group (UK) Ltd, Croydon, CR0 4YY
08/05/2025
01864691-0013